Lifelong management of hypertension

DEVELOPMENTS IN CARDIOVASCULAR MEDICINE

Lancée CT, ed: Echocardiology. 1979. ISBN 90-247-2209-8.

Baan J, Arntzenius AC, Yellin EL, eds: Cardiac dynamics. 1980. ISBN 90-247-2212-8.

Thalen HJT, Meere CC, eds: Fundamentals of cardiac pacing. 1970. ISBN 90-247-2245-4.

Kulbertus HE, Wellens HJJ, eds: Sudden death. 1980. ISBN 90-247-2290-X.

Dreifus LS, Brest AN, eds: Clinical applications of cardiovascular drugs. 1980. ISBN 90-247-2295-0.

Spencer MP, Reid JM, eds: Cerebrovascular evaluation with Doppler ultrasound. 1981. ISBN 90-247-2384-1.

Zipes DP, Bailey JC, Elharrar V, eds: The slow inward current and cardiac arrhythmias. 1980. ISBN 90-247-2380-9.

Kesteloot H, Joossens JV, eds: Epidemiology of arteral blood pressure. 1980. ISBN 90-247-2386-8.

Wackers FJT, ed: Thallium–201 and technetium-99m-pyrophosphate myocardial imaging in the coronary care unit. 1980. ISBN 90-247-2396-5.

Maseri A, Marchesi C, Chierchia S, Trivella MG, eds: Coronary care units. 1981. ISBN 90-247-2456-2.

Morganroth J, Moore EN, Dreifus LS, Michelson EL, eds: The evaluation of new antiarrhythmic drugs. 1981. ISBN 90-247-2474-40.

Alboni P: Intraventricular conduction disturbances. 1981. ISBN 90-247-2483-X.

Rijsterborgh H, ed: Echocardiology. 1981. ISBN 90-247-2491-0.

Wagner GS, ed: Myocardial infarction: Measurement and intervention. 1982. ISBN 90-247-2513-5.

Meltzer RS, Roelandt J, eds: Contrast echocardiography. 1982. ISBN 90-247-2531-3.

Amery A, Fagard R, Lijnen R, Staessen J, eds: Hypertensive cardiovascular disease: Pathophysiology and treatment. 1982. ISBN 90-247-2534-8.

Bouman LN, Jongsma HJ, eds: Cardiac rate and rhythm. 1982. ISBN 90-247-2626-3.

Morganroth J, Moore EM, eds: The evaluation of beta blocker and calcium antagonist drugs. 1982. ISBN 90-247-2642-5.

Rosenbaum MB, ed: Frontiers of cardiac electrophysiology. 1982. ISBN 90-247-2663-8.

Roelandt J, Hugenholtz PG, eds: Long-term ambulatory electrocardiography. 1982. ISBN 90-247-2664-8.

Adgey AAJ, ed: Acute phase of ischemic heart disease and myocardial infarction. 1982. ISBN 90-247-2675-1.

Hanrath P, Bleifeld W, Souquet, eds: Cardiovascular diagnosis by Ultrasound. Transesophageal, computerized, contrast, Doppler echocardiography. 1982. ISBN 90-247-2692-1.

Roelandt J, ed: The practice of M-mode and two-dimensional echocardiography. 1983. ISBN 90-247-2745-6.

Meyer J, Schweizer P, Erbel R, eds: Advances in noninvasive cardiology. 1983. ISBN 0-89838-576-8.

Morganroth J, Moore EN, eds: Sudden cardiac death and congestive heart failure: Diagnosis and treatment. 1983. ISBN 0-89838-580-6.

LIFELONG MANAGEMENT OF HYPERTENSION

edited by

H. MITCHELL PERRY, JR., M.D.

Physician Coordinator for Hypertension
U.S. Veterans Administration
Washington, DC

and

Hypertension Division
Department of Medicine
Washington University School of Medicine
Saint Louis, MO 63106
USA

1983 **MARTINUS NIJHOFF PUBLISHERS**
a member of the KLUWER ACADEMIC PUBLISHERS GROUP
BOSTON / THE HAGUE / DORDRECHT / LANCASTER
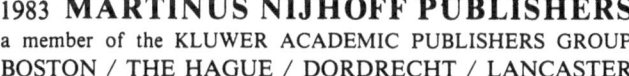

Distributors

for the United States and Canada: Kluwer Boston, Inc., 190 Old Derby Street, Hingham, MA 02043, USA
for all other countries: Kluwer Academic Publishers Group, Distribution Center, P.O.Box 322, 3300 AH Dordrecht, The Netherlands

Library of Congress Cataloging in Publication Data

```
Library of Congress Cataloging in Publication Data
Main entry under title:

Lifelong management of hypertension.

    (Developments in cardiovascular medicine)
    Includes index.
    1. Hypertension--Treatment--Addresses, essays,
lectures.   I. Perry, H. Mitchell (Horace Mitchell),
1923-     .  II. Series.  [DNLM: 1. Hypertension.
2. Hypertension--Therapy.  W1 DE997VME v. 26 / WG 340
L722]
RC685.H8L54  1983     616.1'3206     83-8862
ISBN 0-89838-582-2
```

ISBN-13: 978-94-009-6734-2   e-ISBN-13: 978-94-009-6732-8
DOI: 10.1007/978-94-009-6732-8

Copyright

Preface

In the thirty years since the advent of effective pharmacologic treatment for hypertension, the world of the hypertensive has been transformed beyond recognition. The first change involved only malignant hypertensives with enough residual renal parenchyma to survive. Such a hypertensive could trade inevitable renal failure – unless an intracerebral bleed occurred first – for a rigid regimen which prevented his blood pressure from destroying him but which was associated with nearly intolerable side effects. Over the next 20 years, increasing numbers of patients with hypertension of decreasing severity were treated with drugs that had fewer and fewer side effects. In 1970, with the medical world finally ready to accept the concept, the well-known Veterans Administration Study demonstrated that morbidity and mortality could be diminished in moderately hypertensive patients by antihypertensive therapy that had minimal side effects. As a result there has been a major attempt to bring everyone with elevated blood pressure under lifelong pharmacologic control. It is difficult, however, to know what levels of blood pressure deserve treatment; many who, when therapy first became available, would not have even been considered hypertensive are now candidates for treatment. The lower the pressure, the larger the potential population to be treated, but the smaller the individual risk and hence the smaller the possible benefit. The point where decades of diminished quality of life from treatment begins to outweigh a possible late-life complication is yet to be determined.

From society's point of view, we now have the potential to lower the incidence of several catastrophic cardiovascular complications, and thereby alter the mortality rate for the entire population, by controlling a chronic disease involving millions of asymptomatic patients. To do this, however, requires permanent population-wide maintenance of blood pressure control. Unfortunately, we do not know how to obtain lifelong compliance from the average hypertensive, nor have we decided how far we are justified in pursuing the indifferent or recalcitrant individual whose failure to accept treatment and whose resultant cardiovascular complications constitute a significant burden for society. This book considers therapy for all types of hypertension under the current set of rules, but it particularly concentrates on the lifelong management of mild and moderate hypertensives who make up the vast majority of our hypertensive population.

Finally, I would like to thank Carol H. Jaeger and Elizabeth F. Perry for their assistance in the preparation of the book.

April 1983   H. Mitchell Perry

Contents

List of contributors

Aagaard, George N., M.D., Department of Clinical Pharmacology, University of Washington School of Medicine, Seattle, WA 98195, USA

Bourgoignie, Jacques J., M.D., Division of Nephrology, University of Miami School of Medicine, P.O. Box 016099, Miami, FL 33101, USA

Camel, Greta H., M.D., St. Louis Veterans Administration Medical Center, Washington University School of Medicine, St Louis, MO 63110, USA

Camel, H. Marvin, M.D., Department of Obstetrics and Gynecology, Division of Gynecologic Oncology, Washington University School of Medicine, St Louis, MO 63110, USA

Foerster, James, M.D., Department of Medicine, University of California School of Medicine, Davis, CA 95616, USA

Gast, Michael J., M.D., Ph.D., Department of Obstetrics and Gynecology, Division of Maternal and Fetal Medicine, Washington University School of Medicine, St. Louis, MO 63110, USA

Goldring, David, M.D., Edward Mallinckrodt Department of Pediatrics, Division of Cardiology, Washington University School of Medicine, St. Louis, MO 63110, USA

Julius, Stevo, M.D., Department of Internal Medicine, Division of Hypertension, University of Michigan Medical School, Ann Arbor, MI 48109, USA

Lonigro, Andrew, M.D., Division of Clinical Pharmacology, Saint Louis University School of Medicine, Veterans Administration Medical Center, St. Louis, MO 63110, USA

Neal, William H., M.D., Veterans Administration Medical Center, Dallas, TX

Perry, H. Mitchell, Jr., M.D., Physician Coordinator for Hypertension, U.S. Veterans Administration, Washington, DC; Hypertension Division, Department of Medicine, Washington University School of Medicine, 915 North Grand Boulevard, St. Louis, MO 63106, USA

Schnaper, H., M.D., Department of Medicine, University of Alabama, Birmingham, AL 35294, USA

Sherry, S., M.D., Department of Medicine, Temple University School of Medicine, Philadelphia, PA 19140, USA

Smith, W., McFate, M.D., University of California, Department of Epidemiology and International Health, San Francisco, CA 94143, USA

Stason, W., M.D., Department of Health Services, Harvard School of Public Health, Boston, MA 02115, USA

Introduction

Presently, half of all deaths in industrialized North America and Europe are ascribed to cardiovascular disease, and the majority of that half involves myocardial infarctions, most of which occur in hypertensive individuals. The major changes in the incidence of myocardial infarction during this century in the United States have been the subject of much speculation but no satisfactory explanation. The reported annual incidence rate rose from less than ten per 100,000 in 1920 to a maximum of 300 per 100,000 in the mid-1960s. Since the late 1960s there has been a 30% decrease in incidence. Although confused – and perhaps exaggerated – by four changes in official terminology, both the initial increase and the subsequent decrease seem to be real phenomena. The other major cardiovascular catastrophe is stroke. The pattern of stroke incidence has been generally similar to that of myocardial infarction, although the decrease began much earlier. The decreases suggest that recently some of the right things are being done, but what they are and how important each is remains to be determined.

Sometimes hypertension must seem dull and routine to today's physician: Characteristically he sees a multitude of patients with minimal asymptomatic disease which can easily be controlled by a simple set of algorithms; once controlled, patients must return indefinitely to have prescriptions refilled and to report on usually trivial side effects. This, however, is not the only way of viewing the situation. First, there are fascinating unresolved problems involving hypertension, as indicated in the preceding paragraph. Second, any treatment with the capacity to alter the mortality rate of a whole population has to be exciting. Third, the present stage of chronic widespread pharmacologic treatment of hypertension seems likely to be only temporary, soon to be replaced by prevention, perhaps with an intermediate stage when hypertension can be cured but not yet prevented.

Control of accelerated or malignant hypertension and prevention of its rapidly fatal sequellae by drugs comprise one of the true miracles of modern medicine. The first partially effective antihypertensive treatment became available in the 1940s with a '200-mg sodium diet' or surgical sympathectomy. Although those methods demonstrated that blood pressure could often be controlled and that control slowed or stopped the progress of the disease, most patients refused the diet, while sympathectomy frequently failed to prevent progression and always involved major surgical morbidity. Effective drug therapy was introduced in 1951 and quickly demonstrated that the inexorable downhill course of malignant hypertension – as long as it had not yet progressed to renal failure – could be almost magically halted, immediately extending the median life expectancy of treated patients from less than six months to more than ten years.

The benefits of treatment were much harder to establish for patients with lesser hypertension. In the early days of treatment, some physicians were unwilling to treat patients with so-called benign hypertension of the severe and moderate varieties, because they felt that an elevated pressure must reflect some physiologic need. Their unwillingness to treat was at least partly justified by the very unpleasant and almost universal side effects of the first antihypertensive drugs, including complete autonomic blockade, and by their less common but terrifying toxic effects: fatal hexamethonium pneumonia and hydralazine-induced lupus erythematosus, the latter once involving as many as 10% of exposed patients. Also contributing to the hesitancy to treat was the fact that untreated patients with severe and moderate hypertension were not in the same immediate danger as those with malignant hypertension. Moreover, their morbid events tended to be single unpredictable arteriosclerotic catastropes involving large arteries rather than the predictably rapid and continuous destruction of small vessels, which was the hallmark of malignant hypertension.

Although it is now universally accepted that a diastolic pressure of 105 mmHg or above deserves treatment, two major questions about the treatment of hypertension remain: what level of mild diastolic hypertension justifies treatment and should systolic hypertension in the elderly be treated? The question of whether to treat mild hypertension has become very important, with various studies providing sometimes contradictory data. The answer has tremendous financial implications. The landmark Veterans Administration Trial included subjects with mild hypertension, but they were far too few to provide any answer as to the benefit of treatment. The US Public Health Service Hospital Trial demonstrated that treatment prevented progression to more severe hypertension but did not affect arteriosclerotic complications. As a pilot study, the VA-NIH Mild Hypertension Trial was not designed to show benefit from treatment, but it did raise the question of whether treatment might have undesirable side effects; moreover, it emphasized the difficulty of separating mild hypertensives from normotensives since a third of a rigidly selected mildly hypertensive population became and remained normotensive when given blinded placebo. The Australian Trial indicated benefit from lowering the diastolic pressure to 95 mmHg but no further. Unfortunately, there were markedly divergent results from the two large trials in the United States which compared the effects of intensive treatment by one group of health care providers to presumably less intensive treatment by a different group of providers.

The ultimate hoped-for advantage of treating mild hypertension is obviously to prevent or delay cardiovascular catastrophes. Some of the disadvantages of therapy may seem nebulous or unimportant, certainly they are more difficult to quantify; nonetheless, they can be very real and may have a major impact on the patient. The psychologic effect of merely telling someone that he is 'sick' may alter his quality of life; for instance, it can increase absenteeism. Moreover, the simple lowering of pressure may slow people down and decrease their joie de vivre; certain drugs, particularly some of the centrally acting adrenergic blocking agents, may contribute additionally to this 'slowing.' In addition, any pharmacologically active drug inevitably has some side effects. The hypokalemia associated with thiazide diuretics poses a problem that is currently of considerable concern: is there any significance to the disturbing arrhythmias that sometimes accompany hypokalemia? Are thiazide-treated patients unusually susceptible to sudden death? Finally, it should be emphasized that changes in the quality of life are by no means confined to those resulting from pharmacologic treatment. Although we often recommend major life-style changes with abandon, dietary limitations, exercise requirements and even the cessation of smoking may have a major impact on an individual's happiness.

Although we can treat hypertension, we do not know its cause or even whether it represents a real pathologic entity or simply the upper end of a normal distribution curve of blood pressures. Mild hypertension remains a major risk factor for myocardial infarction, but we do not know whether antihypertensive treatment lowers morbidity and mortality and, if so, to what extent. Moreover, whether or not treatment lowers risk, most patients with mild hypertension will never suffer any major cardiovascular complications from it, and the large majority of those who eventually do will have had many years of trouble-free life before a complication occurs. Under these circumstances, it is reasonable to question whether the whole group of mild hypertensives should be treated or just those at unusually high risks. Should treatment begin when the individual is in his 20s even though the morbidity for the next 30 years is vanishingly small, should it wait 20 years until the danger is more immediate, or should it be postponed indefinitely unless the pressure rises or other risk factors appear? A critical question is whether control of mild hypertension during the 20s, 30s and 40s slows progression of arteriosclerosis and hence delays or prevents arteriosclerotic complications in the 50s and 60s.

Ultimately, our goal is prevention rather than treatment. To this end, a tremendous amount of thus far largely futile effort has been directed toward understanding the pathogenesis of 'essential' hypertension. The role of excess dietary sodium in genetically susceptible individuals is receiving the most attention at the moment. A preventive regimen of low salt intake is currently widely espoused, but there are surprisingly few data on its long-term effects on blood pressure. Potassium, calcium, magnesium and even trace metals like lead or cadmium could be involved in this mechanism. Other factors such as failure of autonomic autoregulation and overactivity of the renin-angiotensin system have also been suggested mechanisms in the causation of hypertension.

One fascinating line of evidence suggests that alkaline earths – and perhaps other water-borne substances that accompany them – could be involved in the pathogenesis of hypertension. An inverse correlation has been repeatedly confirmed between the hardness of drinking water, which reflects dissolved calcium, and cardiovascular mortality, which latter varies markedly from place to place. There is more than a two-fold variation in total 'age-sex-race-standardized mortality' among the 500 plus socioeconomic areas into which the United States has been divided. The entire differences in total mortality are apparently due to differences in cardiovascular mortality, most of them in the incidence of catastrophic morbid events which are considered complications of hypertension. Thus, a tier of 'hard water states' in the middle of the United States from North Dakota to New Mexico include the low mortality socioeconomic areas; whereas, 'soft water states' along the south Atlantic coast include the high mortality areas. South Carolina has twice the death rate that New Mexico or North Dakota has.

There may be a step between the control of hypertension, as we now know it, and prevention, as we hope to know it. There is mounting evidence that either 'cure' or long-term remission of hypertension is possible. Several studies have strongly suggested that after good control for a protracted period of time, about a fifth of patients who discontinue their antihypertensive medication do not have a return of high blood pressure. This topic is currently receiving considerable attention, and several studies have been started to examine the extent of this effect and determine which individuals are likely to develop it. Gradually decreasing severity of hypertension among all well-controlled hypertensive patients was observed in the mid-1950s shortly after the advent of effective treatment, at a time when it was easier to keep track of patients and keep them on a single regimen because there were fewer drugs and fewer therapists. After three years, the average *well-controlled* patient needed only half as much of each antihypertensive agent as had been initially required; no such effect occurred among patients whose blood pressure was not controlled.

In addition to this general effect involving a consecutive series of treated patients, half of a small group with a specific genotype and resultant drug reaction (slow acetylators of hydralazine who developed 'hydralazine'-induced lupus') had complete and long-lasting remissions coupled with significant increases in longevity. The vasculitis, which was a part of this toxicity and which disappeared when the drug was withdrawn, could prove to be a key to understanding how to reverse the hypertensive diathesis. In any case, this sort of observation cries out for further elucidation.

Finally, since we have come to recognize that most hypertension is essential, we can now omit the extensive diagnostic efforts frequently performed in the past, involving a complete workup prior to therapy. The era has passed when all the physician's enthusiasm and all of the patient's money had to be expended in a futile effort at diagnosis, leaving nothing for the effective therapeutic approaches that can prevent morbidity and mortality.

Although the foregoing lists some fascinating questions for future investigation, there are other problems of equal importance, involving the day to day management of hypertension. Therefore, there are chapters in this volume dealing with the available antihypertensive drugs and with nonpharmacologic therapy; with hypertension in pregnancy, childhood and old age; with complications of hypertension; and finally with the economics of hypertension. The sixteen chapters in all, then, represent an attempt to address the immediate concerns of treating hypertension, but at the same time to approach some of the more difficult and less commonly discussed topics associated with the lifelong total management of a condition which has come to be a major part of medical care.

H. Mitchell Perry

1. Epidemiology of mild hypertension

W. McFATE SMITH

The epidemiology of mild hypertension must be understood in terms of the epidemiology of arterial pressure in general. It is the study of the influence of heredity, environment and lifestyle on the susceptibility to and the manifestations of elevated blood pressure. It involves assessing the distribution pattern of elevated arterial pressure in populations according to some characteristic which is believed to influence its occurrence: for example, age, sex, race, body habitus, family history, diet or socioeconomic status. Efforts to identify and understand the causal factors in hypertension have included descriptive studies of entire isolated populations and numerous subsets of large populations, including migrant groups, tribal units and residents of specific geographic locations.

Such studies have not lead to a single etiology or even a unified theory; rather there has emerged a mosaic of factors which are related to the causal process. Those factors which appear to have the strongest association with arterial blood pressure are heredity, age, race, obesity and dietary sodium. Of these factors, only obesity and sodium ingestion are potentially amenable to intervention. Most evidence today indicates that one or more of such environmental factors operate to induce the development of hypertension in genetically susceptible individuals.

Before proceeding further, an attempt must be made to define mild hypertension. Two characteristics of blood pressure have made this somewhat difficult and arbitrary. The first is the wide variability of pressure levels within individual on successive measurements such that they are prone to escape from any narrow class of blood pressure in which they were found initially. This variability is large in comparison to the differences we want to be capable of detecting between populations of groups, making it difficult to recognize small differences between groups. Moreover, as seen in the Hypertension Detection and Follow-up Program, in a two-stage screening program, as many as one-third of those found to have a diastolic blood pressure over 95 mmHg at the initial examination will be below 90 mmHg at the next [1].

The second characteristic is the association of blood pressure levels and blood pressure related risks as continuous variables in the general population (Figure

1). There is no single level of blood pressure which separates normotensives from hypertensives, nor 'milds' from more severe hypertensives.

There is also no evidence for a threshold level for development of complications. Thus, for epidemiologists, it is seldom necessary to define hypertension or 'mild hypertension' except when operationally it becomes desirable to express a prevalence for it. However, as seen in Figure 2, which is a frequency distribution

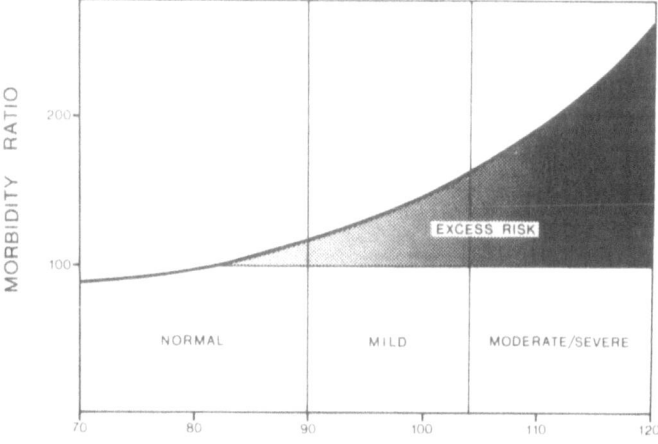

DIASTOLIC   BLOOD   PRESSURE

Figure 1.

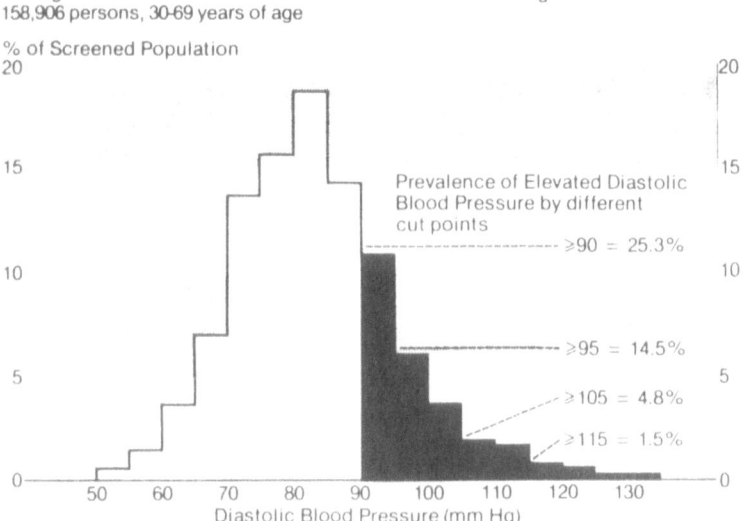

Average of Second and Third Diastolic Blood Pressure Readings at Home Screen
158,906 persons, 30-69 years of age

Figure 2.

of diastolic blood pressures in over 150,000 persons screened at home for the Hypertension Detection and Follow-up Program, it is clearly evident that the prevalence will vary considerably depending upon the arbitrary cutoff point chosen to define it.

LaBarthe illustrated this nicely with data from the U.S. Health Examination Survey of 1960–62 [2]. If mild hypertension is arbitrarily defined as diastolic blood pressure from 90–104 mmHg, the overall prevalence is 15.1% for males and 12.7% for females and, although it varies considerably with age, it is never less than 15% for males over 34 years of age nor for females above age 44 (Table 1).

If one looks at this definition of mild hypertension in relation to the range of pressures below and above it, the prevalence is five times that of levels 105 mmHg or greater. That is, over 80% of hypertensives were in the 90–104 mmHg range (Tables 2 and 3).

The effect on estimates of prevalence of using systolic blood pressure criteria to define mild hypertension can also be seen. For the range of systolic pressures 140–159 mmHg, the prevalence is 193 per thousand, over 30% higher than estimated by diastolic levels exclusively. It should also be noted that, in large measure, these are different individuals. For example, the 140–159 mmHg class of 193 only includes 68 persons from the 90–104 mmHg class. Each class excludes over half from the other (Tables 2 and 3).

Also of interest is the fact that the distribution of diastolic pressures within the 90–104 mmHg range is not symmetrical (Table 4). A majority (57%) were in the interval of 90–94 mmHg range while only 15% were in the 100–104 mmHg category. This simply means that shifting the lower cutoff point upward by

Table 1. Percentage frequencies of diastolic blood pressures from 90–104 mmHg by sex and age, U.S. 1960–1962

Age	Sex	
	Males	Females
18–24	6.9	2.1*
25–34	7.2	4.5
35–44	17.8	11.3
45–54	19.0	17.7
55–64	23.1	22.7
65–74	16.3	22.2
75–79	18.2	17.3
18–79	15.1	12.7

* Includes all values ≥ 90 mmHg.
Source: H.E.S. 1960–1962 (adapted by Labarthe DR, 1977).

Table 2. Prevalence of specified levels of blood pressure per 1000 population, males, 18–79 years

SBP	DBP			
	<90	90–104	≥ 105	Total
≥ 160	32	37	24	93
140–159	118	68	7	193
<140	668	46	0	714
Total	818	151	31	1000

Source: H.E.S. 1960–1962 (adapted by Labarthe DR, 1977).

Table 3. Prevalence of specified levels of blood pressure per 1000 population, DBP 90–104, males, 18–79 years

SBP	DBP			
	90–94	95–99	100–104	Total
≥ 160	13	13	11	37
140–159	34	25	9	68
<140	30	13	3	46
Total	77	51	23	151

Source: H.E.S. 1960–1962 (adapted by Labarthe DR, 1977).

5 mmHg would reduce prevalence a great deal more than shifting the upper boundary downward the same degree. Clearly, the prevalence of mild hypertension is very sensitive to the levels chosen to define it.

If one considers excess risk of mortality in defining the lower boundary of hypertension and includes all those with an excess risk of 50% or more, the definition for men would have to include diastolics at least as low as 85 mmHg (Table 5). Looking at the systolic classes of 138–147 mmHg and higher, even the diastolic sub-class of 83–87 mmHg had a 53% excess risk. But defining mildness in terms of risk should take into account factors other than pressure level. Such factors as age and preexisting target-organ damage not only contribute independently to risk, but also influence the resuls of therapy.

In the Veterans Administration Cooperative Study, the relative efficacy of treatment varied not only by the blood pressure class (those with diastolic blood pressure greater than 105 mmHg clearly having a favorable risk/benefit ratio while those at lower levels did not) but also by age, and presence or absence of target-organ damage [3]. The percent effectiveness of treatment in the 90–104

Table 4. Percentage distributions of clinic readings in relation to home readings in a two-stage screen, white males, HDFP

First screen DBP (home)	Second screen DBP [clinic]			
	<90	90–104	>104	Total
95–104	43.9	49.7	6.3	100.0
105–114	19.1	56.8	24.0	100.0
≥115	8.5	31.4	60.2	100.0
Total	36.8	50.1	13.1	100.0

Source: Hypertension Detection and Follow-up Program, 1977 (adapted by Labarthe DR, 1977).

Table 5. Variations in mortality among men and women, ages 15–69 years, according to systolic and diastolic blood pressures

Systolic blood pressure (mmHg)	Diastolic blood pressure (mmHg)	Mortality ratio (%)*	
		Men	Women
128–137	<83	109	101
	83–87	127	107
	88–92	140	123
	93–97	168	110
	98–102	197	—
138–147	<83	141	118
	83–87	153	122
	88–92	170	120
	93–97	199	195
	98–102	244	220
148–157	<88	180	120
	88–92	191	160
	93–97	224	163
	98–102	269	232
158–167	<88	215	214
	88–92	240	208
	93–97	268	287
	98–102	289	(362)

* Ratios of actual to expected mortality; standard male and female risks, respectively – 100%. Parentheses indicate number of policies terminated by death is 10–34.
Source: Lew EA, 1975 (adapted by Labarthe DR).

mmHg group, age less than 50, and without target-organ damage, was less than one-third what it was for the group 105–114 mmHg, age 50 or *over* and *with* target-organ damage. Even within the 90–104 mmHg group, the percent effectiveness was reduced by 50% in those who were less than age 50 and without target-organ damage.

To summarize these considerations of definition, it must be said that we have arrived at our present one for pragmatic reasons. For therapeutic purposes we use cutoff points based on demonstrated benefit. Mild hypertension is the residual as we move down the pressure scale of demonstrated benefits and up the pressure scale of demonstrated risk. Operationally then, hypertension could be defined as that level of pressure at or above which evaluation and treatment do more good than harm. In a cynical vein, mild hypertension could be considered a euphemism for those pressure levels where we do not know if pharmacologic therapy is indicated or not.

Genetics

Most clinicians have long appreciated that hypertension is common among relatives of hypertensives; the concept that genetic factors play a role in blood pressure regulation is well established. It must be remembered, however, that families share their environment as well as their genes, so that the demonstration of familial correlations does not necessarily require the operation of genetic influences. Recent studies in children, however, lead to the conclusion that familial aggregation of blood pressure, whether between parent and child or between children, is principally the result of heredity [4, 5].

Further powerful support for the important role of heredity has come from studies of twins, the most definitive one involving comparisons of monozygotic and dizygotic twins [6–8]. Monozygotic twins showed clearly higher correlations for both systolic and diastolic pressure than other relatives. Thus, there emerges a clear picture of a major genetic determination of arterial blood pressure and of hypertension as defined at various levels.

Age

Cross-sectional studies in most adult populations show a tendence for the mean values for systolic and diastolic pressure to increase with age (Figure 3). The mean systolic pressure rises slightly during early to mid adult life and then more rapidly after age 40. The mean diastolic pressure shows a small but steady rise through age 60 decreasing thereafter but with no accelerated rise in the forties. Not every individual's pressure rises as he grows older, but it seems that if blood pressure is elevated at any age there's a strong likelihood that it will continue to rise in subsequent years. This is true for whites and blacks alike, but black men and women have higher pressures than whites at each age.

12

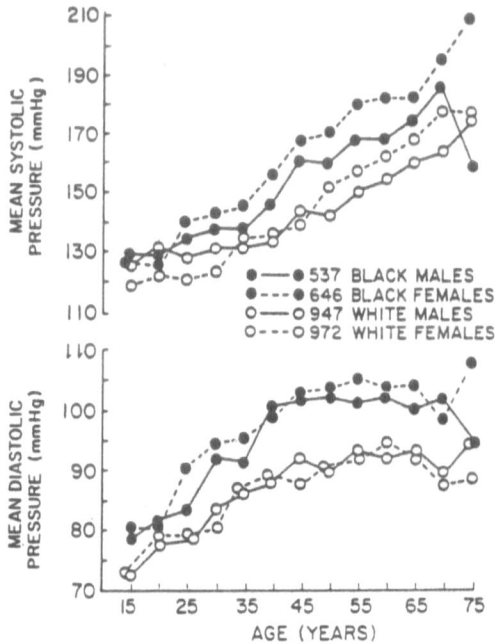

Figure 3. Blood pressure in Evans County Cardiovascular Study, 1960–1962.

Obesity

The positive correlation between blood pressure and obesity is consistent in the community as well as clinical settings and has been documented repeatedly. This association is true for adult men and women and for children. However, obesity is clearly neither a necessary nor a sufficient cause for hypertension, since many obese individuals, including some extremely fat persons, are not hypertensive. Obesity is not only more common in hypertensive than normotensive individuals, normotensive obese subjects are more likely to become hypertensive.

Further strengthening these associations are the observations in large populations that a change in weight over time is associated with a change in blood pressure and this is on the order of a magnitude of 4 mmHg diastolic pressure per 20 pounds change in weight in either direction [9]. In summary obesity is associated with both increased prevalence and incidence of high blood pressure; that is, if overweight, you are more likely to have it and more likely to get it, and a change in weight is associated with a change in blood pressure.

Dietary sodium – the 'salt hypothesis'

The evidence implicating salt in the etiology of hypertension comes from three sources – clinical observations, animal experimentation and epidemiologic studies. Before considering this evidence, it may be useful to review some physiologic and pathophysiologic concepts concerning the regulation of arterial pressure in order to establish credible mechanisms whereby excess dietary salt could be responsible for its elevation.

First of all, blood pressure is the product of the amount of blood pumped by the heart (cardiac output) and the resistance to the flow of this blood by the vascular bed (peripheral resistance). For the majority of patients with established hypertension, including those in whom it is mild, cardiac output is normal and peripheral resistance is increased. However, it has been postulated that an increased cardiac output characterizes the earliest stages of the disease and that an increased peripheral resistance characterizes later stages. It is further suggested that this transition from high output to high resistance occurs because the increased output provides the tissues with more blood than they require. As a consequence, the arterioles contract enough to reduce the flow to match the normal requirement, an auto-regulatory mechanism [10].

Based on both theoretical considerations tested in systems analysis models and experimental data, it has been proposed that an increased central venous pressure resulting from an increased extracellular fluid volume (ECF) leads to the initial increase in cardiac output [11, 12]. This hypothesis holds further that, in those genetically predisposed, some defect in the renal handling of sodium and water is the basis for the increased blood volume. It is suggested that in the early stages of primary hypertension, the kidneys retain only a very small excess of ingested salt and water. As the extracellular fluid volume increases, the cardiac output, and with it the arterial pressure, increases. As the filtration pressure increases, the kidney is able to excrete normal amounts of salt and water. Thus, as postulated in this model, dietary sodium would play an important role in the regulation of blood pressure.

Let us now examine the evidence. First of all, the clinical observations underlying the hypothesis:
1. Over 60% of hypertensives will respond to a very low salt diet (200 mg NaCl) with either normalization or sharp reduction in blood pressure [13].
2. The accelerated removal of salt from hypertensives by diruetics will regularly lower blood pressure. This action is the cornerstone of modern antihypertensive therapy.
3. Patients with renal insufficiency show a direct relationship between salt ingestion and hypertension [14, 15].

In experimental animals, salt ingestion predictably produces hypertension in susceptible species. For example [16, 17]:

1. Rats given salt in drinking water develop hypertension within a few weeks or months. When unselected rats are used, 60–70% will develop elevated pressure in varying degree, the remainder do not.
2. In selected breeding experiments, 'salt sensitive' and 'salt resistant' strains can be quickly separated by selectively inbreeding those rats which do not develop hypertension when given salt.
3. Using genetically 'salt sensitive' rats, it can be shown that young rats are more susceptible to the effects of salt than older rats.
4. Once hypertension develops as a result of feeding salt to these animals, it is permanent.
5. If infant rats of the sensitive strains are given salt for a few weeks, and then the salt is withdrawn, these animals will develop hypertension when they become adults.
6. Even after many generations of inbreeding, the salt sensitive animals will maintain normal blood pressure throughout life if they are never given excessive amounts of salt.

Epidemiological studies provide the principal line of evidence in support of the hypothesis generated by these experimental and clinical observations. One component of this evidence is the absence of hypertension and failure of blood pressure to rise in a number of isolated tribes from widely different parts of the world, whose way of life is marked by a low sodium and a high potassium intake. These include Melanesian tribesman in New Guinea [18] and the Solomon Islands [19], the Easter Islands [20], the Amazon Basin [21], the San Blas Islands off Panama [22], the Kalahari Desert of Africa [23], Australian Aborigines [24], the Highlands of Malaysia [25], Polynesians from isolated islands in the Pacific [26] and rural Uganda [27].

Studies of migratory populations originally unacculturated and free from hypertension, but who have adopted modern ways of life, reveal that their blood pressure rises and hypertension is present. Associated with this invariably is a marked increase in salt consumption [28].

These between-population comparisons are nicely summarized in Dahl's famous graph comparing the prevalence of hypertension and salt intake [29] (Figure 4). Although these data are neither age nor sex adjusted, the concept of a linear relationship between the sodium intake and blood pressure of populations appears generally valid.

In conclusion, a role for sodium in the pathogenesis of hypertension is generally accepted and is fostered by the observations that by increasing dietary salt intake, hypertension is produced in laboratory animals and in some people with renal insufficiency. Conversely, the notion that excessive use of salt by normal persons leads to hypertension remains controversial. Man's appetite for salt clearly exceeds his physiological needs. It is postulated that this excess results in high blood pressure in some individuals which could be prevented by a chronic

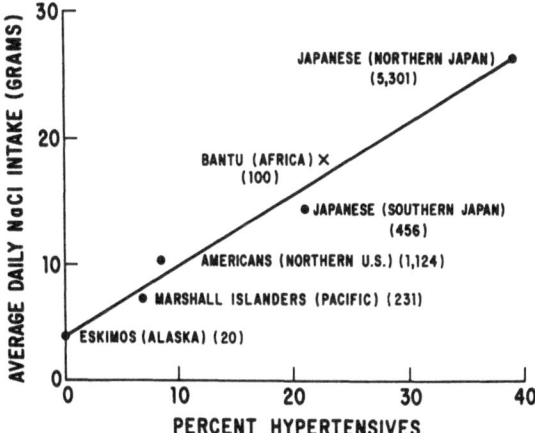

Figure 4.

reduction in salt intake. Although the epidemiological studies are, in general, supportive of the dietary salt-hypertension hypothesis, they fail to be conclusive due to the difficulty in discriminating between salt, per se, and other environmental and genetic factors.

So much then for the factors associated with the development of hypertension. Let's turn our attention now to the consequences or risks which are associated with elevated blood pressure. As noted at the outset, blood pressure and blood pressure risks are related as continuous variables in the general population. The greatly increased risk of experiencing stroke, heart attacks and heart failure among hypertensives is always present despite the fact that at any given time the majority of them are asymptomatic. Actuarial data from life insurance companies clearly demonstrate that the risk of dying prematurely from cardiovascular complications is increased even for persons with only slight elevations of blood pressure and that this risk rises sharply in proportion to blood pressure levels throughout their range with no cutoff point or threshold [30].

In addition to the actuarial data, similar information has been accumulated in a number of prospective epidemiologic studies in different parts of the United States in recent years. The best known among these is the Framingham Heart Study, in which over 20 years of follow-up at biennial intervals has occurred [31]. Shown in Figure 5 is the age adjusted risk of cardiovascular morbidity by WHO blood pressure classification.

Figure 6 demonstrates the rising incidence of clinical manifestations of coronary heart disease in accordance with this same blood pressure classification.

Figure 7 simply illustrates the well-known role of other risk factors, such as cholesterol, glucose intolerance, cigarette smoking and LVH on the electrocardiogram. For these calculations, systolic blood pressure is held constant at 165 mmHg and we note the rising risk based upon the presence of one or more of the other factors.

16

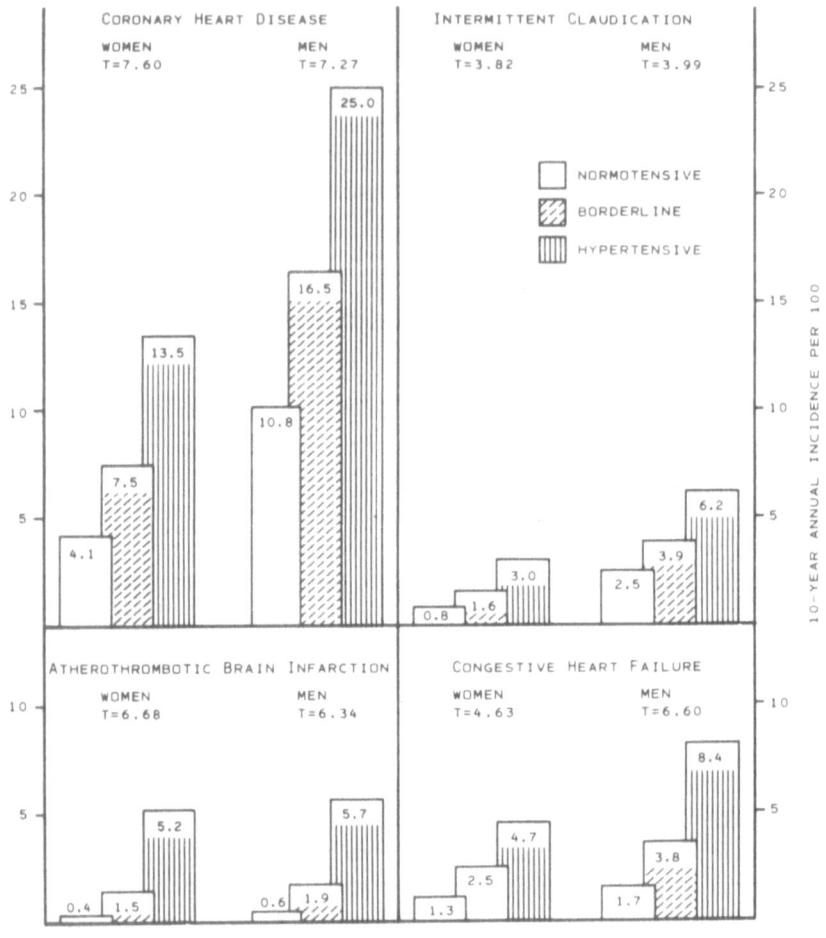

AGE ADJUSTED RISK OF CARDIOVASCULAR MORBIDITY
ACCORDING TO HYPERTENSIVE STATUS AT EACH BIENNIAL EXAM

Figure 5.

The National Cooperative Pooling Project combined the findings of six such investigations [32]. Follow-up was for ten years and included 6640 white men, ages 30–59 at first examination, who were considered to be free from clinical coronary heart disease at that time (Table 6). Most (53% of the 40–49 group) had diastolic pressures below 85 mmHg; and only 5% in the 105 mmHg or greater level. Major coronary events included 325 nonfatal myocardial infarctions and 213 deaths from coronary disease including sudden death. These were expressed as rates per 10,000 in the next table (Table 7). The range of increased risk from lowest to highest diastolic pressure categories varied from more than double for

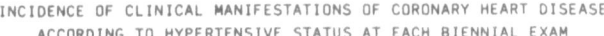

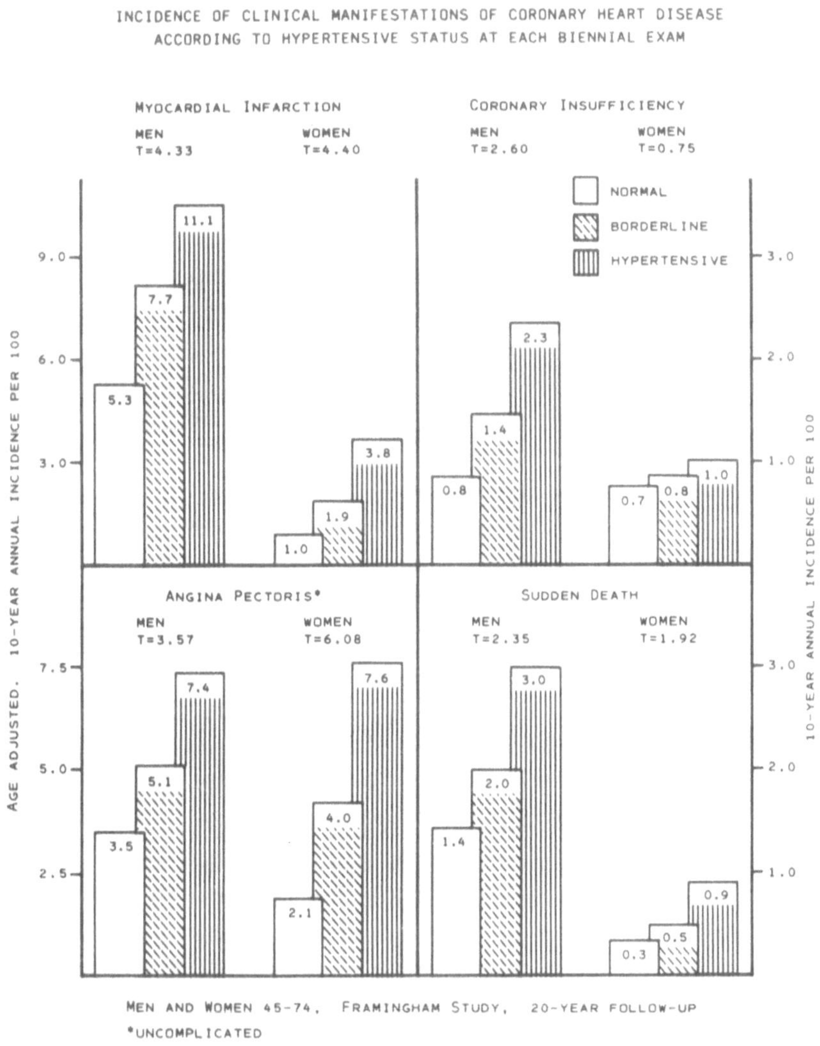
INCIDENCE OF CLINICAL MANIFESTATIONS OF CORONARY HEART DISEASE
ACCORDING TO HYPERTENSIVE STATUS AT EACH BIENNIAL EXAM
MYOCARDIAL INFARCTION
MEN
T=4.33
WOMEN
T=4.40
CORONARY INSUFFICIENCY
MEN
T=2.60
WOMEN
T=0.75
NORMAL
BORDERLINE
HYPERTENSIVE
11.1
7.7
5.3
3.8
1.9
1.0
2.3
1.4
0.8
1.0
0.8
0.7
9.0
6.0
3.0
3.0
2.0
1.0
AGE ADJUSTED. 10-YEAR ANNUAL INCIDENCE PER 100
10-YEAR ANNUAL INCIDENCE PER 100
ANGINA PECTORIS*
MEN
T=3.57
WOMEN
T=6.08
SUDDEN DEATH
MEN
T=2.35
WOMEN
T=1.92
7.4
5.1
3.5
7.6
4.0
2.1
3.0
2.0
1.4
0.9
0.5
0.3
7.5
5.0
2.5
3.0
2.0
1.0
MEN AND WOMEN 45-74, FRAMINGHAM STUDY, 20-YEAR FOLLOW-UP
*UNCOMPLICATED

Figure 6.

ages 50–59 to over tenfold for ages 30–39. When the rates for all levels are considered, the effect of age is also evident.

Finally, it should be pointed out that excess deaths are not the only problem. Disability resulting from hypertension and its complications and the associated great economic cost to the individuals, society and government ranks at the top of the list for causes for all of the major sex and race groups in the labor force.

These facts have challenging implications for prevention and must be considered at several levels. At one level, it is reducing complications and death in subjects at high risk. Pressure-lowering drugs are effective in this regard. On the

18

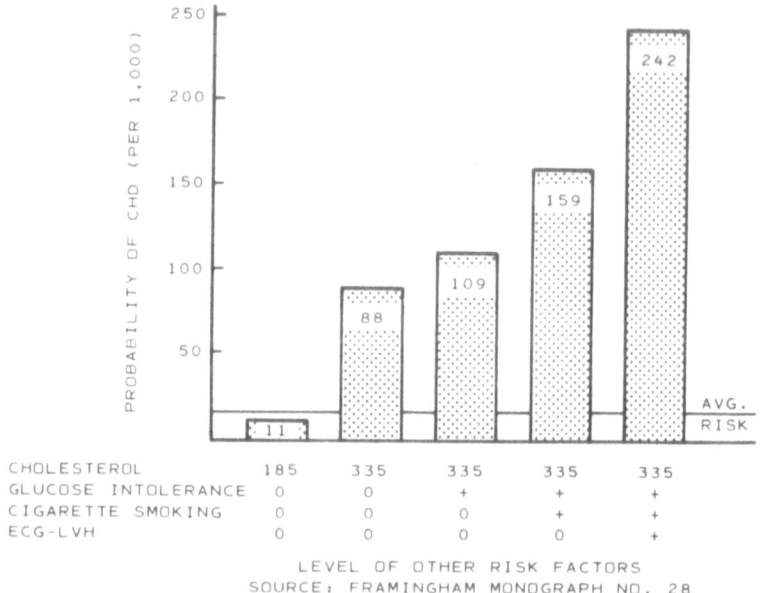

Figure 7.

other hand, if we consider those with mildly elevated pressures without target-organ damage, the risk/benefit ratio for drug treatment is not so clearly favorable.

Primary prevention is the control of those factors which, when present, may lead to elevated pressures in a normotensive individual. It is the most attractive and exciting approach, the logic of which is suggested by population studies, but neither its feasibility nor its efficacy has been tested.

In conclusion, it is worth noting that during the past ten years, when considerable national attention has been focused on the problem of hypertension, with widespread community screening activities and intensive public and pro-

Table 6. Distribution of men by age and diastolic blood pressure at baseline

Diastolic pressure (mmHg)	Age		
	30–39 (N = 1211)	40–49 (N = 3460)	50–59 (N = 1969)
	%	%	%
<85	61	53	50
85–94	26	29	29
95–104	10	13	13
>104	3	5	8

Source: Pooling Project of the Council on Epidemiology of the American Heart Association.

Table 7. Total non-fatal myocardial infarction and all coronary deaths (ten-year rates/10,000)

Diastolic pressure (mmHg)	Age		
	30–39	40–49	50–59
<85	106	603	858
85–94	538	680	1431
95–104	576	707	1896
>104	1463	1907	2116
Combined rate	335	715	1299

Source: Pooling Project of the Council on Epidemiology of the American Heart Association.

fessional information programs, substantial improvement has taken place in both the levels of awareness and the percentage under treatment and controlled. Figure 8 illustrates the situation as it existed over 15 years ago, at which time nearly half were unaware of their hypertension, and of those aware and under treatment, only 16% were well controlled. The situation had not changed a decade later as seen in the Health and Nutrition Examination Survey, which preceded the National High Blood Pressure Education Program [33]. However, two separate surveys since that time, the Community Hypertension Evaluation Clinics (CHEC) and the Hypertension Detection and Follow-up Program, a study of 14 communities which revealed as many as 37% of nonhypertensives to be controlled on therapy, indicate that we have begun to make progress [34, 1].

PERCENT OF HYPERTENSIVES AWARE, TREATED, AND CONTROLLED:
NATIONAL HEALTH EXAMINATION SURVEYS, 1960–62 AND 1971
AND THE HYPERTENSION DETECTION AND FOLLOW–UP STUDY, 1973–74

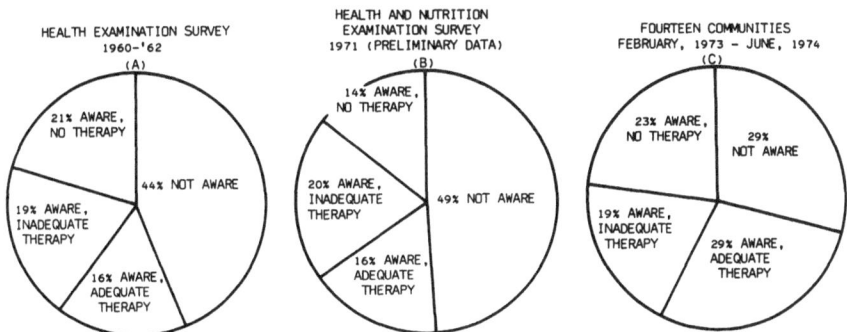

(A) COMPUTED FROM DATA PUBLISHED IN VITAL AND HEALTH STATISTICS, SERIES 2, NUMBER 22, MARCH, 1967, NATIONAL CENTER FOR HEALTH STATISTICS.

(B) COMPUTED FROM UNPUBLISHED PRELIMINARY DATA FURNISHED BY THE NATIONAL CENTER FOR HEALTH STATISTICS.

(C) HYPERTENSION DETECTION AND FOLLOW–UP STUDY, NATIONAL HEART AND LUNG INSTITUTE.

Figure 8.

20

References

1. Hypertension Detection and Follow-up Program Cooperative Group. Blood pressure studies in 14 communities. A two-stage screen for hypertension. JAMA 237:2385, 1977.
2. Labarthe DR: Problems in definition of mild hypertension. In: Perry HM, Jr, Smith WM (eds) Mild hypertension: to treat or not to treat. Ann N Y Acad Sci 304:3, 1978.
3. Veterans Administration Cooperative Study Group on Antihypertensive Agents. Effects of treatment on morbidity in hypertension. III. Influence of age, diastolic pressure, and prior cardiovascular disease; further analysis of side effects. Circulation 45:991, 1972.
4. Zinner SH, Levy PS, Kass EH: Familial aggregation of blood pressure in childhood. N Engl J Med 284:401, 1976.
5. Biron P, Mongeau J, Bertrand D: Familial aggregation of blood pressure in adopted and natural children. In: Paul O (ed) Epidemiology and control of hypertension. Miami, Symposia Specialists, 1975.
6. Hines EA Jr, McIlhaney M, Gage R: A study of twins with normal blood pressures and with hypertension. Trans Assoc Am Physicians 70:282, 1957.
7. Mathers J, Osborne R, DeGeorge F: Studies of blood pressure, heart rate and the electrocardiogram in adult twins. Am Heart J 62:634, 1961.
8. Vander Molen R, Brewer G, Honeyman MS et al: A study of hypertension in twins. Am Heart J 79:454, 1970.
9. Tyroler HA, Heyden S, Hames CG: Weight and hypertension: Evans County studies of blacks and whites. In: Paul O (ed): Epidemiology and control of hypertension. Miami, Symposia Specialists, 1975, p 177.
10. Guyton AC, Coleman TG, Cawley AW et al: A systems analysis approach to understanding long-range arterial blood pressure control and hypertension. Circ Res 35:159, 1974.
11. Floyer MA, Richardson PC: Mechanism of arterial hypertension. Role of capacity and resistance vessels. Lancet 1:253, 1961.
12. Ledingham JM, Cohen RD: The role of the heart in the pathogenesis of renal hypertension. Lancet 2:979, 1963.
13. Kempner W: Treatment of hypertensive vascular disease with rice diet. Am J Med 4:454, 1948.
14. Brown JJ, Dusterdieck G, Fraser R et al: Hypertension and chronic renal failure. Br Med Bull 27:128, 1971.
15. Onesti G, Kim KE, Fernandes M et al: Hypertension of renal parenchymal disease. Proc 6th Int Cong Nephrol, 1975, p 284.
16. Dahl LK: Salt and hypertension. Am J Clin Nutr 25:231, 1972.
17. Dahl LK: Effects of chronic excess salt ingestion – experimental hypertension in the rat: correlation with human hypertension. In: Stamler J, Stamler R, Pullman TN (eds) The epidemiology of hypertension. New York, Grune & Stratton, 1967, p 218.
18. Maddocks I: Blood pressures in Melanesians. Med J Aust 1:1123, 1967.
19. Page LB, Danion A, Moellering RC Jr: Antecedents of cardiovascular disease in six Solomon Island societies. Circulation 49:1132, 1974.
20. Cruz-Coke R, Etcheverry R, Nagel R: Influence of migration on blood pressure of Easter Islanders. Lancet 1:697, 1964.
21. Lowenstein FW: Blood pressure in relation to age and sex in the tropics and subtropics. A review of the literature and an investigation in two tribes of Brazil Indians. Lancet 1:389, 1961.
22. Kean BH: The blood pressure of the Cuna Indians. Am J Trop Med 24:341, 1944.
23. Kaminer B, Lutz WPW: Blood pressure in Bushmen of the Kalahari Desert. Circulation 22:289, 1960.
24. Abbie AL, Schroder J: Blood pressure in Arnhem Land Aborigines. Med J Aust 2:493, 1960.
25. Burns-Cox CJ, Maclean JD: Splenomegaly and blood pressure in an Orang Asli community in

West Malaysia. Am Heart J 80:718, 1970.

26. Prior IAM, Evans JG, Harvey HPB et al: Sodium intake and blood pressure in two Polynesian populations. N Engl J Med 279:515, 1968.

27. Shaper AG: Cardiovascular disease in the tropics. III. Blood pressure and hypertension. Br Med J 3:805, 1972.

28. Scotch N: A preliminary report on the relation of sociocultural factors to hypertension among the Zulu. Ann NY Acad Sci 84:1000, 1960.

29. Meneely GR, Dahl LK: Electrolytes in hypertension: the effects of sodium chloride. The evidence from animal and human studies. Hypertension and its treatment. Med Clin North Am 45:271, 1961.

30. Society of Actuaries: Build and Blood Pressure Study, Chicago, 1959.

31. Kannel WB, Dawber TR: Hypertension as an ingredient of a cardiovascular risk profile. Br J Hosp Med 508: April, 1974.

32. Paul O: Risk of mild hypertension: A ten-year report. Br Heart J 33 (Suppl):116, 1971.

33. National Health Survey. Blood pressure levels of persons 6–74 years, United States, 1971–1974. National Center for Health Statistics, Vital and health Statistics, Series 11, No 203, Sept 1977.

34. Stamler J, Stamler R, Riedlinger WF et al: Hypertension screening of 1 million Americans: Community Hypertension Evaluation Clinic (CHEC) Program, 1973 through 1975. JAMA 235:2299, 1976.

2. Childhood precursors of adult hypertension

DAVID GOLDRING

Introduction

There is little question that untreated childhood hypertension secondary to renal disease, coarctation of the aorta and hormonal disorders may persist into adulthood; however, whether primary hypertension in infants and children may be the antecedent of adult hypertension has not been answered, because no longitudinal blood pressure studies from infancy into adulthood have been done. This was probably due to the impression which most physicians had that primary hypertension was relatively rare in childhood, and therefore, blood pressures were not measured routinely in infants and children before 1970. As a result of the educational campaign which was mounted by the American Heart Association and the National Institute of Health about ten years ago, more and more physicians are measuring blood pressure in infants and children, and primary hypertension will probably be diagnosed with greater frequency. Indeed, recent studies by Londe [1] and Loggie [2] contend that primary hypertension is the most common form of hypertension in children, contrary to the previously held notion that most hypertension in childhood was secondary to renal disease, as reported by Haggerty [3].

Primary hypertension

Blood pressure measurement in children

The sphygmomanometric method for the measurement of blood pressure has been described very thoroughly by a study committee of the American Heart Association [4], and accurate measurements can be made if the instructions are carefully followed. It is important to be aware of the many factors which may affect the accuracy of the measurement as shown by Londe and Goldring [5] (Table 1). The width of the cuff is especially important in measuring the blood pressure of the pediatric patient because of the changing arm size with growth.

Table 1. Possible sources of error in measuring blood pressure

---

Equipment
    Defective sphygmomanometer, tubing, cuff, stethoscope

Use of equipment
    Arm cuff not at heart level
    Improper cuff size
    Too slow inflation, too rapid deflation
    Mercury column not at eye level

Examiner
    Imperfect knowledge of technique
    Hearing deficiency
    Variations in use of single or multiple determinations of blood pressure
    Terminal digit preference

Variations in condition of subject
    Sitting position
    Supine position
    Presence of pain
    Time after exercise
    Time after meal
    Bladder distention
    Alcohol ingestion
    Anxiety
    Infection
    Smoking
    Coffee or tea ingestion
    Drug therapy (sympathomimetic drugs, contraceptive pill)
    Fever

Environment
    Diurnal variation
    Ambient temperature
    Noise pollution

Reprinted with permission [5].

However, all one has to remember is that the cuff width should be 20% wider than the diameter of the arm, and the cuff should encircle the arm. If the cuff is too narrow, a falsely elevated blood pressure will result. Two popular misconceptions deserve mention. An elevated blood pressure in an obese child is often dismissed as an artifact of the obesity. However, if the proper size cuff is used, the pressure measurement will be accurate; and if an elevated pressure is found, the patient deserves continued observation. Another false notion held was that an elevated blood pressure during the pubertal years was a normal finding. Londe et al. [6] pointed out a number of years ago that there was no correlation between the blood pressure and sexual maturational development as judged by serum levels of follicular stimulating and luteinizing hormones and the stage of sexual development (pubic hair, breast development and onset of menarche). Therefore, an elevated blood pressure in an adolescent boy or girl should not be considered a normal finding.

Blood pressure measurement in infants

The sphygmomanometric method is too difficult to use in infants and children up to the age of two years and probably accounts for the relatively few studies on blood pressure in infants. The 'flush' method introduced about 30 years ago by Goldring and Wohltman [7] was useful in the diagnosis of coarctation of the aorta in infants. This method measured the mean pressures as shown by Goldring et al. [8] and provided a means of comparing the gradient in pressure between the upper and lower extremities. The 'flush' method has been replaced by the more popular and accurate Doppler technique as reported by Hernandez et al. [9] and provides a relatively easy way for measuring blood pressure in infants.

Blood pressure standards

Shortly after the article by Londe et al. [1] pointed out that primary hypertension was the most common form of hypertension in childhood, studies of children's blood pressure began to appear. Unfortunately, there were marked variations in the suggested values for the 50th and 95th percentiles (Figures 1, 2 and 3) [2, 7, 10–25]. This can be explained by the different methodologies used by the investigators. Some of the authors measured the blood pressure in the sitting position; others in the supine position. Some averaged the second and third pressures as the pressure of record; some averaged the pressures of both upper extremities. Some used the fourth Korotkoff sound; other the fifth Korotkoff phase as the diastolic signal.

Racial differences in blood pressure were examined by Londe et al. [26], who found no significant difference in the blood pressure of black and white children between the ages of three and 15 years. Goldring et al. [16] found that white adolescents 14–18 years of age had significantly higher pressures at the 50th percentile than did the black subjects, whereas Kilcoyne [18] found that the black adolescents had higher pressures at the 50th percentile than did the white subjects.

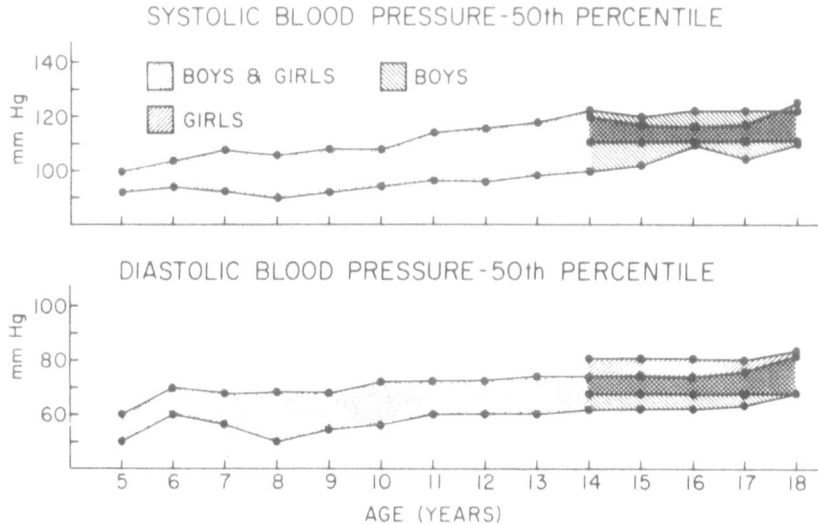

Figure 1. Spread of blood pressures at the 50th percentile as reported in literature [2, 7, 10-25].

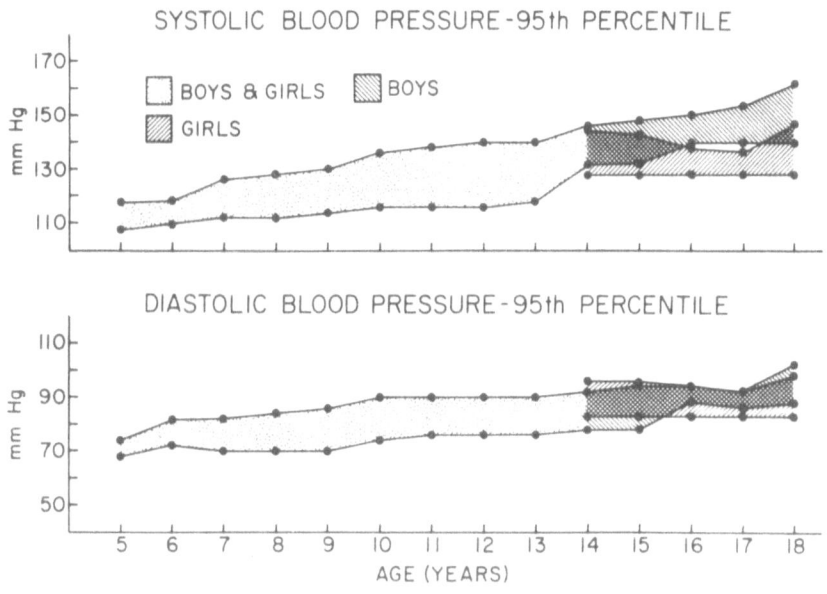

Figure 2. Spread of blood pressures at the 95th percentile as reported in the literature [2, 7, 10-25].

SYSTOLIC BLOOD PRESSURE

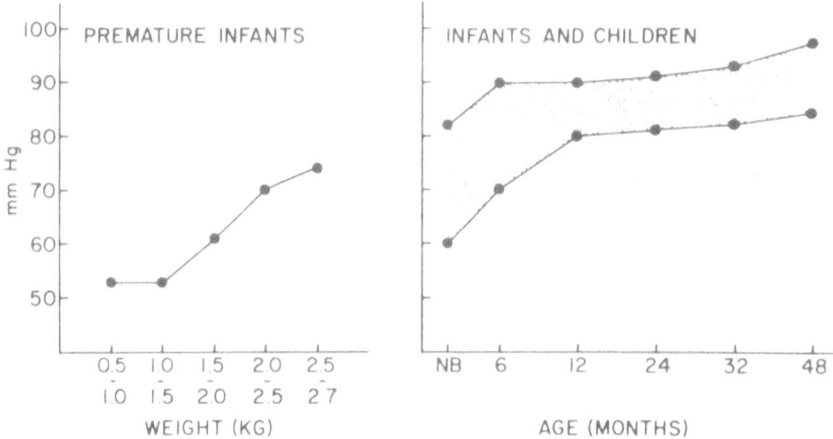

Figure 3. Spread of blood pressures as reported for premature infants and full-term infants from birth to two years of age as reported in the literature (boys and girls) [2, 7, 10–25].

Incidence of primary hypertension

There are relatively few studies of blood pressure in infants. Therefore, the incidence of primary hypertension in this age group is unknown. Adelman [27] and Plumer [28] feel that most instances of hypertension in infants are secondary to aortic thrombosis because of umbilical artery catheterization. Since the advent of the Doppler technique for measuring blood pressure in infants, more studies of blood pressure in this age group will be appearing; and it will not be surprising to find that in infants, as in older children, primary hypertension may be the most common form of hypertension.

The reported incidence of primary hypertension from three to 18 years of age ranges from 1.4% to 11%, undoubtedly because the investigators did not use a uniform definition of hypertension, and the method of measuring blood pressure varied from investigator to investigator [2].

Tracking phenomenon

An important question is whether the childhood hypertensives will remain hypertensive as adults. As yet, no answer is available to this question except from some limited tracking studies of blood pressure, which suggest that the tracking correlation is higher in adulthood than in childhood.

Tracking correlation is defined as the relationship between blood pressure measurements obtained at two points in time for the same individual. Tracking correlations for adults 35–70 years have been reported by McKeown [29] and Feinlieb [30] as 0.6 for systolic pressure and 0.5 for diastolic pressure. Zinner [31] reported tracking correlation of only 0.025 for systolic pressure and 0.14 for diastolic pressure for children 2–14 years of age. However, Londe et al. [1] found that 65% of hypertensive children 3–15 years of age remained hypertensive after three to nine years of follow-up.

Definition of childhood primary hypertension

Master [32] suggested that adults whose blood pressures (systolic, diastolic or both systolic and diastolic) are between the 90th and 95th percentiles be classified as suspect hypertensives, and those whose blood pressures are above the 95th percentile be considered hypertensives. We feel that this is a reasonable definition of hypertension and is the one which we use in children. In addition, we feel that before a diagnosis of hypertension is made, the child's blood pressure should remain elevated for at least one year, during which time the pressure has been measured every three to four months. Blood pressures which we consider as suspect hypertension in our geographic area are shown in Table 2. A popular notion has been that it is the elevation of the diastolic pressure which is the important predictor of morbidity and mortality. However, the study of Dustan and Tarazi [33] stresses that an elevated systolic pressure is just as important a determinant of future morbidity and mortality as the diastolic pressure.

Table 2. Approximate guidelines for suspect blood pressure values (boys and girls)

| Age in years | Supine position (average of second and third readings): | | | |
	Birth–2	3–5	6–9	10–13
Blood pressure mmHg	100 >—— 70	110 >—— 74	116 >—— 76	120 >—— 80
	Seated position (average of second and third readings):			
Age in years	Girls	Boys		
	14–18	14–15	16–18	
Blood pressure mmHg	125 >——— 80	130 >——— 80	135 >——— 85	

Diagnostic evaluation

The child who should be selected for referral to a pediatric cardiologist for thorough evaluation is one whose systolic, diastolic or both systolic and diastolic pressures have been elevated at or above the 95th percentile for about one year and are based upon four to five measurements during that year. The present evaluation which we recommend is more abbreviated than the comprehensive evaluation which our group did some years ago [1]. In this early study of 74 childhood hypertensives, after a comprehensive evaluation we found only five whose elevated pressure may have been secondary to renal disease. Important findings were that 50% of the children were obese, and one or both of their parents had primary hypertension. In the light of our early experience, we now recommend the following abbreviated work-up: a careful history and physical examination including a funduscopic examination as well as measurement of blood pressure in the upper and lower extremities, urinalysis, serum determination of fasting glucose, sodium, potassium, urea nitrogen, creatinine, chest roentgenogram, an electrocardiogram, echocardiogram, systolic time intervals and an exercise stress test. The reasons for the last five cardiac examinations are to establish baselines for future evaluations and to see if the hypertensive patient demonstrates the characteristic cardiovascular dynamics described below. Secondary causes of hypertension such as renal disease and endocrine disorders and coarctation of the aorta are usually easily ruled out after the above limited evaluation as shown by Goldring et al. [34].

Clinical profile of juvenile hypertensive

There is great need for a specific test to identify the child with primary hypertension. Recently, two interesting studies by Garay et al. [35] and Canessa et al. [36] reported that they could distinguish primary from secondary hypertensives by significant differences in sodium-potassium flux ratios of red blood cells. If this finding can be verified by other investigators, it should prove to be a very important contribution.

We studied a group of 114 adolescent primary hypertensives and compared them with 71 normotensive age and sex-matched controls [34]. The results of the study are summarized in tabular form. Table 3 presents the range of blood pressures in the hypertensives. There were significant differences between the hypertensives and normotensives in the systolic time–interval studies (Table 4) and the echocadiographic evaluation (Table 5). The blood pressure and heart rate response of the hypertensives to the bicycle stress test are shown in Tables 6 and 7. Note that there was no rise in the diastolic pressure with this type of exercise. There was no significant difference in the slopes or the blood pressure

Table 3. Juvenile hypertensives (population sample: 3494)

Number of students whose systolic or diastolic or both systolic and diastolic pressures persistently exceeded the 95th percentile	266 (7.6%)
	Range of blood pressure (mmHg)
Girls 14–18 years	128–164 / 82–96
Boys 14 years	134–164 / 80–88
15 years	136–164 / 86–94
16–18 years	140–174 / 88–100

Table 4. Systolic time intervals

	Female					Male				
	Normotensive (27)		Hypertensive (38)			Normotensive (27)		Hypertensive (71)		
	Mean	S.D.	Mean	S.D.	'P' less than	Mean	S.D.	Mean	S.D.	'P' less than
LVET	278	25.5	273	38.4	N.S.	278	21.0	285	30.1	N.S.
Q-S_2	394	23.4	373	42.6	0.05	398	24.8	382	27.5	0.01
PEP	116	15.8	101	20.6	0.005	120	17.0	97	22.8	0.001
PEP/ LVET	0.4	0.08	0.38	0.11	N.S.	0.34	0.08	0.35	0.10	0.001

LVET = Left ventricular ejection time (m/sec); Q-S_2 = Electro-mechanical systole (m/sec); PEP = Pre-ejection period (m/sec); ( ) = Number of subjects. Reprinted with permission [34].

curves except that the systolic and diastolic pressures of the hypertensives were higher. However, the hypertensives showed a slower return of the heart rate to the pretest level when compared with the normotensives. Two other interesting findings were that a significant number of hypertensives showed basilar cardiac hypertrophy on the electrocardiograms and vectorcardiograms, and the hypertensive boys showed significantly higher serum levels of triglycerides and low density lipoprotein fractions than did the normotensives. The hypertensive girls had higher serum concentrations of the very low density lipoprotein fraction as compared with the normotensive girls. A summary of the findings in the hypertensive patients is given in Table 8. One finding in the above study deserves

Table 5. Echocardiographic evaluation, mean arterial pressure and systemic resistance

| | Female | | | | | Male | | | | |
| | Normotensive (31) | | Hypertensive (42) | | | Normotensive (35) | | Hypertensive (67) | | |
	Mean	S.D.	Mean	S.D.	'P' less than	Mean	S.D.	Mean	S.D.	'P' less than
EDVI	62	29.2	48	16.3	0.05	76	37.3	48	20.8	0.001
ESVI	22	14.4	17	14.1	N.S.	30	18.1	14	7.4	0.001
SVI	40	17.1	33	10.3	0.05	46	21.6	34	14.0	0.010
CI	3	3.03	2	1.03	0.05	3	1.9	2	1.1	0.010
EF	66	8.8	69	9.7	N.S.	63	9.3	70	5.8	0.001
Vcf	1	0.25	1	0.33	N.S.	0.9	0.25	1	0.2	0.001
SID	31	6.7	33	6.7	N.S.	29	6.8	34	4.5	0.001
MAP mmHg	78	8.9	93	10.8	0.001	80	8.9	91	9.0	0.001
R (units)	28	13.5	40	13.5	0.01	31	22.6	48	28.3	0.001

EDVI = end-diastolic volume index (ml/M^2); ESVI = end-systolic volume index $(ml = M^2)$; SVI = stroke volume index (ml/M^2); CI = $L/m/M^2$; EF = ejection fraction; Vcf = velocity of circumferential fiber shortening (cir/sec); SID = % shortening of left ventricular internal diameter; MAP = mean arterial pressure; R = resistance.
Reprinted with permission [34].

Table 6. Peak blood pressures during exercise

| | Female | | | | | Male | | | | |
| | Normotensive (31) | | Hypertensive (40) | | | Normotensive (35) | | Hypertensive (71) | | |
	Mean	S.D.	Mean	S.D.	'P' less than	Mean	S.D.	Mean	S.D.	'P' less than
Peak systolic pressure during exercise	145.81	16.20	174.1	23.69	0.001	161.43	24.25	192.37	25.00	0.001
Peak diastolic pressure during exercise	60.45	17.64	77.60	13.20	0.001	59.83	12.95	74.74	10.96	0.001

Reprinted with permission [34].

Table 7. Heart rate response to exercise

	Female Normo- tensives (31)		Hyper- tensives (40)			Male Normo- tensives (35)		Hyper- tensives (71)		
	Mean	S.D.	Mean	S.D.	'P' less than	Mean	S.D.	Mean	S.D.	'P' less than
Baseline heart rate	84.6	16.43	88.65	19.89	N.S.	76.11	15.90	73.61	13.60	N.S.
Peak heart rate during exercise	174.13	13.46	180.90	18.22	0.05	173.94	14.43	183.15	17.54	0.05
Heart rate 10 min after exercise	94.84	12.52	100.10	19.41	N.S.	87.66	14.48	97.10	16.83	0.01

Reprinted with permission [34].

Table 8. Characteristics of juvenile essential hypertensives

1. Obesity
2. Basilar hypertrophy (ECG/VCG)
3. Normal chest x-ray, normal physical findings, normal blood electrolytes and urine
4. Elevated serum triglyceride (LDL, VLDL)*
5. Abnormal blood pressure and pulse response to exercise stress test
6. Systolic time intervals

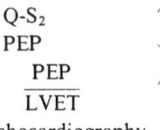

    Q-S_2 ↑
    PEP ↓
    $\dfrac{\text{PEP}}{\text{LVET}}$ ↑

7. Echocardiography
    Volume indices ↓
    EF ↑
    VCF ↑
    SID ↑
    CI ↓
8. MAP ↑
9. R ↑

* LDL = Low density lipoprotein; VLDL = Very low density lipoprotein.

emphasis. The cardiac index was significantly lower and the peripheral systemic resistance was elevated in the hypertensives when compared with the normotensive controls. Therefore, the popular conception that early hypertensives are characterized by a hyperkinetic circulation, i.e., increased cardiac output and normal peripheral systemic resistance, was not observed in the above study. We believe, as do Dustan and Tarazi [33] and Davignon et al. [37] that young primary hypertensives are a heterogeneous group, as is true of adult hypertensives; some have a hyperkinetic circulation; others have a depressed cardiac output and an elevated peripheral systemic resistance.

Thus, if one has a pediatric patient with persistent hypertension whose history and physical examination do not support a diagnosis of renal disease, coarctation of the aorta or hormonal disorder and whose blood chemistries and urine examination are normal, one should consider the diagnosis of primary hypertension. This presumptive diagnosis is further strengthened if, in addition, the patient has the findings shown in Table 8. If this clinical profile is substantiated in studies by other investigators, it should be of value in making the diagnosis of primary hypertension and in the evaluation of therapeutic intervention.

Treatment

The decision about treatment with antihypertensive drugs is a very difficult one to make because of a number of considerations. We do not know how many of these young hypertensive patients will remain hypertensive. We also are aware of the untoward reactions of all antihypertensive drugs in adults, as well as in children, who are being treated for hypertension secondary to renal disease as reported by Sinaiko [38]. We have very little information about the long-term effects of these drugs upon a developing individual. The beneficial effect of drug therapy is that there is the possibility that treatment of the young hypertensive may arrest the disease. Even mild hypertensive individuals may benefit from treatment according to the reports of the Veterans Administration studies which showed significant reduction in morbidity and mortality in severe as well as mild hypertensive adults [39, 40]. Does this finding justify drug therapy for the young, mild and asymptomatic primary hypertensive subject? After careful consideration of the above, we feel that the preferred therapy should be non-pharmacologic, such as weight reduction for the obese, moderate dietary salt restriction, and a regular regimen of dynamic exercise. This treatment poses no health threat to the child.

Weight reduction

Chiang [41] pointed out the association of obesity and hypertension when he suggested that weight gain was an environmental stress which might cause hypertension in genetically predisposed individuals. Kannel, in the Framingham study [42], and Levy [43] showed that the risk of developing hypertension was significantly greater in the obese.

The pathogenesis of hypertension in the obese person is incompletely understood, but is felt to be upon the basis of increased cardiac output as noted by Alexander [44] and Whyte [45].

Reduction of arterial pressure by caloric restriction is possible in the obese as well as in the nonobese individuals. Recently, Reisin [46] showed significant reduction of systolic and diastolic pressures in obese, hypertensive patients who lost weight due to caloric restriction with no significant change in the intake and output of salt. To date, there have been no such studies in obese, hypertensive pediatric patients, but a trial is warranted even though compliance may be difficult to achieve.

It is well known that psychological factors play an important role in weight control [47–49]. Prior to the start of a weight reduction program, psychiatric and social assessment are needed to identify factors which might interfere with a weight control program. This evaluation should include the family when their support should be stressed. Also, ongoing psychiatric consultation is important to help the subjects and their families cope with the changes in lifestyle and patterning which necessarily are associated with successful weight reduction. A team approach is needed and should include the primary physician, a nutritionist, social worker and psychiatrist. What is most important are family support and frequent visits to the physician, preferably the same physician, once or twice a month, to help the patient adhere to the regimen.

Diet modification

Moderate dietary salt restriction. The NIH Report of the Hypertension Task Force [50] noted that there is considerable circumstantial evidence linking dietary salt intake to blood pressure in experimental animals and humans. Other ions such as calcium, chloride and potassium may also play a role, as reported by Kotchen et al. [51] and the NIH Task Force Report [50]. The degree of sodium restriction necessary to effect a significant reduction in pressure is unknown, although it is believed that a reduced intake to 50 mEq of salt per day is necessary to achieve a reduction in blood pressure. This degree of salt restriction will be unpalatable and compliance will undoubtedly be difficult. Therefore, what may be more acceptable to children may be achieved by not using salt in cooking and not adding salt to food at the table, and restricting foods with high salt content as enumerated by Carter [52]. Again, compliance will be difficult to achieve. Tactful emphasis, family support and guidance by frequent visits to the physician may help the patient adhere to the regimen.

Reduction of blood lipid concentration. The prospective and retrospective studies of Wilmore [53] enumerated certain risk factors such as hypertension, elevated blood lipids, cigarette smoking, diabetes mellitus, obesity, anxiety, inadequate physical activity and family history of coronary heart disease, which he claimed predisposed individuals to premature development of coronary artery disease in adults. The subject remains controversial. Recently, Lauer [54] and Blumenthal [55] have identified some of these factors in children and suggested that these children may be the individuals who are at risk of developing coronary artery disease as adults. This conclusion is highly speculative, because there are no longitudinal studies of children with these risk factors. Martz [56] has suggested that diet modification by the reduction of high cholesterol content foods and the use of drug therapy such as clofibrate, cholestyramine and nicotinic acid to further lower blood cholesterol may reduce the risk of developing coronary artery disease in adults. These results are also controversial. In light of this controversy, one is not justified in using this type of diet modification and drug therapy in the pediatric patient with primary hypertension as a means of reducing the risk of developing coronary artery disease as an adult. Enthusiastic proponents of this type of dietary manipulation have suggested this approach for all infants and children. Advising radical changes in the diet of all infants and children as a means of lowering blood lipids by reducing the intake of high cholesterol-containing foods is not justified as pointed out by Schubert [57], because we do not have enough information about what serious harm may come from drastic modification of the diet. However, the practitioner is justified in determining the blood level of cholesterol, triglyceride and lipoprotein fractions in a child with primary hypertension. This is important, especially if after a careful history and physical examination, he suspects Type II hyperlipoproteinemia. An aggressive approach with diet modification and drugs is then indicated in this disorder as shown by Levy and Rifkind [58].

Exercise

A number of investigators [59–64] have shown that dynamic exercise of a few months' duration lowers blood pressure in some primary hypertensive patients. This kind of therapy, i.e., a regimen of running, bicycling or swimming, might have special appeal for the young patient. It is also possible that weight reduction of the obese primary hypertensive patient and an exercise regimen may have synergistic effects in normalizing the blood pressure.

Ekbloom [65] and Saltin [66] have provided an explanation for the physiologic processes involved in lowering the blood pressure by showing that dynamic exercise results in an adaptive decrease in heart rate in normal individuals, both at rest and during submaximal exercise. They also showed that cardiac output at rest and during work requiring a given submaximal oxygen uptake is often lower in the trained as compared with the untrained state. Pulse wave and arterial pressure analyses have provided evidence that tension-time index and ejection-time index are reduced after training, as noted by Hanson [67]. The relatively hypokinetic circulatory state produced by exercise-training is probably caused by the negative inotropic effect of the reduction in heart rate, and to adaptations in the neuroendocrine system which result in increased vagal tone and decreased release of norepinephrine and epinephrine as described by Hartley [68]. The exercise regimen should be tailored to the patient's interest. For the adolescent group we suggest that they exercise for 45 min a day, and the exercise should be strenuous enough to increase the heart rate to approximately 150 beats/min for 45 min. If the subjects select running, then they should build up their endurance so that they run about three to five miles a day four times a week. If they select bicycling, they should build up their endurance so that they ride 10–15 miles a day four times per week. If they select swimming, they should build up their endurance so that they swim one to two miles four times per week.

Isometric exercises, such as some forms of weight lifting and hand-grip exercise, are not recommended for adult hypertensive patients who may have known or silent coronary artery disease or compromised cardiac function, because of greater stress placed upon the heart muscle, thus requiring increased coronary blood flow as shown by Bradfield [69]. This form of exercise may be beneficial and safe for the pediatric primary hypertensive whose heart and coronary circulation are known to be normal.

The safety of the dynamic exercise regimen has been demonstrated by Fixler [70] and Nudel [71] who did not detect significant electrocardiographic abnormalities in juvenile primary hypertensive patients during exercise stress tests on the stationary bicycle or treadmill. We have given bicycle stress tests to more than 200 adolescent hypertensive patients [34] and have observed no electrocardiographic abnormalities (significant T wave, ST segment changes or arrythmias). However, as an extra precaution, we do recommend either a bicycle or treadmill stress test with electrocardiographic and blood pressure monitoring on hypertensive patients before starting exercise regimens.

Another possible benefit of a dynamic exercise regimen is the lowering of the serum triglyceride concentration and an increase in the serum high density lipoprotein fraction, according to Lampman [72] and Hartung [73]. The higher concentration of this lipoprotein fraction may be a protective factor against coronary heart disease, according to Gordon [74].

Other forms of therapy

Smoking and the use of contraceptive pills should be prohibited. Behavior modification methods, such as biofeedback, relaxation techniques and psychotherapy, have been tried with questionable benefit. According to the NIH Report of the Task Force on Hypertension [75], there is insufficient evidence of benefit at this time to warrant their trial.

Step-care therapy

There may be some patients who do not respond to the nonpharmacologic approach, whose blood pressure progressively rises to life-treatening levels, and who, therefore, might have to be placed upon antihypertensive drug therapy. Before taking this step, the physician should review the circumstances carefully and make certain that the lack of response is not upon the basis of noncompliance. If noncompliance is the reason for the therapeutic failure, drug therapy may also fail. However, if the patient is compliant and still fails to respond, the step-care approach, which has been advocated for adults and described elsewhere in this text, should be given a trial. The step-care approach is also described in the report of the National Committee on Detection, Evaluation, and Treatment of High Blood Pressure [76]. Most of the drugs used for adults have not been approved for children under 12 years of age and dosage schedules have been constructed by extrapolation from adult standards according to Sinaiko [38]. The recommended drug dosages are set forth in Table 9.

As discussed in the report mentioned above [76], the first step is to try a thiazide diuretic. In a recent article, Mongeau [77] suggested the use of propranolol as a Step I drug in place of a diuretic. The study was done on only ten patients who were classified as 'labile hypertensive patients' because of fluctuations in blood pressures. No information was given about cardiac output and peripheral systemic resistance. Therefore, we do not know whether these patients had a hyperkinetic circulation. However, propranolol was effective in lowering their pressure. More studies are needed before the use of beta-blocking agents should be recommended as a first-step drug.

Secondary hypertension

If untreated, hypertension in children due to renal disease, coarctation of the aorta and hormonal disorders will persist into adulthood. It is beyond the scope of this chapter to present these subjects in detail. Therefore, the following discussion will be brief, and the reader is referred to the references noted in the bibliography for more comprehensive treatment.

Table 9. Recommended drug dosages for use in pediatric antihypertensive therapy

Drug	Initial daily dose[a] (mg/kg)	Maximum therapeutic response (days)[b]	Maximum daily dose mg/kg	total
Diuretic agents				
Chlorothiazide	10	14	20	2 gm
Hydrochlorothiazide	1	14	2	200 mg
Chlorthalidone	1	14	2	200 mg
Furosemide	0.5 to 1	14	#	#
Spironolactone	0.1	14	2	200 mg
Agents acting on adrenergic nervous system				
Propranolol	0.5 to 1	3 to 5		2 gm
Methyldopa	10	7	40	2 gm
Guanethidine	0.2 to 0.5	14	#	#
Reserpine	0.02	7	#	#
Clonidine		5 to 7	#	#
Vasodilator agents				
Hydralazine	1	3 to 4	#	200 mg
Minoxidil[c]	0.1 to 0.2	2 to 4	#	#
Prazosin[c]	#	3 to 4	#	#

[a] Per 24-hr period. With the exception of guanethidine, these drugs should be administered approximately every 12 hr.
[b] Period of time required to achieve maximal therapeutic response at a given dosage instituted with greater frequency may cause an exaggerated pharmacologic response.
[c] Not approved for use as an antihypertensive agent in children by the FDA.
 # Recommended dosages for pediatric patients not firmly established. Use governed by therapeutic response and adverse reactions.
Reprinted with permission [38].

Renal disease

Chronic glomerulonephritis and chronic pyelonephritis account for most of the patients with hypertension according to Robson [78], and the common renal causes of chronic hypertension are listed in Table 10.

The diagnostic approach to the child with hypertension upon the basis of renal disease is outlined by Robson [78] and will be discussed briefly. A careful history and thorough physical examination should be done. The patient's history should have information about recurrent urinary tract infections, unexplained fever, hematuria and trauma to the abdomen or back.

A careful urine analysis should be done, and a cleanly voided, mid-stream urine specimen should be obtained for culture. Renal function should be assessed by the glomerular filtration rate, by the determination of blood urea

Table 10. Common renal causes of chronic hypertension in children

Disease state	Relative incidence (%)		
	Ooi et al [46]	Rance et al [46]	Gill et al [47]
Intrinsic renal lesions			
Acquired diseases			
Chronic glomerulonephritis	46	7	49
Chronic pyelonephritis	25	42	18
Obstructive uropathy		4	7
Tumors		1	
Trauma			
Papillary necrosis			1
Radiation nephritis			
Following renal transplantation		10	
Congenital lesions			
Renal cystic disease	6	9	7
Hypoplastic and dysplastic kidneys (total or partial)	3	1	6
Metabolic disorders such as cystinosis			
Other disorders such as ectopic, duplex kidneys	3		1
Renovascular			
Renal artery stenosis	17	19	7
Renal artery thrombosis		1	
Renal arteritis		3	
Renal vein thrombosis		3	

Reprinted with permission [78].

nitrogen and serum creatinine. It may be necessary to do a creatinine clearance. Excretion urography should be done to demonstrate the structural anatomy of the urinary tract. A plasma renin activity should be determined to evaluate renal parenchymal or renovascular disease.

If the diagnosis is not made after the preceding tests are carried out, it may be necessary to do a renal biopsy as well as renal arteriography, ultrasonography and radionuclide studies.

If one suspects renal artery stenosis, the determination of the concentration ratio of peripheral vein renin in venous blood obtained from the kidneys by selective cannulation of the renal veins may have to be done.

These patients should first be tried upon a nonpharmacologic therapeutic regimen. If this fails, the step-care approach should be initiated. The drugs and dosages are shown in Table 9. Most of the information about drug therapy for hypertension in children during the last 20 years has been gathered as a result of treating children with hypertension secondary to renal disease, undoubtedly because renal disease is probably the principal cause of morbidity and mortality from hypertension in childhood. According to the NIH Task Force Report on Hypertension [50], it is because of this that drug therapy is more justified in renal hypertension than in primary hypertension in children.

Coarctation of the aorta

This is a congenital malformation which is a narrowing of the aorta, usually just distal to the origin of the left subclavian artery. The incidence has been estimated as one in 12,000 children, according to Keith et al. [82].

The diagnosis is made by measuring the blood pressure in the upper and lower extremities, and the diagnostic finding is hypertension in the upper extremities and hypotension in the lower extremities; the gradient in pressure is usually 20 mmHg or more. According to Wiggers and Gupta [83], the cause of the hypertension is felt to be upon the basis of anatomic obstruction, although the role of the renin-angiotensin system has not been ruled out.

Coarctation of the aorta is curable when treated surgically by resection of the stenotic portion of the aorta and anastomosing the two cut ends.

When this malformation is seen in infants with congestive heart failure, the patient usually has, in addition, one or more left-to-right shunts (interventricular septal defect, patent ductus arteriosus). At present, most physicians are in agreement that surgical therapy is preferable to conservative medical management and provides a higher salvage rate of infants according to Hartmann et al. [84].

The older child with coarctation of the aorta is usually asymptomatic, but the defect should be repaired, preferably between the ages of five and eight years. At that age the aortic lumen has already achieved 50% of the size of the adult aorta, so that even if the anastamotic site does not grow with age, no gradient in pressure will result according to Rosenberg et al. [85].

About 10–15% of patients who have had successful surgical repair remain hypertensive and no explanation is available for this. However, on the brighter side, a cure is achieved in 90% of the patients.

Hormonal disorders

Causes of juvenile hypertension secondary to hormonal disorders are listed in Table 11 as reported by New and Levine [86]. The diagnosis may be suspected after a careful history is taken and a thorough physical examination is done. The diagnosis can then by confirmed by a number of laboratory tests noted in Table 11.

Table 11. Endocrine disorders associated with hypertension [86]

Endocrine disorder	Common presenting signs and symptoms	Treatment
1. 11β-hydroxylase deficiency	Virilization, rapid growth, advanced bone age, decreased plasma renin activity and aldosterone, elevated urinary 17-ketosteroids, 17-hydroxysteroids, plasma DOC, compound S and androgen	Glucocorticoid treatment will suppress the hormones noted to normal levels
2. 17-hydroxylase deficiency	Hypogonadism, male pseudohermaphroditism, amenorrhea and hypocalcemia, decreased plasma renin activity, urinary aldosterone excretion, 17-ketosteroid and 17-hydroxysteroids, plasma cortisol and androgens, poor response to ACTH stimulation	Elevated plasma DOC concentration decreases with glucocorticoid treatment
3. Cushing's syndrome [87]	Obesity, poor growth, plethora, muscular weakness, elevated peripheral vein renin, normal urinary aldosterone excretion, elevated plasma and urinary 17-hydroxysteroids	Total bilateral adrenalectomy and replacement therapy with glucocorticoid and mineral corticoids; 25% develop chromophobe adenoma of pituitary gland which requires irradiation for control
4. Pheochromocytoma [88]	Sustained hypertension, headache, sweating, nausea and vomiting, weight loss, visual disturbances, palpitation and abdominal or chest pains, increased concentrations of catecholamines and their metabolites in urine and serum, roentgenogram of abdomen and intravenous pyelography are of value if a large adrenal tumor is present	Surgical removal after alpha and beta adrenergic blockade
5. Hyperthyroidism [89]	Emotional lability, nervousness, irritability, increased sweating, increased appetite with or without change in weight, increased height with age, heat intolerance, weakness, tremors, tachycardia, increased systolic pressure with widened pulse pressure, moist skin, exophthalmus LAG, and diffusely enlarged firm thyroid gland, elevated serum T_4, T_3, FT_4 and RT_3U, TSH levels are normal, low or undetectable	Surgical excision of thyroid gland or medical treat- with propylthiouracil or methimazole (Tapazole)

Although hypertension secondary to hormonal disorders is relatively rare in the practice of the general pediatrician, the recommendation of the NIH Hypertension Task Force [75] is to screen juvenile hypertensive patients for endocrine abnormalities, because there is a possibility that there may be an unidentified hormone which may be a specific biochemical marker for the hypertension.

Summary

1. The pathogenesis of primary hypertension remains unknown.
2. There is mounting evidence that primary hypertension may have its inception in infancy or childhood.
3. Non-pharmacologic treatment (weight reduction for the obese, moderate salt restriction and a dynamic exercise regimen) should be the first approach to the pediatric patient with primary hypertension, because the long-term effects of the antihypertensive drugs upon the growing individual are unknown.
4. Drastic alteration of the child's diet with the goal of lowering the cholesterol blood level is not justified, because we do not have enough information about the possible untoward effect(s) of such severe diet modification on the maturing individual.
5. More blood pressure standards are needed from infancy through 16 years of age with blood pressure measurements performed according to the guidelines set forth by the American Heart Association, so that there is better agreement of the blood pressure values for the 50th, 90th and 95th percentiles according to age and sex.
6. Longitudinal studies extending from infancy through adulthood are needed to see if the young hypertensive becomes the adult hypertensive.
7. A physiologic or chemical marker is needed to identify the individual with primary hypertension.
8. Studies are needed for the evaluation of nonpharmacologic therapeutic intervention in the young hypertensive and to determine if such therapy may possibly arrest the disease in the early stages.
9. The study of primary hypertension at its inception in infancy and childhood may more likely provide an understanding of the pathogenesis of primary hypertension.

Acknowledgments

The author gratefully acknowledges the help of Miss Linda Mabry in typing the manuscript, as well as the invaluable editorial assistance of his wife, Evelyn. This

42

research was supported in part by the Alpha Phi Sorority Fund and U.S. Public
Health Grant HL 21578–03.

References

1. Londe S, Bourgoignie JD, Robson AM et al: Hypertension in apparently normal children.
   J Pediatr 78:569, 1971.
2. Loggie JMH: Essential hypertension in adolescents. Postgrad Med 56:133, 1974.
3. Haggerty RJ, Maroney MW, Nadas AS: Essential hypertension in infancy and childhood. Am
   J Dis Child 92:535, 1956.
4. Kirkendall WM, Feinlieb M, Freis ED, et al: Recommendations for human blood pressure
   determination by sphygmomanometers. Circulation 62:1146, 1980.
5. Londe S, Goldring D: High blood pressure in children: problems and guidelines for evaluation
   and treatment. Am J Cardiol 37:650, 1976.
6. Londe S, Johanson A, Kronomer NS, et al: Blood pressure and puberty. J Pediatr 87: 896, 1975.
7. Goldring D, Wohltman H: Flush method for blood pressure determinations in newborn infants.
   J Pediatr 40: 284, 1952.
8. Goldring D, Strauss A, Urrutia H, et al.: Flush blood pressure and mean intraaortic pressure.
   Pediatr Res 14:445, 1980.
9. Hernandez A, Goldring D, Hartmann AF Jr: Measurement of blood pressure in infants and
   children by the Doppler ultrasonic techniques. J Pediatr 148:788, 1971.
10. Moss AJ, Adams FH: Flush blood pressure and intraarterial pressure. Am J Dis Child 107:489,
    1954.
11. Hernandez A, Meyer DA, Goldring D: Blood pressure in neonates. Contemp Obstet Gynecol
    5:34, 1975.
12. Levinson HJ, Kidd BSL, Gemmell PA et al: Blood pressure in normal full-term and premature
    infants. Am J Dis Child 111:374, 1966.
13. Swiet de M. Fayers P, Shinebourne EA: Value of repeated blood pressure measurements in
    children – the Brompton Study. Br Med J 219:1567, 1980.
14. Swiet de M, Fayers P, Shinebourne EA: Systolic blood pressure in a population of infants in the
    first year of life. The Brompton Study. Pediatrics 65:1028, 1980.
15. Schachter J, Lachin JM, Wimberly FC: Newborn heart rate and blood pressure: relation to race
    and socioeconomic class. Psychosom Med 38:390, 1976.
16. Goldring D, Londe S, Sivakoff M, et al: Blood pressure in a high school population. I. Standards
    for blood pressure and the relation of age, sex, weight, height and race to blood pressure in
    children 14–18 years of age. J Pediatr 91:884, 1977.
17. Aschinberg LC, Zeis PM, Miller RA et al: Essential hypertension in childhood. JAMA 238:322,
    1977.
18. Kilcoyne MM, Richter RW, Alsup PA: Adolescent hypertension. Circulation 50:758, 1974.
19. Londe S: Blood pressure in children as determined under office conditions. Clin Pediatr 5:71–78,
    1966.
20. Lauer RM, Connor WE, Leaverton PER et al: Coronary heart disease risk factors in school
    children. The Muscatine Study. J Pediatr 86:697, 1975.
21. McCue CM, Miller WW, Mauck HP et al: Adolescent blood pressure in Richmond, Virginia
    schools. Va Med 106:210, 1979.
22. Kotchen JM, Kotchen TA, Echwertmein NC et al: Blood pressure distribution of urban
    adolescents. Am J Epidemiol 99:315, 1974.
23. National Health Survey: Blood pressure levels of children 6–11 years, publication (HRA) 74–

1617. US Department of Health, Education and Welfare, Dec 1972.

24. Voors AW, Forster TA, Frerichs RR et al: Studies of blood pressure in children, ages 5–14 years, in a total biracial community. The Bogalusa Study. Circulation 54:319, 1976.

25. Miller RA, Shekelle RB: Blood pressure in tenth grade studients. Circulation 54:993, 1976.

26. Londe S, Gollub S, Goldring D: Blood pressure in black and white children. J Pediatr 90:93, 1977.

27. Adelman RD: Neonatal hypertension. Pediatr Clin North Am 25:99, 1978.

28. Plumer LB, Mendoza SA, Kaplan GW: Hypertension in infancy: the case for aggressive management. J Urol 113:555, 1975.

29. McKeown T, Reewin RG, Whitfield AGW: Variations in casual measurements of arterial pressure in two populations (Birmingham and South Wales) reexamined with intervals of 3–4½ years. Clin Sci 24:437, 1963.

30. Feinlieb M, Halperin M, Garrison RJ: Relationship between blood pressure and age. Read before the 97th Annual Meeting of the American Public Health Association, Philadelphia, Nov 1969.

31. Zinner SH, Martin LF, Sachs F et al: A longitudinal study of blood pressure in childhood. Am J Epidemiol 100:437, 1975.

32. Master AM, Dublin L, Marks H: The normal blood pressure range and its clinical implications. JAMA 143:1464, 1950.

33. Dustan HP, Tarazi RC: Hemodynamic abnormalities of adolescent hypertension. In: New MI, Levine LS (eds) Juvenile hypertension. New York, Raven Press, 1977, pp 1, 81.

34. Goldring D, Hernandez A, Choi S et al: Blood pressure in a high school population. II. Clinical profile of the juvenile hypertensive. J Pediatr 95:298, 1979.

35. Garay RP, Elghogi JL, Dagher G et al: Laboratory distinction between essential and secondary hypertension by measurement of erythrocyte cation fluxes. N Engl J Med 302:769, 1980.

36. Canessa M, Adragna H, Solomon HS et al: Increased sodium-lithium countertransport in red cells of patients with essential hypertension. N Engl J Med 302:772, 1980.

37. Davignon A, Rey C, Payot M et al: Hemodynamic studies of labile essential hypertension in adolescents. In: New MI, Levine LS (eds) Juvenile hypertension. New York, Raven Press, 1977, p 189.

38. Sinaikio AR, Mirkin BL: Clinical pharmacology of anatihypertensive drugs in children. Pediatr Clin North Am 25:137, 1978.

39. Veterans Administration Cooperative Study Group on Antihypertensive Agents: Effects of treatment on morbidity in hypertension: results in patients with diastolic blood pressures averaging 115 through 129 mmHg. JAMA 202:1028, 1967.

40. Veterans Administration Cooperative Study Group on Antihypertensive Agents: Effects of treatment on morbidity in hypertension: results in patients with diastolic blood pressure averaging 90 through 114 mmHg. JAMA 213:1143, 1970.

41. Chiang BN, Perlman LV, Epstein FH: Overweight and hypertension. Circulation 39:403, 1969.

42. Kannel W, Brand N, Skinner J, Dawber T, McNamara P: Relation of adiposity to blood pressure and development of hypertension. The Framingham Study. Ann Intern Med 67:48, 1967.

43. Levy RL, White PD, Stroud WD et al: Overweight: its prognostic significance in relation to hypertension and cardiovascular-renal diseases. JAMA 131:12, 951, 1946.

44. Alexander JK: Obesity and the circulation. Mod Concepts Cardiovasc Dis 32:799, 1963.

45. Whyte H: Behind the adipose curtain. Am J Cardiol 15:66, 1965.

46. Reisin E, Abel R, Modan M: Effect of weight loss without salt restriction on reduction of blood pressure in overweight hypertensive patients. N Engl J Med 298:1, 1978.

47. Gross I, Wheeler M, Hess K: The treatment of obesity in adolescents using behavioral self-control. Clin Pediatr 15:920, 1976.

48. Carrera F III: Obesity in adolescence. In: Kiell N (ed) The psychology of obesity: dynamics and treatment. Springfield, Ill, Thomas, 1973.

49. Stunkard AJ, Ruch J: Dieting and depression reexamined. A critical review of reports of untoward responses during weight reduction for obesity. Ann Intern Med 81:526, 1974.

50. Report of the Hypertension Task Force. Salt and water. National Institutes of Health Publication, 79–1630, 1979.

51. Kotchen TA, Gall HJ, Guthrie GP Jr et al: Regulation of renin release by chloride. Cardiovasc Med 4:475, 1979.

52. Carter GA, Lauer RM, Loggie JMH: Coronary heart disease risk factors: identification and management. In: Shen JYT (ed) The clinical practice of adolescent medicine. New York, Appleton Century Crofts, 1980, p 240.

53. Wilmore JH, McNamara JJ: Prevalence of coronary heart disease risk factors in boys 8 to 12 years of age. J Pediatr 84:527, 1974.

54. Lauer RM, Connor WE, Leaverton PE, Reiter RS et al: Coronary heart disease factors in school children. J Pediatr 86:697, 1975.

55. Blumenthal S, Jese MJ, Hennekens CH et al: Risk factors for coronary artery disease in children of affected families. J Pediatr 87:1187, 1975.

56. Martz BL: Drug management of hypercholesterolemia. Am Heart J 97:389, 1979.

57. Schubert WK: Fat nutrition and diet in childhood. Am J Cardiol 3:581, 1973.

58. Levy RI, Rifkind BM: Diagnosis and management of hyperlipoproteinemia in infants and children. Am J Cardiol 31:547, 1973.

59. Hanson JS, Nedde WH: Preliminary observations on physical training for hypertensive males. Circ Res 27 (Suppl):49, 1970.

60. Boyer JL, Kasch FW: Exercise therapy in hypertensive men. JAMA 211:1668, 1970.

61. Choquette G, Ferguson RJ: Blood pressure reduction in borderline hypertensives following physical training. Can Med Assoc J 108:699, 1973.

62. Sannerstedt R, Wasir H, Henning R et al: Systemic hemodynamics in mild arterial hypertension before and after physical training. Clin Sci Mol Med 45 (Suppl 1):145, 1973.

63. Sannerstedt R: Hemodynamic response to exercise in patients with arterial hypertension. Acta Med Scand 180 (Suppl):458, 1966.

64. Hagberg JM, Ehsani AA, Heath GW et al: Beneficial effects of endurance exercise training in adolescent hypertension. Am J Cardiol 45:489, 1980.

65. Ekbloom B, Astrand PO, Saltin B et al: Effect of training on circulator response to exercise. J Appl Physiol 24:518, 1968.

66. Saltin B, Blomquist G, Mitchell JH et al: Response to exercise after bedrest and artery training. Circulation 38 (Suppl 7):1, 1968.

67. Hanson JS, Tabakin BS, Levy AM et al: Longterm physical training and cardiovascular dynamics in middle aged man. Circulation 38:783, 1976.

68. Hartley HL, Mason JW, Hogan RP et al: Multiple hormonal responses to graded exercise in relation to physical training. J Appl Physiol 33:602, 1972.

69. Bradfield N: Exercise and the heart: a rational approach to cardiac rehabilitation. Primary Cardiol 14:July–Aug, 1977.

70. Fixler DE, Pennek L, Browne R et al: Response of hypertensive adolescents to dynamic and sometric exercise stress. Pediatrics 64:579, 1979.

71. Nudel DB, Gootman N, Brinson SC et al: Exercise performance of hypertensive adolescents. Pediatrics 65:1073, 1980.

72. Lampman RM, Santanya JT, Hodge MF et al: Comparative effects of physical training and diet in normalizing serum lipids in men with Type IV hypoproteinemia. Circulation 55:652, 1977.

73. Hartung GE, Fareyt JP, Mitchell RE et al: Relation of diet to high density-lipoprotein cholesterol in middle aged marathon runners, joggers and inactive men. N Engl J Med 302:357, 1980.

74. Gordon T, Casteli WP, Hjortland MC et al: High density lipoprotein as a protective factor against coronary heart disease. Am Heart J 62:707, 1977.

75. Report of the Hypertension Task Force, US Department of Health, Education and Welfare, Public Health Service, National Institutes of Health. NIH Publication No 79–1631, Vol IX, Sept, 1979.
76. Report of Joint National Committee on Detection, Evaluation and Treatment of High Blood Pressure. US Department of Health, Education and Welfare, Public Health Service, National Institutes of Health. DHEW Publications No (NIH) 78–1088.
77. Mongeau JG, Biron P, Picardo LM: Propranol efficacy in adolescent essential hypertension. In: New MI, Levine LS (eds) Juvenile hypertension. New York, Raven Press, 1977, p 219.
78. Robson AM: Special diagnostic studies for the detection of renal and renovascular forms of hypertension. Pediatr Clin North Am 25:83, 1978.
79. Ooi BS, Chen BTM, Roih CCS et al: Causes of hypertension in the young. Br Med J 2:744, 1970.
80. Rance CP, Arbus GS, Balfe JW et al: Persistent systemic hypertension in infants and children. Pediatr Clin North Am 2:801, 1974.
81. Gill DG, Mendes da Costa B, Cameron JS, Cameron MC, Joseph MC, Ogg CS, Chantler C: Analysis of 100 children with severe and potential hypertension. Arch Dis Child 51:951, 1976.
82. Keith JD, Rowe RD, Vlad P: Coarctation of the aorta. Heart disease in infancy and childhood, 2 Ed. New York, Macmillan, 1967, p 210.
83. Gupta TC, Wiggers CJ: Basic hemodynamic changes produced by aortic coarctation of different degrees. Circulation 3:17, 1951.
84. Hartman AF Jr, Goldring D, Strauss A et al: Coarctation of the aorta. In: Moss AJ (ed) Heart disease in infants, children and adolescents. Baltimore, Williams & Wilkins, 1976.
85. Rosenberg HS, Lima T, Henderson SR et al: Maturation of the aortic isthmus. Cardiovasc Res Cent Bull 47:Oct–Dec, 1971.
86. New MI, Levine LS: Adrenocortical hypertension. Pediatr Clin North Am 25:67, 1978.
87. Hung W, August GP, Glasgow AW: Pediatric Endocrinology. Garden City, Medical Examination Publishing, 1978, pp 249–252.
88. Ibid, pp 267–269.
89. Ibid, pp 157–159.

3. Therapeutic decisons in management of borderline hypertension

STEVO JULIUS

In this chapter the thesis will be developed that for patients with very mild hypertension, antihypertensive therapy is not mandatory, but some of these patients are heading for trouble and it would be useful if they could be recognized in advance in order to single them out for early treatment.

Remarks will be organized around the area of borderline hypertension. These are patients whose blood pressure occasionally is above 140 systolic and/or 90 mmHg diastolic, but whose readings are sometimes in the normal range. Such patients are most perplexing to the clinician. Should they be treated? The answer can be found only if one uses data on the natural history of borderline hypertension. Is borderline hypertension a pathologic condition that eventually leads to a more severe, established hypertension?

Figure 1 is an illustration of the course of hypertension in one patient. In 1953, as a student he had a systolic blood pressure of 160. During his student days he continued to have systolic readings between 140 and 160. At that time, his diastolic blood pressure was always under 90. No one was concerned about the readings. Later, when the patient was 30 years old, the diastolic for the first time reached a value of 90 mmHg. By then he was a practicing physician, but in spite of his qualifications he did not perceive this reading as a change from the levels he had as a student. When he was 35, the systolic reading was 200 and the diastolic reading reached 110 mmHg, but again he did not consider this a big change and nothing was done. A few years later he was admitted as an emergency case with nosebleeds, headaches, readings of 200/140 and funduscopic changes of accelerated hypertension. Note that this patient's heart rate was always elevated. This was considered to be a good sign, as it convinced the patient and his physicians he had 'only anxiety' and 'only a nervous blood pressure elevation.' Obviously, their optimism was not justified.

How representative is the course of this patient in the majority of persons with borderline hypertension? It was shown as early as 1945 that patients with transient (borderline) hypertension had twice the chance of developing hypertension within five years as people who had a normal blood pressure [1]. Furthermore, the kind of hypertension that develops in these patients is sufficiently severe

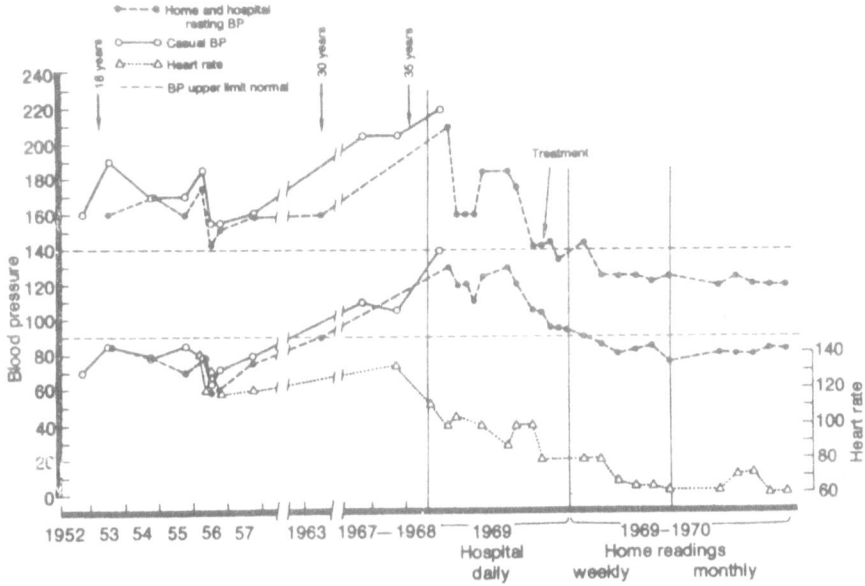

Blood pressures and heart rates from a patient's records at the University of Michigan.

Figure 1. The record of a 'minor' blood pressure problem.

to cause complications. Mortality and hypertension-related morbidity are increased in borderline hypertension. An average ratio of development of sustained hypertension, morbidity, and mortality in hypertensive and normotensive subjects is shown in Figure 2. More detailed information about studies that provide the basis for this figure can be obtained in a published review of borderline hypertension [2].

Before dire predictions are made from the fact that there is an excess of mortality and cardiovascular morbidity in patients with borderline hypertension, it should not be forgotten that these are *relative* ratios, that is, borderline hypertensive patients have a higher incidence than the general population. But how much higher is the incidence? Figure 3 shows a review of literature regarding the absolute levels of eventual development of more severe forms of hypertension in individuals with borderline hypertension (for details see [2]). It can be seen that after ten or 20 years only 20% of patients with borderline hypertension will develop sustained hypertension. That is not a large number. The risk is higher than in the general population but certainly not overwhelming. Therefore, we have a real therapeutic dilemma. Should one be alarmed by the increased relative risk and treat all patients with borderline hypertension, or should one be pacifed with the low absolute risk and forego treatment? In the absence of hard data, one can try to project what would happen if all patients with borderline hypertension

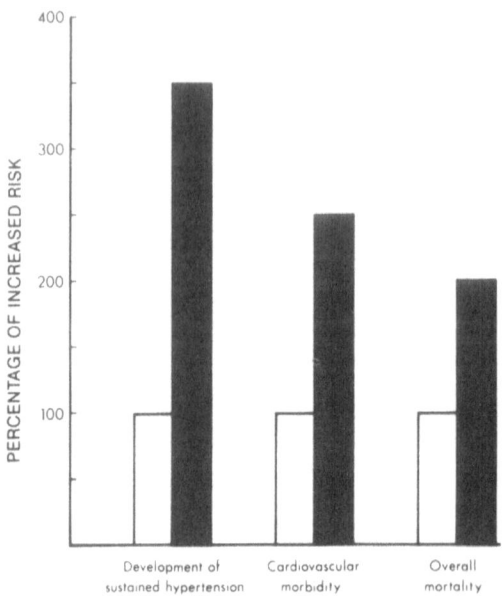

Figure 2. Occurrence of hypertension, cardiovascular morbidity, and overall mortality. Open bars (= 100%) = normotensive subjects; shaded bars = patients with borderline hypertension.

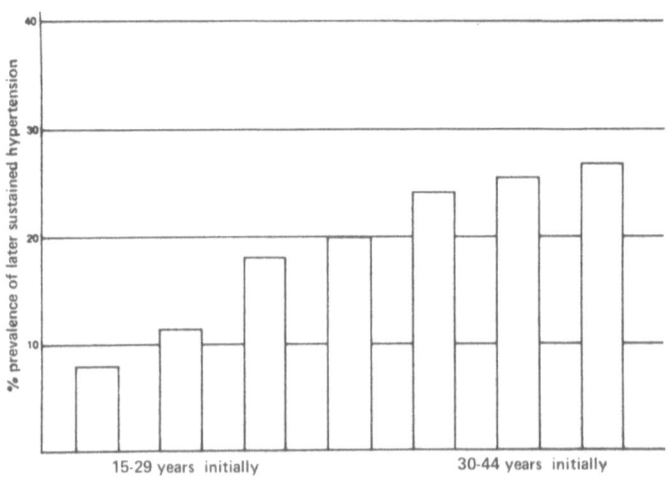

Figure 3. Development of hypertension in previous borderline hypertensives. In all studies patients were followed longitudinally for 10–20 years. Columns represent results from various studies. Details can be found in [2].

were treated – starting with the well-known Veterans Administration Cooperative Study on the treatment of hypertension, using their data to make statistical assumptions.

It is assumed that (a) the period of treatment will be the same as in the VA Study; (b) the lower the blood pressure, the less effective treatment will be; and (c) over that period of time about 10% of borderline hypertensive patients will develop hypertension of similar severity as that considered in the VA Study. Finally it is assumed that the treatment will be effective only in this 10% and not in the other 90% who will not develop hypertension. We can then calculate the percentage of patients 'saved' if everybody with borderline hypertension were treated (Figure 4).

In the VA Study, if 100 patients with diastolic blood pressures between 90 and 115 mmHg were not treated, 55 developed complications. In those who were treated, the treatment was 6% effective in preventing complications. So, a number can be construed, percentage 'saved' from an event. There are 100 patients treated for five years and 36 are 'saved' from a complication, the study suggests; that clearly makes sense. It is reasonable to treat 100 patients for the benefit of 36 persons.

What happens with borderline hypertension using these assumptions? There are 100 patients with borderline hypertension, and over five years ten of them

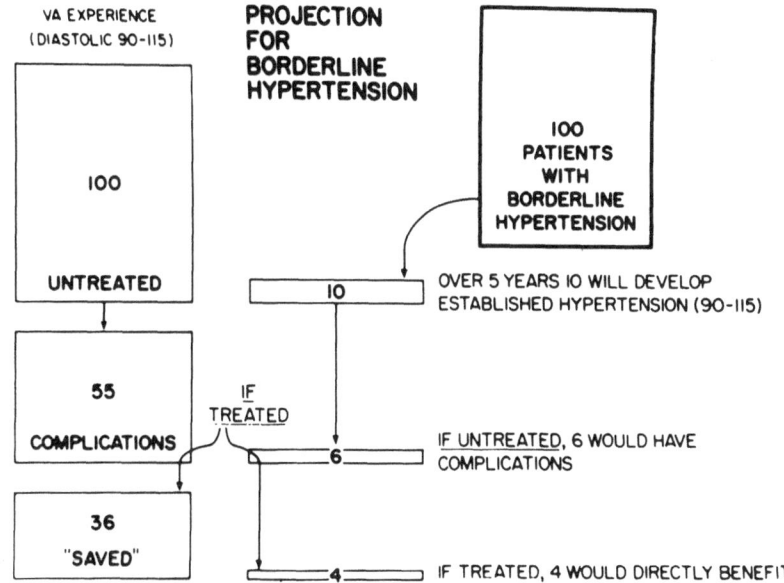

Figure 4. A graphic presentation of the experience of the Veterans Administration Study on effects of treatment in mild hypertension (left panel). The Veterans Administration data are used in the right panel to project the effectiveness of treatment in borderline hypertension.

will develop the kind of hypertension observed in the VA. If there is no treatment, six will develop complications; and if there is treatment, four individuals may be 'saved.' There would be 100 patients treated for the benefit of four. That is not a meaningful proposition.

The projections are even less favorable if recently published data of the large HDFP Study on mild hypertension [4] are perused. Without going into details, it is fair to say that the study was not designed to check effect of no treatment versus treatment. Instead, it tested aggressive treatment ('special care') versus usual treatment ('referred care'). This complicates the analysis a great deal. The study was so designed that the mortality was the only endpoint for evaluation. Although there are attempts to report on the cardiovascular morbidity, because of the study design conclusions from such reports cannot be accepted without reservations. The study found less mortality in the special care group, but in addition to cardiovascular mortality, mortality from all causes was also reduced in the special care group. Consequently, the question of whether the improved prognosis in the special care group stems only from the antihypertensive treatment or also from other nonspecific effects of good medical care remains open. Nevertheless, one tends to accept the results of the HDFP Study – a 20% reduction in mortality in very mild hypertension (diastolic 90–95 mmHg). If the HDPF Study is projected as for the VA Study, the results are dismal. If 100 patients with borderline hypertension were to be treated aggressively by the special care approach, after five years less than one (0.75%) would be saved from an event. It really does not make sense to treat 100 individuals for a possible benefit to one of them. What should be done? Attempts should be made to find those individuals among patients with borderline hypertension who are heading for trouble. Factors predicting hypertension and its complications must be identified. How can future hypertension be predicted, and even more difficult, how can future hypertension leading to an event be predicted?

A number of provocative tests have been proposed on the theory that increased blood pressure responsiveness to stress may be predictive of a tendency to future hypertension. Cold pressor tests, response to exercise, and response to mental stress have been investigated. A general assessment of all of these tests is that they have been unsuccessful in predicting hypertension [5].

Some other provocative tests may hold promise, but have not yet been investigated in prospective studies. Sodium loading and testing the vascular reactivity [6] and response to tilt [7] may be altered in borderline hypertension. It has also been shown that patients with borderline hypertension and youngsters in families of patients with hypertension are hyperresponders to mental stress [8, 9]. However, the crucial question, whether increased blood pressure responsiveness to a test is representative of an individual's overall blood pressure variability and ultimately of his prognosis, has not been resolved. Furthermore, even the basic assumption for these tests, that repeated temporary increases of blood pressure lead eventually to established hypertension, has never been proved. Attempts have been made [10, 11], but I am not aware of any study where repeated pressor episodes caused permanent blood pressure elevation in animals.

If provocative tests are not reliable, what else can be done to predict whether an individual will become hypertensive in the future? There are some descriptive characteristics which predict the future development of hypertension. Of particular interest are elevated initial blood pressure levels, obesity, tachycardia, family history and then combinations of these.

Of all of these characteristics, in clinical practice the most important ones are the initial blood pressure level and initial heart rate. It may seem redundant to again discuss blood pressure. Borderline hypertension has already been discussed. The point, however, is that blood pressure measurement in the office is not sufficient to characterize the extent of the blood pressure elevation in a patient with borderline hypertension.

The point is illustrated in Figure 5. In this study in East Berlin [12], 98 patients with borderline hypertension were seen in 1968 and again in 1970: 20% had become normotensive, 50% remained borderline and around 30% were hyper-

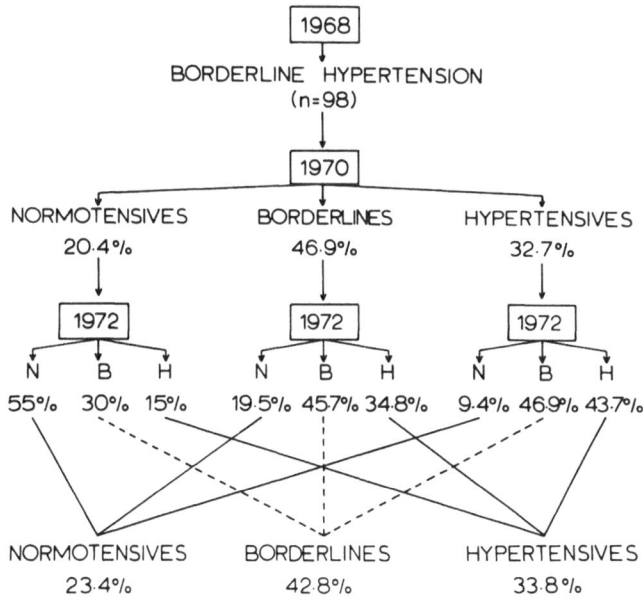

Figure 5. Experience with three blood pressure measurements performed in the same individual over a period of four years in East Berlin. Lowest of two sitting casual readings is reported. Borderline hypertension = systolic blood pressure of 140–158 mmHg and/or diastolic pressure of 90–94 mmHg; hypertension = blood pressure less than or equal to 160/96 mmHg (courtesy of Dr KH Günther).

tensive. These patients were studied again in 1972. At that time the percentages of normotensive, borderline and hypertensive subjects were similar to those in 1970, but different individuals comprised the subgroups. Persons previously hypertensive were normotensive, some normotensive subjects were hypertensive, and many of the borderline subjects changed their classification.

There is no way of telling from repeated blood pressure readings in a clinic whether someone has progressed and developed more severe hypertension; utilization of home blood pressure measurements, however, or some other kind of frequent repeated assessment, is helpful in determining blood pressure trends in borderline hypertension.

In a study in Michigan [13], subjects who were normotensive or had borderline hypertension in the clinic were taught to measure their own blood pressure and asked to obtain two readings a day for seven consecutive days. The distribution of home blood pressure readings in normotensive subjects followed the pattern of a bell-shaped curve. When means and standard deviation of home blood pressure in these normotensive individuals were considered, about 30% of the patients with borderline hypertension in the clinic became normotensive at home, 40% remained borderline and 30% could be called hypertensive with blood pressure more than two standard deviations above the normal mean. Consequently the home blood pressure technique provides a possible tool to find out which patient has a more serious problem. It seems very likely that those people who have higher blood pressures at home are at higher risk for future hypertension. Interestingly, the upper limit for two standard deviations above the normal mean at home proved to be almost exactly 140/90 mmHg.

The other risk factor deserving special comment is tachycardia, chiefly because the significance of tachycardia is misunderstood. If a patient has a fast heart rate in the physician's office, it is considered a good sign. The assumption is that tachycardia reflects 'only anxiety' and that under other less tense circumstances the blood pressure in all likelihood will be normal. This simply is not true. In our study [13], the clinic heart rates of those patients who became normotensive were as fast as in those whose blood pressure at home was in the hypertensive range. Furthermore, epidemiologic studies show that a faster heart rate at youth is a predictor of later hypertension. An example is given in Figure 6 [14]. Findings such as these have been reconfirmed in other studies [15, 16]. It can be seen that fast heart rate *without* high blood pressure in youth leads to future hypertension. The risk for future hypertension is particularly high if both transient blood pressure elevation and tachycardia are present in a youth. So, tachycardia is not a benign sign and should not be used as a convenient excuse to neglect an individual's blood pressure elevation.

After these two factors have been singled out, it should not be forgotten that there are also other risk factors such as family history, race and obesity. How can all these factors be used in a rational way to select patients with borderline

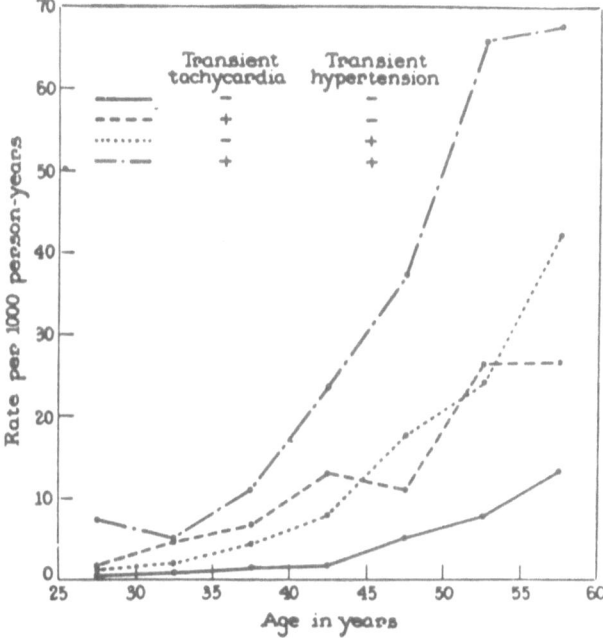

Figure 6. Rates of developing sustained hypertension by age according to the presence or absence of transient tachycardia and transient hypertension. Each age group was followed for five years (courtesy of JAMA).

hypertension who might need antihypertensive treatment? With the help of Dr. M. Anthony Schork in Michigan, we made some predictions about the usefulness of antihypertensive treatment in patients with borderline hypertension if we were to choose those individuals who are in the upper quintile of risk, that is, have almost all the risk factors for future hypertension. The data for the assumptions came from the VA Study [3] and from the Chicago Epidemiologic Study report [16]. Details of these projections can be found in another paper [5], but the basic message is that if we were to treat 100 patients with borderline hypertension who are in the upper quintile risk group, after five years of treatment 12 patients might be saved from a complication. Such a yield is sufficiently high to recommend treatment for the whole upperquintile-of-risk group.

Using this background, some practical guidelines on antihypertensive treatment in borderline hypertension may be worked out. Some principles underlying those guidelines are are follows: First, it is necessary to differentiate between management and treatment. Management consists of all nonpharmacologic measures; treatment means giving drugs. Second, treatment should not be given to all patients with borderline hypertension and must be reserved for those individuals considered to be at highest risk. Third, only small does of antihypertensive drugs should be used, and they should be continued only if (a) they cause no side effects, and (b) such doses lower the average home diastolic blood pressure at least 5 mmHg. Fourth, before treatment is initiated, good baseline blood pressures are needed in order to follow future blood pressure trends.

With these principles considered, a scheme to handle patients with borderline hypertension has been developed. All patients without an exception must be managed. Management consists of determining baseline blood pressures and following blood pressure trends every six months. The preferred way of obtaining baselines is by the use of home blood pressure self-determination. Further aspects of management are (a) dietary sodium restriction (2–3 gm NaCl/day), (b) weight control and (c) moderate exercise.

An adequate physical examination is the first step in deciding whether a patient with borderline hypertension might need antihypertensive treatment. The examination aims at factors related to severity of hypertension. If there is an abnormal funduscopic examination or signs of left ventricular hypertrophy, even if the blood pressure is in the borderline range, this is not borderline hypertension. All such patients have hypertension and should be treated. Moreover, if the laboratory examination shows left ventricular hypertrophy or increased serum creatinine, the patient has a more advanced disease and needs to be treated. Determining risk factors for atherosclerosis such as abnormal lipids, fasting blood sugar and uric acid also assists in the therapeutic decision. Finally, measurement of weight and height and obtaining a good family history are also very important.

When the history, the physical examination and the laboratory evaluation have been completed, the next step is to take home blood pressure readings, two readings a day for seven consecutive days. The decision-making process is described in Table 1. In essence, a combination of home blood pressure measurements and risk factor assessment is used to initiate the antihypertensive treatment. The treatment is continued if effective, and need for treatment is periodically reassessed. Those who did not respond or who developed unacceptable side effects are closely followed; if the blood pressure increases, they are then subjected to aggressive antihypertensive therapy.

The point that treatment is attempted but not forced deserves underscoring. This is different from the usual stance in patients with established hypertension. The risk in borderline hypertension is not sufficient to warrant the usual aggressive antihypertensive therapeutic strategy of adding antihypertensive drugs until normotension is attained.

When accepting this approach, one has the responsibility to manage and periodically reexamine *all* patients with borderline hypertension. For them the decision to treat has been postponed, but their risk of hypertension and its complications is higher than normal and some time in the future treatment may be necessary.

Table 1. Flow sheet for treatment of borderline hypertension

Step I	a. Physical examination
	Funduscopy
	Signs of left ventricular hypertrophy
	b. Laboratory examination
	ECG
	Chest x-ray
	Urine, creatine
	Lipids, FBS
	c. Obtain home blood pressure readings seven
	days, each morning and evening

	Attempt treatment	*Observe* BP *trends one a year if . . .*
Step II	a. Average home BP > 140/90	a. Average home BP < 130/80
	b. Average home BP 130–140/80–90	b. Average home BP 130–140/80–90
	Patient under age 50	
	Family history positive, *or*	
	Family history negative but	
	two other risk factors	
Step III	a. If no side effects and BP-5 mm	a. If after a year BP up 10 mmHg,
	– continue for two years	attempt treatment
	– reassess	
	b. If no response or side effects,	b. If after a year BP up 5 mmHg,
	follow semiannually; if BP	repeat readings in six months up
	5 mmHg, treat more vigorously	

In summary, patients with borderline hypertension represent a pool of potential hypertensive patients. Not all of them will develop future, more severe hypertension. A proportion of patients with borderline hypertension is at particularly high risk. The known risk factors for later hypertension are obesity, black race, positive family history, tachycardia and transient elevation in blood pressure level. Among those, the the blood pressure level is the strongest predictor. Antihypertensive treatment is not mandatory for all patients with borderline hypertension. In those at highest risk, a mild antihypertensive treatment is indicated. The rest of the patients need to be followed and their blood pressure should be managed by nonpharmacological means.

Since this paper was written, two new studies on the effect of treatment on mild hypertension have been published [17, 18]. The author reviewed these studies and made similar projections as with the VA study. These studies reinforce the author's belief that not all patients with borderline hypertension should be subjected to life long drug treatment. A recent WHO recommendation [19] takes even a more conservative attitude toward initiation of antihypertensive therapy.

References

1. Levy RL, Hillman CC, Stroud WD, et al: Transient hypertension: its significance in terms of later development of sustained hypertension and cardiovascular-renal diseases. JAMA 126: 829–833, 1944.
2. Julius S, Schork MA: Borderline hypertension – a critical review. J Chron Dis 23:723–754, 1971.
3. Veterans administration Cooperative Study Group on Antihypertensive Agents (1977): Propranolol in the treatment of essential hypertension. JAMA 237:2303–2310, 1977.
4. The Hypertension Detection and Follow-up Cooperative Group: Mild hypertensives in the hypertension detection and follow-up program. Ann NY Acad Sci 304:254–266, 1978.
5. Julius S, Schork MA: Predictors in hypertension. In: Perry HM Jr, Smith WM (eds) Mild hypertension: to treat or not to treat. Ann NY Acad Sci 304:38–52, 1978.
6. Mark AL, Lawton WJ, Abboud FM, Fitz AE, Connor WE, Heistad DD: Effects of high and low sodium intake on arterial pressure and forearm vascular resistance in borderline hypertension. Circ Res 36–37 (Suppl I):I-194 – I-198, 1975.
7. Hull DH, Wolthuis RA, Cortese T, Longo MR Jr, Triebwasser JH: Borderline hypertension versus normotension: differential response to orthostatic stress. Am Heart J 94:414–420, 1977.
8. Hollenberg NK, Williams GH, Adams DF: Essential hypertension: abnormal renal vascular and endocrine responses to a mild psychological stimulus. Hypertension 3:11–17, 1981.
9. Falkner B, Onesti C, Angelakos ET, Fernandes M, Langman C: Cardiovascular response to mental stress in normal adolescents with hypertensive parents. Hemodynamics and mental stress in adolescents. Hypertension 1:23–30, 1979.
10. Folkow B, Rubinstein EH: Cardiovascular effects of acute and chronic stimulation of the hypothalamic defense area in the rat. Acta Physiol Scand 68:48–57, 1966.
11. Cowley AW Jr, Liard JF, Guyton AC: Role of the baroreceptor reflex in daily control of arterial blood pressure and other variables in dogs. Circ Res 32:564–576, 1973.
12. Linss GH, Bothig S: Normotension and hypertension, part 3 (in German). Dtsch Gesundheitsw 29:635, 1974.
13. Julius S, Ellis CN, Pascual AV, Matice M, Hansson L, Hunyor SN, Sandler LN: Home blood pressure determinations: values in borderline ('labile') hypertension. JAMA 229:663–666, 1974.
14. Levy RL, White PD, Stroud WD et al: Transient tachycardia: prognostic significance alone and in association with transient hypertension. JAMA 129:585–588, 1945.
15. Paffenbarger RS Jr, Thorne MC, Wing AL: Chronic disease in former college students. VIII. Characteristics in youth predisposing to hypertension in later years. Am J Epidemiol 88:25–32, 1968.
16. Stamler J, Berkson DM, Dyer A, Lepper MH, Lindberg HA, Paul O, McKean H, Rhomberg P, Schoenberger JA, Shekelle RB, Stamler R: Relationship of multiple variables to blood pressure – findings from four Chicago epidemiologic studies. In: Paul O (ed) Epidemiology and control of hypertension. Miami, Symposia Specialists, 1975, pp 307–352.
17. Hypertension Detection and Follow-up Program Cooperative Group: Five-year findings of the Hypertension Detection and Follow-up Program. 1. Reduction in mortality of persons with high blood pressure, including mild hypertension. JAMA 242:2562–2571, 1979.
18. Australian National Blood Pressure Study: Tha Australian therapeutic trial in mild hypertension. Lancet 1:1261–1267, 1980.
19. Bulletin of the World Health Organization. 61(1):53–56, 1983.

4. Salt, diuretics and resistance to treatment

JACQUES J. BOURGOIGNIE

Sodium occupies a central place in the pathogenesis and treatment of hypertension. This was recognized many years ago before chemotherapy for the treatment of hypertension was available. Kempner [1] used a rice diet providing 8 mEq of sodium to treat 500 patients. The diet was ineffective in 178 patients. In the patients successfully treated, the average blood pressure fall was 47 mmHg systolic and 21 mmHg diastolic. Today, diuretics constitute the first line of antihypertensive treatment.

After an overview of normal sodium homeostasis, I shall review the role of sodium in blood pressure regulation and in the development and maintenance of hypertension, before considering the contribution of diuretics to treatment and the mechanisms underlying the development of resistance to antihypertensive regimens.

This review is selective and I apologize to the many authors whose contribution is not cited.

A. Normal sodium homeostasis

Sodium is obligated to the extracellular fluid (ECF) and only 5–10% of total body sodium in intracellular. Thus, sodium that leaks into the intracellular fluid (ICF) from the ECF is transported back into the ECF. Since sodium plus an electrically equivalent number of anions constitute over 90% of the osmotically active particles in the ECF, addition of sodium to the ECF, from ICF or external sources, also obligates to that compartment an equivalent amount of water, from ICF or other sources, to maintain ECF tonicity constant. Therefore, sodium controls ECF volume, the aim of which is to preserve the integrity of circulatory performance and organ perfusion.

These considerations give sodium ions a central role in the relationship of total ECF volume, i.e., plasma plus interstitial volumes, to overall vascular capacitance that determines such fundamental indices of cardiovascular performance as mean arterial blood pressure and left ventricular filling volume.

The range over which normal individuals maintain sodium balance varies from essentially zero to as much as 1500 mEq/day [2]. The ability to regulate sodium balance over this wide range of intake suggests the existence of a precise control system that is sensor oriented and feedback regulated with a responsive end-organ, the kidney, ultimately responsible for adjusting the rate of sodium excretion. The control system and the feedback mechanisms adjusting urinary sodium excretion to ECF volume and circulatory capacitance are very complex and poorly integrated. Nevertheless, the continuous interaction between various sensor and effector mechanisms serves to ensure near-constancy of the ECF volume [3].

B. Sodium and blood pressure regulation

The maintenance of blood pressure within relatively narrow limits in health results from the interaction of multiple factors no less complicated than those regulating sodium homeostasis. While short-term regulation seems to be the responsibility of the autonomic nervous system, long-term regulation involves the kidney in several ways [5]:

1. As already mentioned, the kidney is responsible for sodium excretion and balance. Increases in sodium excretion negatively affect sodium balance, ECF volume and arterial pressure while increases in ECF or blood pressure positively affect sodium excretion. The connection between pressure and sodium excretion involves physical and humoral factors. An increased excretion by nonautoregulated juxtamedullary nephrons in which perfusion pressure and single nephron filtration rate correlate directly may contribute [4]. A humoral connection has also been postulated that involves a natriuretic factor (vide infra).
2. The kidney is also responsible for renin secretion. A decrease in blood pressure positively affects renin secretion; the subsequent increase in angiotensin raises blood pressure to restore it to its original value. The converse occurs when blood pressure increases. This pressure-renin-pressure system is a powerful blood pressure regulator.
3. Renin secretion is also under sodium control. Sodium depletion positively affects renin secretion and ECF volume expansion inhibits renin synthesis. Conversely, an increase in renin secretion and angiotensin formation negatively affects sodium excretion. Thus, the kidney balances factors that interplay in the control of both ECF volume and vascular resistance, two major determinants of vascular capacitance.

When dietary sodium intake is low, ECF volume contracts, renin and angiotensin activities are high and sodium excretion is low; blood pressure remains normal or decreases slightly. When dietary sodium intake is high, ECF volume expands, renin and angiotensin activities are low and sodium excretion is high; blood pressure remains normal or increases slightly. Hence blood pressure normally stays constant when renin and body's sodium stores change in a reciprocal manner.

C. Sodium and hypertension

The evidence linking sodium and hypertension is considerable and based on several sources [6]: (a) Epidemiological studies show that the prevalence of hypertension correlates inversely with salt intake; (b) the ECF volume of 'salt eaters' is expanded in comparison to that of 'no-salt eaters'; (c) hemodynamic studies suggest that the development of chronic experimental hypertension is a homeostatic response to a chronic increase in ECF volume; (d) finally, experience indicates that hypertension can be decreased by eliminating sodium from the diet or by continuous diuretic therapy. Either of these therapeutic manipulations results in a lowering of blood pressure that correlates with a reduction in ECF volume. It must be emphasized, however, that a greatly reduced amount of sodium, to about 1 gm or 17 mEq, is necessary to produce more than a minimal reduction in blood pressure.

A direct correlation between ECF volume and blood pressure is best seen in anephric patients or in patients with end-stage renal failure. A correlation has also been demonstrated between changes in ECF volume and changes in blood pressure in patients with essential or renovascular hypertension, or with primary aldosteronism undergoing either sodium loading or deprivation or diuretic therapy [7]. On the other hand, an absolute increase in ECF volume exists only in a minority of patients with essential hypertension. This absence of demonstrable volume expansion is explained by a secondary autoregulatory rise in total peripheral resistance which reduces volume expansion and normalizes systemic flow while maintaining blood pressure high. In normal and in hypertensive subjects a negative correlation exists between total peripheral resistance and circulating blood volume: the higher the peripheral resistance, the lower the blood volume. The similarity of this relationship in normal and in hypertensive subjects reflects an appropriate peripheral blood flow regulation. However, in comparison to normal subjects, at an equivalent total peripheral vascular resistance, many patients with essential hypertension have an expanded blood volume [8].

The evidence that involves sodium in the pathogenesis of hypertension is far from absolute. Indeed, studies in man and in animals indicate that, in addition to sodium per se, a genetic constitution is a decisive determinant of the vascular and blood pressure responses to salt [9]. This was elegantly shown by Dahl, Heine and Tassinari [10] who used selective inbreeding to produce a substrain of rats that become hypertensive when placed on a sodium-rich diet but remain normotensive when maintained on a diet of normal sodium content. These observations clearly demonstrate that environmental influences can have a dramatic effect on the blood pressure of genetically predisposed individuals. Subsequent studies in this and other species of rats showed that the kidney had a critical role in the development of the hypertension. Renal crosstransplantation studies demonstrated a fall in blood pressure to normal when a genetically hypertensive rat was nephrectomized and given a kidney from a normotensive donor. Conversely, hypertension rapidly developed when a normotensive rat was given a kidney from a genetically hypertensive animal [11–14]. Tobian et al. [15] reported that the kidneys of these hypertensive rats exhibit a reduced intrinsic natriuretic capacity with a blunted pressure–sodium excretion relationship.

Thus, the evidence that a high dietary sodium exerts deleterious effects by promoting hypertension is considerable. The latter is expressed largely only when an underlying genetic predisposition develops that appears to involve some defects in the kidney's ability to excrete sodium.

The defect in essential hypertension is unknown. Experimentally, it often is reflected in an inability of the kidney to excrete sodium. Thus, the normal relationship between arterial pressure and sodium excretion is altered. In conditions that produce hypertension such as during renal vasoconstriction, increased tubular sodium reabsorption secondary to DOCA administration or when functional nephron mass is decreased, an increased arterial pressure is needed to reestablish a normal sodium excretion rate [5] (Figure 1).

Total ECF volume is the critical factor that correlates best with the increase in

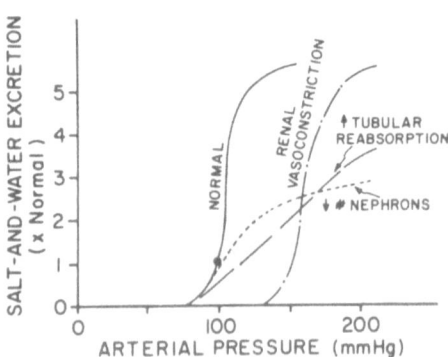

Figure 1. Schematic arterial pressure–sodium excretion relationships for normal conditions and three interventions that produced hypertension. Increased arterial pressure is needed to reestablish normal sodium excretion in the cases of renal vasoconstriction and increased tubular reabsorption. In the case of decreased number of nephrons, increased arterial pressure is required only at higher-than-normal sodium intake (reproduced with permission from [5]).

blood pressure in hypertensive subjects. The fact that an increased ECF volume is not consistently measured in hypertensives may indicate that blood pressure is elevated as a compensatory mechanism necessary to enhance sodium excretion and restore a normal ECF volume. In this context hypertension is a disease of maladjustment of sodium homeostasis. This regulatory mechanism in patients with primary aldosteronism or in excessive licorice ingesters explains why edema does not develop. Natriuresis develops as the ECF volume expands and hypertension ensues. This escape phenomenon is believed to result rom the effects of a natriuretic hormone [3, 16].

The suggestion has recently been made that essential hypertension in man also results from an inherited variability in the kidney to eliminate sodium. The difficulty in eliminating sodium would increase the concentration of a circulating sodium potassium ATPase inhibitor which affects sodium transport in all cells. In the kidney, it acts as a natriuretic hormone to correct urinary sodium excretion. In the arteriole, it causes a rise in intracellular sodium, and consequently calcium concentration, thereby increasing vascular reactivity. These changes give rise to a gradual increase in arterial pressure (Figure 2). This provocative hypothesis has some experimental support and is under vigorous investigation [17–24].

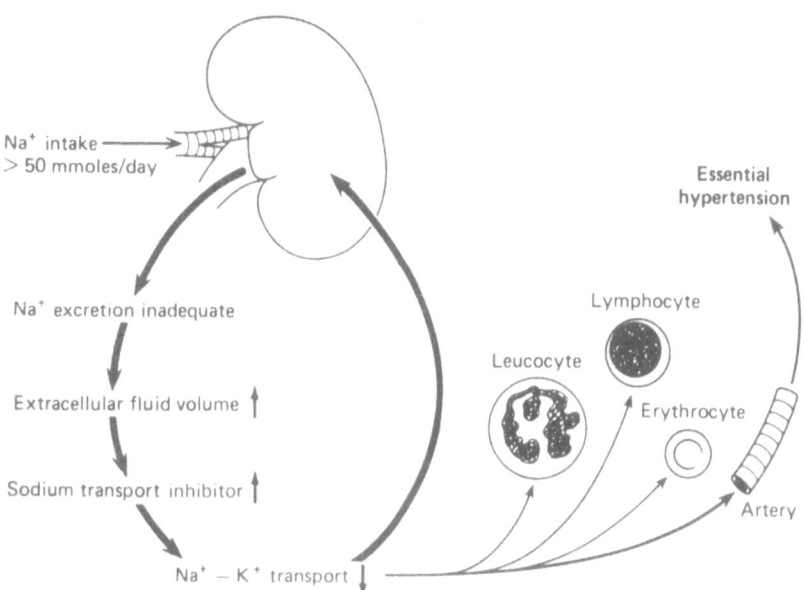

Figure 2. Hypothesis for the possible role of a circulating sodium-transport inhibitor in the etiology of essential hypertension (reproduced with permission from [20]).

D. Diuretics

In the preceding context, it is not surprising that diuretics are useful in the treatment of hypertension. The action of diuretics results from their capacity to inhibit tubular reabsorption and increase urinary excretion of solute, primarily sodium and chloride [25, 26]. Since filtered water is reabsorbed by the kidneys as a consequence of solute reabsorption, agents that inhibit solute reabsorption in turn inhibit water reabsorption and induce a diuresis. Thus, diuretic-induced urinary losses result in ECF volume contraction.

Since the proximal tubule is the site where the majority of the filtered sodium is reabsorbed, one might have expected that those agents inhibiting proximal sodium reabsorption would induce the greatest natriuresis. This is not the case, however, because reabsorption in the more distal tubular segments is load-dependent; the loop of Henle, in particular, compensates and increases its reabsorptive rates of solutes that have escaped proximal tubular reabsorption. Thus, acetazolamide inhibits carbonic anhydrase but is only a weak diuretic.

The most potent diuretics are the loop diuretics. They inhibit, in a dose-dependent fashion, the medullary thick ascending limb of Henle. With these agents, in excess of 25% of the filtered load of sodium may appear in the final urine. Since sodium chloride reabsorption in the ascending limb is responsible for an effective countercurrent concentrating mechanism that generates a hypertonic medullary interstitium, the loop diuretics also impair the renal capacity to concentrate urine and conserve water. Furosemide initially increases glomerular filtration rate. It also increases urinary calcium excretion.

The thiazide diuretics act in the cortical diluting segment of the loop of Henle and early distal tubule. These diuretics inhibit only the urinary diluting ability and not the concentrating capacity because they decrease sodium reabsorption in the cortical, but not the medullary, portion of the ascending limb. All thiazide diuretics have comparable effects. They differ from each other primarily in duration of action. Metolazone is more potent and its synergistic effects with furosemide may result in dangerous natriuresis. In contrast to furosemide, thiazides tend to decrease glomerular filtration rate and decrease urinary calcium excretion.

Triamterene, amiloride and spironolactone act in the distal nephron where potassium secretion takes place. The former two drugs inhibit sodium reabsorption and block potassium secretion independently of the presence of aldosterone; while spironolactone is a steroid antagonist of aldosterone and is ineffective in the absence of circulating aldosterone. These diuretics are potassium-sparing, whereas the diuresis of thiazides and other diuretics which act proximally to the site of potassium secretion are associated with a kaliuresis.

The natriuretic effects of chronic diuretic administration are self-limited. Indeed, intrarenal adjustments in response to diuresis and natriuresis tends to slow down or brake the urinary excretion of salt. This 'braking phenomenon' of diuretic action is illustrated in Figure 3. Normal subjects given a diuretic and a fixed sodium intake quicky develop a negative sodium balance. After the initial phase of diuretic action, the amount of sodium appearing in the urine progressively diminishes to match sodium intake, a point of sodium balance. There is then compensation by other tubular nephron segments, proximal and/or distal, to offset the inhibition of sodium chloride reabsorption in nephron segments affected by the diuretic; balance for sodium is then reestablished albeit at a lower level of total ECF volume. This 'braking phenomenon' to diminish net sodium excretion has been viewed as the mirror image of the 'escape' phenomenon seen in patients on a high salt intake and exogenous mineralocorticoid. Natriuretic factor may be important in establishing the new steady state in each case [25].

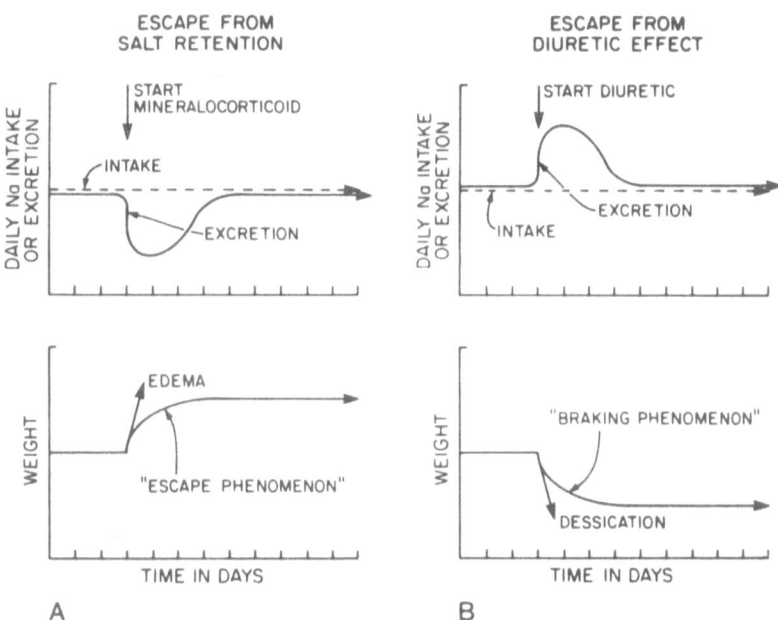

Figure 3. Illustration of the 'escape phenomenon' (A) in subjects given a large salt load and excess mineralocorticoid, and the 'braking phenomenon' (B) in subjects placed on a limited salt intake and given a loop diuretic. In both situations, salt balance is reestablished after a short period of imbalance. In the new steady state there is (A) positive salt balance and weight gain in the subjects given excess sodium chloride and (B) negative salt balance and weight loss in the subjects receiving the diuretic. It is postulated that a natriuretic factor, increasing in A and decreasing in B, is important in establishing the new steady state in each case (reproduced with permission from [25]).

E. Diuretics in hypertension

All diuretics have been used in chronic hypertension. A common response develops with any and all of them with common side effects resulting from their ability to decrease ECF volume. As a consequence of the 'breaking' natriuresis of chronic diuretic use, the antihypertensive effects of diuretics are also self-limited. Moreover, because of the reciprocal balance between sodium and the renin-angiotensin system, as sodium and water are lost, ECF volume contracts and the renin-angiotensin system is activated; the consequent increase in renin and angiotensin levels substitute for the sodium and water deficits and sustain the hypertension, albeit at a lower level of pressure.

For the same reason, the antihypertensive effects of different diuretics are by and large similar. This stems from the fact that, whereas potent diuretics result in a greater contraction of ECF volume, they also stimulate renin-angiotensin more vigorously than weak diuretics, through induction of greater ECF volume contraction and stimulation of renal prostaglandin. Therefore, no net chronic antihypertensive gain is seen with potent diuretics whereas the prevalence and intensity of acute side effects increases markedly.

The effects of thiazide diuretics on blood pressure are illustrated in Figure 4. In this experiment, Dahl's salt-resistant and salt-sensitive rats were maintained on a high sodium diet with or without chlorothiazide. In salt-resistant animals sodium had little effect on blood pressure, and chlorothiazide had no effect. In salt-sensitive animals, sodium was hypertensinogenic resulting in the death of

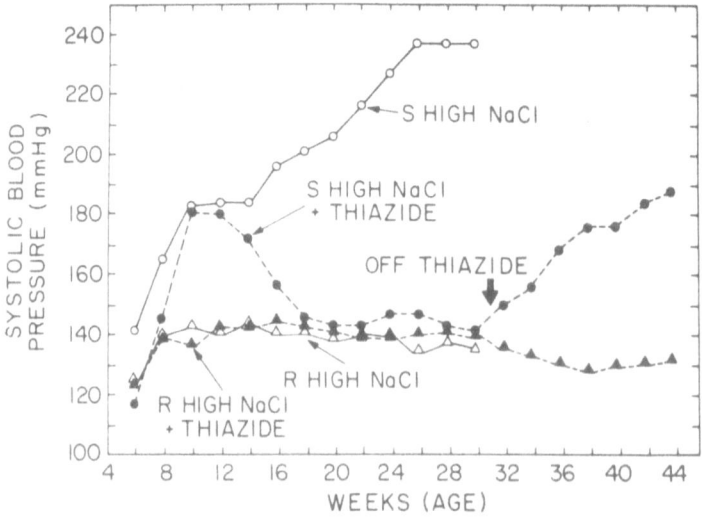

Figure 4. Effect of chlorothiazide on blood pressure in hypertension-resistant (R) and hypertension-sensitive (S) rats on a high salt diet (reproduced with permission from [27]).

80% of the animals at week 31. In contrast, whereas salt-sensitive rats given chlorothiazide initially developed the same degree of hypertension with sodium administration, starting at week 12 they exhibited a rapid fall in blood pressure to levels undistinguishable from those of salt-resistant rats or from those of salt-sensitive rats maintained on a low sodium diet (not shown). Rats on chlorothiazide also showed no mortality. This lowering of blood pressure was associated with an increase in urinary sodium excretion only in salt-sensitive rats. Despite administration of chlorothiazide, blood pressure and natriuresis remained normal in equivalent groups maintained on a low sodium diet (not shown). The lack of chlorothiazide effects in rats on a low sodium diet was a consequence of a low ECF volume which was reflected in a high plasma renin activity. A unique aspect of this study is the finding that chlorothiazide failed to prevent the development of hypertension by high sodium diet but reduced blood pressure only at a later stage [27].

These observations with chlorothiazide in rats resemble the antihypertensive effects of chronic diuretic therapy in man. The greatest antihypertensive effects occur in sodium-replete subjects with low plasma renin activity, whereas little antihypertensive effect is seen in volume-contracted patients with high plasma renin activity.

The initial natriuresis accounts for the acute antihypertensive action of thiazide diuretics whereas a direct vasodilator effect is often postulated to explain the decrease in peripheral vascular resistance that is associated with chronic thiazide administration. There is little evidence to support a dual mechanism in the antihypertensive action of thiazide diuretics. Shah, Khatri and Freis [28] performed sequential hemodynamic studies in hypertensive patients before and during eight weeks of thiazide therapy. Their results clearly show that the long-term effects of thiazides, like their short-term effects, are associated with a chronic contraction of the ECF volume, though plasma volume tends to return to baseline values. The fall in blood pressure with thiazides occurs only after an effective diuresis in induced and is maintained as long as the ECF volume remains contracted. All studies, except one [29], indicate that plasma and ECF volumes remain reduced during long periods of treatment. A dual mechanism of action, therefore, need not be postulated. The fact that salt-free dextran usually will not restore the hypertension, whereas sodium chloride will, indicates that re-expansion of total ECF, rather than plasma volume alone, is required to overcome the antihypertensive effects of the thiazides. Moreover, after discontinuation of long-term thiazide treatment, there is a prompt rebound in plasma volume, ECF volume and blood pressure providing further evidence that the thiazides continue to maintain their volume-reducing effect during chronic administration. The lack of antihypertensive action of thiazides in anephric animals and in anuric patients also mitigate against a direct vasodilator effect [30, 31].

Another, albeit indirect, argument against a vasodilator action of thiazides may also be found in the importance of the ECF volume status that commands the response to exogenous or endogenous pressor or depressor stimuli.

Indeed, whereas ECF volume expansion (and inhibition of the renin-angiotensin system) augments the pressor responsiveness to angiotensin or catecholamines, it blunts the vasodepressor response to vasodilating agents including β-adrenergic blocking drugs and angiotensin antagonists. In this situation, the depressor response of thiazides is enhanced. Conversely, when ECF volume is contracted (and the renin-angiotensin system activated), pressor responsiveness is blunted whereas depressor responses are enhanced. Resistance to diuretic action is then common (Figure 5).

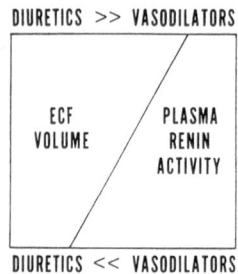

Figure 5. Diagram of relative blood pressure sensitivity to diuretic vs vasodilator agents as a function of ECF volume and plasma renin activity.

F. Resistance to antihypertensive treatment

Clinical experience has demonstrated that, so called resistance to anti-hypertensive drug therapy is, nowadays, more apparent than real [32]. In my opinion, truly resistant hypertension defined as blood pressure that cannot be adequately controlled with a suitable drug regimen no longer exists, provided that the medication is prescribed and taken appropriately. An acquired apparent resistance, however, is not uncommonly observed.

1. Resistance to vasodilators

A common feature to all vasodilating drugs is the induction of sodium retention with time. This salt-retaining effect is proportional to the potency of the drug. It is most apparent with agents like diazoxide or minoxidil. As a consequence of progressive salt retention, the ECF volume expands and the renin-angiotensin system's activity is attenuated. This, as indicated in Figure 5, progressively abrogates the antihypertensive effect of any vasodilating drug. Resistance sets in and blood pressure returns to pretreatment hypertensive values. Such a course is

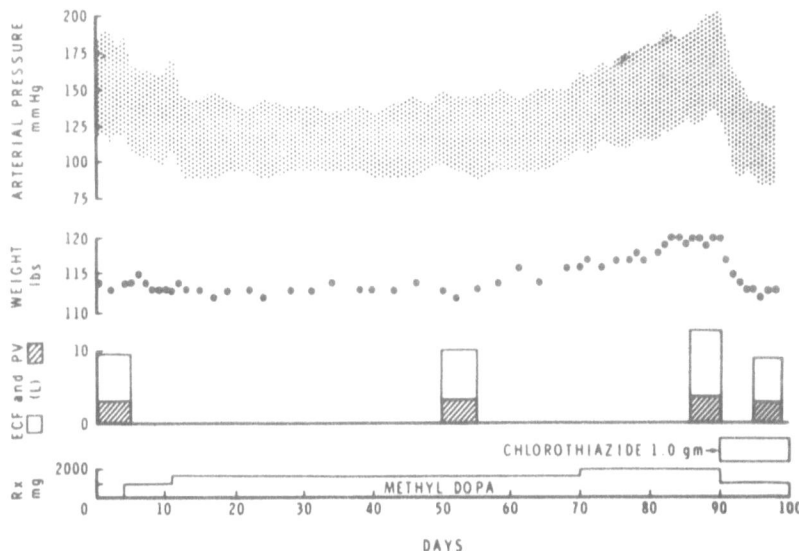

Figure 6. Chart of arterial pressure and ECF volume changes in a patient receiving methyldopa over a three-month period (reproduced with permission from [33]).

illustrated in Figure 6 for a patient treated with methyldopa. Changes in ECF volume did not accompany a satisfactory antihypertensive response to methyldopa; but, resistance to methyldopa was associated with weight gain and progressive increase in total ECF volume. At this point, administration of a diuretic resulted in weight loss, ECF volume reduction and blood pressure control [33].

Observations, in patients treated with diazoxide indicate that changes in total ECF volume, rather than plasma volume, are critical to effect changes in blood pressure. Administration of dextran, a plasma volume expander, does not increase blood pressure significantly in patients with diazoxide-controlled blood pressure [33].

Thus, the diuretics ability to contract ECF volume chronically is used to enhance the hypotensive effects of other agents as well as to prevent the development of resistance to vasodilators.

2. Resistance to diuretics

Many clinical factors modify the response to diuretics in general or to specific diuretics in particular (Table 1). When resistance to diuretics develops, one must question the patient's compliance and his level of sodium intake. Ideally, sodium

Table 1. Clinical factors influencing the response to diurects

Compliance	Renal disease
Diet	Acid-base status
Site of action	Hyperaldosteronism
Dose	Volume status
Age	Drug interaction
Bedrest	

intake should not exceed about 75 mEq/day for two purposes: (a) a heavier sodium intake may overwhelm the diuretic's antihypertensive potency; and (b) when sodium intake is decreased from 180 to 75 mEq/day, diuretic-induced potassium losses are halved [34]. When blood pressure responds poorly, an overnight urine should be analyzed for sodium content; only if less than 50 mEq of sodium are present should the dose of the diuretic be increased or another antihypertensive agent be added [35].

As already discussed the tubular site of action of the drug is important for its diuretic response. A large dose–response is useful to titrate the effects of any drug. Such exists only for furosemide with an effective dose range varying from 10–20 mg to about one gram. In fact, unless some specific indication exists, only thiazide diuretics should be used in the treatment of hypertension and less diuretic than is often prescribed will usually provide all the antihypertensive action that diuretics are capable of providing while diminishing the hypokalemia. For most patients with good renal function 25–50 mg of hydrochlorothiazide or 25 mg of chlorthalidone once a day is enough. Tweeddale, Ogilvie and Reudy [36] have shown that 25 mg of chlorthalidone has the same antihypertensive effect as 50–200 mg/day.

Young adults are less sensitive to the antihypertensive effects of thiazide diuretics than elderly patients who often exhibit an enhanced hypotensive response and, therefore, require a reduction of diuretic dosage. It is possible that the enhanced antihypertensive effect of thiazides in elderly patients with non-compliant arteries is due to an inadequate baroreceptor compensation for the reduced ECF volume and cardiac output [28].

Doses of diuretics, that were ineffective in the ambulatory patient, may bring an excellent diuretic response after hospitalization and bedrest.

The most important determinant to influence the response to diuretics is the underlying disease, particularly the volume status associated with it and the level of renal function. Perhaps, because most diuretics act from the luminal side of the tubule and need to be secreted in the proximal tubule to reach their site of action, their efficacy decreases rapidly as renal function decreases. Because of its potency and dose-dependent effect, high doses of furosemide may remain effective in patients with advanced renal insufficiency and a GFR of 10 ml/min.

Metolazone also has been shown to be effective in patients with a GFR of less than 25 ml/min but not in patients with a GFR of 10 ml/min. When renal function is impaired (serum creatinine greater than 2 mg percent), multiple daily doses of furosemide or a single dose of metolazone may be needed.

Whereas metabolic acidosis classically enhances the diuretic response to mercurials and blunts the response to acetazolamide, the acid-base status is not a determinant of effectiveness for thiazide or loop diuretics.

Aldosterone per se is not important, except for spironolactone action. Rather the volume status associated with changes in aldosterone secretion dictates the diuretic response. Sensitivity to diuretics correlates positively with the effective arterial blood volume. Thus, in primary aldosteronism with ECF volume expansion or in primary volume expansion (from excess salt ingestion) associated with a decrease in aldosterone secretion, sensitivity to diuretics is enhanced; in contrast, in edematous patients with a decreased effective intravascular volume (nephrotic syndrome, cirrhosis with ascites) and secondary hyperaldosteronism, resistance to thiazides and loop diuretics is common. The same is seen in non-edematous patients with malignant hypertension whose ECF volume is often markedly contracted and plasma renin activity and aldosterone extremely high. Moreover, in these patients vasoconstriction may be so intense that the hypertension may resist even the administration of nitruprusside unless sodium chloride is first administered. These conditions of hyperaldosteronism secondary to increased renin-angiotensin stimulation may be exquisitely sensitive to inhibitors or antagonists of the renin-angiotensin system (Figure 5) [37, 38].

A common complication of diuretic therapy is volume depletion as a result of overdiuresis. Beside hypokalemia, this is another reason to use the least amount of drug that is effective in removing fluid slowly. When volume depletion occurs or when renal excretion of solute and water exceeds the rate of mobilization of interstitial fluid, intravascular volume contraction and azotemia result with stimulation of renin, angiotensin and aldosterone and resistance to further diuretic action (Figure 5). Thus, overdiuresis will render resistant to diuretics a patient who was initially sensitive to the drug.

Finally, an antagonism between diuretics and drugs that inhibit prostaglandin synthesis has been demonstrated. Such antagonism has been reported with aspirin or indomethacin and furosemide, ethacrynic acid, spironolactone, chlorthalidone, hydrochlorothiazide in rat, dog and man on renal blood flow, sodium excretion, renin release or blood pressure [39–49]. In the study of Patak et al. [39], whereas 240 mg/day of furosemide alone for four days resulted in a negative sodium balance that averaged 90 mEq/day with a 13 mmHg decline in mean arterial pressure, administration of furosemide and indomethacin together resulted in a markedly blunted natriuresis and no change in blood pressure. The ability of nonsteroidal antiinflammatory drugs to blunt or even neutralize the antihypertensive effects of diuretics may be the sum of three actions, all of which involve prostaglandin inhibition. The marked reduction in renin secretion works to lower blood pressure. However, this effect is evidently more than offset by sodium and water retention from intrarenal prostaglandin inhibition and by a loss of systemic vasodilator capacity which normally buffers the effects of angiotensin during diuretic therapy [46]. These drug interactions must be kept in mind in clinical situations where patients may require both these type of drugs.

Acknowledgments

Dr. Bourgoignie is supported with funds from the National Institutes of Health (USPHS Grant AM 19822) and from the Florida Heart Association.

References

1. Kempner W: Treatment of hypertensive vascular disease with rice diet. Am J Med 4:545–577, 1948.
2. Pratt JH, Luft F: The effect of extremely high sodium intake on plasma renin activity, plasma aldosterone concentration, and urinary excretion of aldosterone metabolites. J Lab Clin Med 93:724–729, 1979.
3. Bourgoignie JJ, Pennell JP, Jacob AI: Sodium metabolism and volume homeostasis. In: Gonick HC (ed) Current nephrology, Vol 3. Boston, Houghton Mifflin, 1979, p 1–40.
4. Stumpe KO, Lowitz HD, Ochwadt B: Function of juxtamedullary nephrons in normotensive and chronically hypertensive rats. Pflugers Arch 313:43–52, 1969.
5. Coleman TG, Holl JE, Norman RA Jr: Regulation of arterial blood pressure. In: Brenner BM, Stein JH (eds) Contemporary issues in nephrology. 8. Hypertension. New York, Churchill Livingstone, 1981, p 1–20.
6. Freis ED: Salt, volume and the prevention of hypertension. Circulation 53:589–595, 1976.
7. Dustan HP, Tarazi RC, Bravo EL, Dart RA: Plasma and extracellular fluid volumes in hypertension. Circ Res 22:I 73–I 31, 1973.
8. Tarazi RC: Hemodynamic role of extracellular fluid in hypertension. Cir Res 25:II 73–II 183, 1976.
9. Mark AL, Gordon FJ, Takeshita A: Sodium, vascular resistance and genetic hypertension. In: Brenner BM, Stein JH (eds): Contemporary issues in nephrology. 8. Hypertension, New York, Churchill Livingstone, 1981, pp 21–39.
10. Dahl LK, Heine M, Tassinari L: Role of genetic factors in susceptibility to experimental hypertension due to chronic excess salt ingestion. Nature 194:480–482, 1962.
11. Dahl LK, Heine M, Thompson K: Genetic influence of renal homografts on the blood pressure of rats from different strains. Proc Soc Exp Bio Med 140:852–855, 1972.
12. Dahl LK, Heine M, Thompson K: Genetic influence of the kidneys on blood pressure. Evidence from chronic renal homografts in rats with opposite predispositions to hypertension. Circ Res 34:94–101, 1974.
13. Bianchi G, Fox U, DiFrancesco GF, Giovanetti AM, Pagetti D: Blood pressure changes produced by kidney cross-transplantation between spontaneously hypertensive rats and normotensive rats. Clin Sci Mol Med 47:435–448, 1974.
14. Kawabe K, Watanabe TX, Shione K, Sokabe H: Influence on blood pressure of renal isografts

between spontaneously hypertensive and normotensive rats, utilizing the F hybrids. J Heart J 19:886–894, 1978.

15. Tobian L, Lange J, Azar S, Iwai J, Koop D, Coffee K, Johnson MA: Reduction of natriuretic capacity and renin release in isolated, blood-perfused kidneys of Dahl hypertension-prone rats. Circ Res 43:192–198, 1978.

16. Favre H: Role of the natriuretic factor in the disorders of sodium balance. Adv Nephrol 11: 3–25, 1982.

17. Overbeck HW: The sodium pump in cardiovascular muscle in hypertension: whose hypothesis? Clin Exp Hypertens 1:551–556, 1979.

18. Gruber KA, Whitaker JM, Buckalew VM Jr: Endogenous digitalis-like substance in plasma of volume-expanded dogs. Nature 287:743–745, 1980.

19. Haddy FJ: Mechanism, prevention and therapy of sodium-dependent hypertension. Am J Med 69:746–758, 1980.

20. de Wardener H, MacGregor GA: Dahl's hypothesis that a saluretic substance may be responsible for a sustained rise in arterial pressure. Its possible role in essential hypertension. Kidney Int 18:1–9, 1980.

21. de Wardener HE: The natriuretic hormone. Proc 8th Int Congr Nephrol, Athens, 1981, pp 47–53.

22. Buckalew VM: Salt, natriuretic hormone and hypertension. Ann Int Med 95:511–512, 1981.

23. Overbeck HW: Elevated arterial pressure, vascular wall 'waterlogging' and impaired cardiac growth in rats chronically receiving digoxin. Proc Soc Exp Biol Med 167:506–513, 1981.

24. Gruber KA, Whitaker JM, Rudel LL, Bullock BC: Increased circulating levels of an endogenous digoxin-like factor in hypertensive non-human primates. Hypertension (in press).

25. Grantham JJ, Chonko AM: The physiological basis and clinical use of diuretics. In: Brenner BM, Stein JH Contemporary issues in nephrology, Vol 1. New York, Churchill Livingstone, 1978, pp 178–211.

26. Dirks JH: Mechanisms of action and clinical uses of diuretics. Hosp Pract 14:99–110, 1979.

27. Iwai J, Ohanian EV, Dahl LK: Influence of thiazide on salt hypertension. Circ Res 40:I131–I134, 1977.

28. Shah S, Khatri I, Freis ED: Mechanism of antihypertensive effect of thiazide diuretics. Am Heart J 95:611–618, 1978.

29. Conway J, Lauwers P: Hemodynamic and hypotensive effects of long-term therapy with chlorothiazide. Circulation 21:21–27, 1960.

30. Orbison JL: Failure of chlorothiazide to influence tissue electrolytes in hypertensive and non-hypertensive nephrectomized dogs. Proc Soc Exp Biol Med 110:161–164, 1962.

31. Bennett WM, McDonald WJ, Kuehnel E: Do diuretics have antihypertensive properties independent of natriuresis? Clin Pharmacol Ther 22:499–504, 1977.

32. Tarazi RC: Management of the patient with resistant hypertension. Hosp Pract 16:49–57, 1981.

33. Finnerty FA, Davidov M, Mroczek WJ, Gavrilovich L: Influence of extracellular fluid volume on response to antihypertensive drugs. Circ Res 26:I71–I80, 1970.

34. Ram CVS, Garrett BN, Kaplan NM: Moderate sodium restriction and various diuretics in the treatment of hypertension. Effects on potassium wastage and blood pressure control. Arch Intern Med 141:1015–1019, 1981.

35. Kaplan NM: Management strategies in hypertension. In: Brenner BM, Stein JH (eds) Contemporary issues in nephrology, Vol 8. New York, Churchill Livingstone, 1981, pp 339–369.

36. Tweeddale MG, Ogilvie RI, Reudy J: Antihypertensive and biochemical effects of chlorthalidone. Clin Pharmac Ther 22:519–527, 1977.

37. Romero JC, Holmes DR, Strong CG: The effect of high sodium intake and angiotensin antagonist in rabbits with severe and moderate hypertension induced by constriction of one renal artery. Circ Res 40:I17–I23, 1977.

38. Atlas SA, Case DB, Sealey JE, Laragh JH, McKinstry DN: Interruption of the renin-angiotensin system in hypertensive patients by captopril induces sustained reduction in aldosterone secretion, potassium retention and natriuresis. Hypertension 1:274–280, 1979.

39. Patak RV, Mookerjee BK, Bentzel CJ, Hysert PE, Babej M, Lee JB: Antagonism of the effects of furosemide by indomethacin in normal and hypertensive man. Prostaglandins 10:649–659, 1975.

40. Williamson HE, Bourland WA, Marchand GR: Inhibition of ethacrynic acid induced increase in renal blood flow by indomethacin. Prostaglandins 8:297–301, 1974.

41. Tweeddale MD, Ogilvie RI: Antagonism of spironolactone-induced natriuresis by aspirin in man. N Engl J Med 289:198–200, 1973.

42. Bailie MD, Barbour JA, Hook JB: Effects of indomethacin on furosemide-induced changes in renal blood flow. Proc Soc Exp Biol Med 148:1173–1176, 1975.

43. Williamson HE, Bourland WA, Marchand GR: Inhibition of furosemide induced increase in renal blood blow by indomethacin. Proc Soc Exp Biol Med 148:164–167, 1975.

44. Hoffman LM, Garcia HA: Interaction of spironolactone and indomethacin at the renal level. Proc Soc Exp Biol Med 141:353–355, 1972.

45. Berg KJ, Loew D: Inhibition of furosemide-induced natriuresis by acetylsalicylic acid in dogs. Scand J Clin Lab Invest 37:125–131, 1977.

46. Lopez-Ovejero JA, Weber MA, Droyer JIM, Sealey JE, Laragh JH: Effects of indomethacin alone and during diuretic or β-adrenoreceptor blockade therapy on blood pressure and the renin system in essential hypertension. Clin Sci Mol Med 55:203–207, 1978.

47. Attalah AA: Interaction of prostaglandins with diuretics. Prostaglandins 18:369–375, 1979.

48. Patak RV, Fadem SZ, Rosenblatt SG, Lifschitz MD, Stein JH: Diuretic induced-changes in renal blood flow and prostaglandin E excretion in the dog. Am J Physiol 236:F 494–F 500, 1979.

49. Smith DE, Brater DC, Lin ET et al: Attenuation of furosemide's diuretic effect by indomethacin: pharmacokinetic evaluation. J Pharmacokinet Biopharm 7:265–274, 1979.

5. Autonomic drugs used in the treatment of the hypertensive patient with particular reference to beta-receptor blocking agents

ANDREW J. LONIGRO

I. Introduction

Controversy over whether or not to treat the patient with essential hypertension was effectively quelled by the initial reports in 1967 and 1970 of the 'Veterans Administration Cooperative Study' that subjects with sustained elevations of diastolic blood pressure greater than 104 mmHg, showed marked improvement in both morbidity and mortality when compared to placebo-treated control groups [1, 2]. Once the diagnosis of essential hypertension has been established in the individual patient, however, the practicing physician, as an integral part of formulation of therapeutic objectives, is confronted with an imposing list of pharmacological agents from which to choose – all of which will reduce blood pressure. Rational selection of one or more of these agents in terms of efficacy and safety is dependent not only upon knowledge of the pharmacology of the compounds to be used, but also upon an evaluation of the patient to define the degree of target-organ damage and to assess physiologic derangements. In this chapter autonomic contributions to blood pressure control will be reviewed briefly, followed by a more complete discussion of those agents which interfere with autonomic mechanisms with particular reference given to beta-receptor blocking agents.

II. Blood pressure regulation

Blood pressure is generally described as a function of cardiac output and total peripheral resistance. To understand the interrelationships of blood pressure, cardiac output and resistance, it must be clearly recognized that blood pressure is the variable being regulated; viz., changes in cardiac output and/or total peripheral resistance are subservient to the imperative of arterial pressure maintenance. For every individual, blood pressure is regulated around a fixed value often referred to as the 'set-point.' This 'set-point' is higher in patients with hypertension than it is in normotensive individuals. Thus, when blood pressure is altered by positional change, state of activity, medications or other factors in either hypertensive or normotensive individuals, compensatory mechanisms will be set into motion to return blood pressure to the 'set-point' for that individual. Compensation is effected through alterations in cardiac output and/or total peripheral resistance. Hence, an awareness of the determinants of cardiac output and total peripheral resistance is fundamental to the understanding of blood pressure regulation under physiologic as well as pathologic conditions. Moreover, pharmacological intervention in hypertensive disease can be understood only in terms of its interaction with one or more of these regulatory systems.

Autonomic contributions to the regulation of cardiac output are considerable and multifaceted. Although the amount of blood expelled by the heart is dependent, in large part, on the extent of ventricular filling during diastole ('Frank-Starling mechanism'), 'completeness' of emptying during systole (ejection fraction) can be increased by sympathetic stimulation or decreased by parasympathetic stimulation. Moreover, the nervous system can influence the degree to which the heart fills during diastole by altering the amount of blood returned to the heart through effects on venous tone and intravascular volume. When the veins, which serve as the reservoir of blood volume are constricted or dilated as a result of nervous activity, the amount of blood returned to the heart will, perforce, be increased or decreased, respectively. In addition, the nervous system modulates the renal contribution to the regulation of intravascular volume by affecting sodium and water excretion. Thus, nervous influences on intrarenal blood flow distribution can have profound effects on glomerular filtration and tubular function; moreover, the disposition of sodium is influenced by the activity of the renin-angiotensin-aldosterone system, which is regulated, in part, by the autonomic nervous system.

Similarly, autonomic activity is a major determinant of total peripheral resistance. Although blood viscosity, as well as the length of the vessel through which blood is pumped are considerations in any estimate of total peripheral resistance, the largest and most important contributor to total peripheral resistance is the diameter of the arteriole. In addition to some degree of intrinsic control, arteriolar diameter is affected by circulating hormones such as angiotensin and catecholamines, and by the state of autonomic activity.

III. The autonomic nervous system

A. *Anatomical considerations*

Langley proposed the term 'Autonomic Nervous System' for the '... sympathetic system and the allied nervous system of the cranial and sacral nerves, and for the local nervous system of the gut' [3]. Although there has been much confusion over the terminology applied to the autonomic nervous system through the years, today two great divisions are recognized: the 'parasympathetic' or 'craniosacral' division and the 'sympathetic' or 'thoracolumbar' division. The following discussion will focus primarily on the sympathetic division of the autonomic nervous system.

As suggested by Gaskell in the early part of this century [4], the autonomic nervous system is understood best when it is considered as a reflex arc, consisting of three components; namely, the afferent limb, the central connections and the efferent limb. The afferent limb of the reflex begins in specialized structures referred to as 'cardiovascular-receptors,' discrete, specialized cells or structures capable of detecting changes in pressure, volume or blood gas composition (they must not be confused with pharmacologic 'receptors' which are molecular structures at or near cellular membranes and represent the chemical entity of the cell with which drugs interact). This term encompasses systemic arterial baroreceptors, pulmonary arterial baroreceptors, cardiac mechanoreceptors, arterial chemoreceptors and lung inflation receptors. The cell bodies of afferent nerves from these receptors lie either in the dorsal root ganglia of the spinal nerves or in the sensory ganglia of several cranial nerves. The latter enter the vasomotor centers in the *medulla oblongata* and the former synapse directly with the cell bodies of the preganglionic autonomic motorneurons in the intermediomedial and intermediolateral regions of the spinal cord. Ascending projections from segmental spinal inputs terminate mainly in the bulbar pressor area in the lateral reticular formation. Areas of blood pressure control have been identified within the *medulla oblongata* as well as in the hypothalamus and cortex. Several descending tracts, both stimulatory and inhibitory, from these areas have been shown to influence the activity of spinal autonomic motorneurons. The preganglionic autonomic motorneurons send projections out of the spinal cord via the anterior horn to sympathetic ganglia located in the sympathetic chain or in or near the organ which is innervated. Within the ganglia, the preganglionic neurons form synapses around the cell bodies of the postganglionic neurons. These postganglionic sympathetic neurons extend to effector organs, such as the heart, the resistance vessels and the kidney.

B. Neurochemical transmission

Transmission of nervous impulses at each synapse occurs through the release of one or more chemical substances. These chemical substances traverse the synaptic cleft and stimulate the postsynaptic neuron or effector cell by stimulating one or more pharmacological 'receptors.' The concept of chemical transmission of nerve impulses was convincingly demonstrated by Otto Loewi in 1921 when he showed that Ringer's solution removed from the ventricle of an isolated perfused frog's heart which had been arrested through stimulation of the vagal-sympathetic truck, would produce arrest of another heart when introduced into its ventricle [5]. He concluded that a chemical substance had been released into the ventricle of the first heart which produced cardiac slowing and arrest and which could be transferred to the second heart to produce similar effects. It is now recognized that all synaptic sites, whether in the central nervous system or peripheral to it, are associated with neurochemical transmission. The neurohumoral transmitter of all preganglionic autonomic fibers, all postganglionic parasympathetic fibers and a few postganglionic sympathetic fibers is acetylcholine. Norepinephrine is the transmitter for the majority of the postganglionic sympathetic fibers. The terms cholinergic and adrenergic are used to describe neurons that liberate acetylcholine and norepinephrine, respectively. Until recently, relatively few substances were considered as candidates for synaptic transmitters within the central nervous system. Now there are many including amino acids, acetylcholine, catecholamines, 5-hydroxy-tryptamine, histamine and peptides.

Norepinephrine is synthesized within the nerve. Through the action of tyrosine hydroxylase, tyrosine is converted to dopa, which is acted upon by dopa decarboxylase to form dopamine, which is converted to norepinephrine by dopamine-beta-hydroxylase. The adrenal medulla is analogous to a postganglionic sympathetic nerve in that it is innervated by preganglionic sympathetic neurons, which elaborate acetylcholine. The acetylcholine, in turn, stimulates the release of catecholamines from the adrenal medulla. Eighty-five percent of the catecholamine released by the adrenal gland is epinephrine and the remainder norepinephrine.

C. Adrenergic receptors

A pharmacologic receptor is usually pictured as a macromolecule within the cell membrane which displays high affinity for a limited range of organic structures. More than 70 years ago Langley introduced the term 'receptive substance' to designate the specific hypothetical material in or on a cell with which a given active agent had to react in order to evoke its response [6]. It was largely the work of A.J. Clarke which influenced numerous investigators to characterize the receptors for different endogenous agonists in a variety of effector organs or cells [7].

Initial descriptions of the sympathetic nervous system and the release of neurotransmitters proved to be extremely confusing because of the diversity of effects produced by exogenously applied epinephrine and adrenergic nerve stimulation. Considerable insight was gained into adrenergic mechanisms when, in 1948, Ahlquist concluded that sympathetic nerve stimulation released one transmitter, namely, norepinephrine, and that all adrenergic responses could be explained on the basis of that transmitter acting on two different receptors [8]. According to this concept, the adrenergic cardiovascular responses produce vasoconstriction through stimulation of 'alpha' receptors, whereas both cardiac stimulation and vasodilation occur through stimulation of 'beta' receptors.

It is now recognized that these adrenergic receptors can be subdivided further into beta-1 and beta-2 receptors [9] as well as alpha-1 and alpha-2 receptors [10]. Beta-1 receptors are found mainly in the heart and, when stimulated, produce an increase in both heart rate and force of contraction; whereas beta-2 receptors are found primarily in the periphery and, when stimulated, produce vasodilatation. Beta-1 receptors in fat cells, which are not innervated, produce lipolysis when stimulated. Beta-2 receptors in bronchial and intestinal smooth muscle, when stimulated, produce relaxation. The recognition of alpha-adrenergic receptor subtypes was suggested by the observation that alpha-adrenergic agonists suppressed the amount of catecholamine released from nerve terminals. It is now recognized that there are alpha receptors located at presynaptic sites which regulate, in an autoinhibitory fashion, the release of norepinephrine from the nerve ending. Thus, when high concentrations of norepinephrine are present, subsequent impulses release less norepinephrine. These presynaptic alpha receptors have been termed alpha-2 receptors to distinguish then from the post-synaptic or alpha-1 receptor. The latter, when stimulated, produce constriction of the blood vessel.

IV. Drugs which interfere with adrenergic mechanisms

A. Beta-adrenergic blocking agents

1. Introduction
Beta-adrenergic blocking agents, originally introduced as antianginal compounds, were soon found to possess antihypertensive properties as well [11]. Because of their efficacy and their paucity of untoward effects, beta-adrenergic blocking agents have increased in popularity and, at present, represent a major component of all antihypertensive therapy. The first beta-adrenergic antagonist to be used extensively was propranolol. Recently, several others have become available for general clinical use; it is anticipated that many more will be available within the next several years.

2. Properties
Beta-receptor blocking agents are distinguished one from the other on the basis of several pharmacological properties, such as the presence or absence of sympathomimetic (agonist) activity, membrane-stabilizing (local anesthetic, or

quinidine-like) effects or selectivity for one beta-receptor subtype over the other. Although these properties may account for some untoward effects and may give some insight into mechanisms of action, it must be clearly recognized that the sole pharmacological property of these compounds which correlates well with antihypertensive activity is the capacity to block beta-adrenergic receptors.

Prichard [12] suggested that beta-receptor blocking agents should be classified into three 'Divisions' based upon the type(s) of receptor blocked by the agent (Table 1). Division I drugs are nonselective and block both beta-1 and beta-2 adrenergic receptors. Division II drugs are cardioselective, exhibiting a much larger affinity for the beta-1 receptor than for the beta-2 receptor. Division III drugs block beta as well as alpha receptors (Table 1). Each 'Division' has been subdivided further into Groups I–IV based upon the other pharmacologic properties of these compounds [13]. Group I drugs possess both membrane stabilizing, as well as intrinsic sympathomimetic activity; Group II, solely membrane stabilizing activity; Group III, solely intrinsic sympathomimetic activity; and Group IV, neither intrinsic sympathomimetic activity nor membrane stabilizing effects (Table 1).

3. Proposed mechanisms of action

Several hypotheses have been proposed to explain the mechanism of the antihypertensive action of beta-receptor blocking agents, however, no single theory has been adequate to explain the antihypertensive properties of *all* the beta-

Table 1. Classification of beta-receptor blocking agents

Division	Group I MSE[a] ISA[b]	Group II MSE[a] No ISA[b]	Group III No MSE[a] ISA[b]	Group IV No MSE[a] No ISA[b]
I (Nonselective)	Pronethalol Oxprenolol Alprenolol Bunitrolol Penbutolol	Propranolol	Pindolol	Sotalol Timolol Nadolol Bunolol
II (Selective)	Acebutolol	Metoprolol Tolamolol	Practolol	Atenolol
III (Alpha & Beta)		Labetalol		

[a] MSE = membrane stabilizing effects.
[b] ISA = intrinsic sympathomimetic activity.

receptor blocking agents and, indeed, more than one mechanism may contribute to this effect.

a. Effect on cardiac output. Although cardiac output is reduced promptly after administration of beta-receptor blocking agents, the hypotensive effects are usually delayed. Since cardiac output falls in the face of an unchanged blood pressure, the first response to beta-adrenergic receptor blockade is actually an increase in total peripheral resistance. It is only after several days of therapy that peripheral resistance and blood pressure decrease [14]. In addition, patients who do not respond to beta-receptor blockade with a reduction of blood pressure still exhibit significant decreases in cardiac output similar in magnitude to that observed in responders. Therefore, the reduction in cardiac output, which is an immediate response to the application of beta-receptor blocking agents, cannot account for the eventual reduction in blood pressure since the two events are separated in time. There is some experimental evidence to suggest that the lack of blood pressure reduction as an initial response to beta-adrenergic blockade is caused by increased baroreceptor reflex activity consequent to the fall in cardiac output [15].

b. Effects on renin secretion. Inhibition of the release of renin from the juxta-glomerular apparatus because of blockade of beta-2 receptors has been proposed as the mechanism of action of beta-receptor blocking agents [16]. In patients with high renin hypertension, this may, indeed, be a major mechanism to account for the lowering of blood pressure in response to therapy with beta-receptor blockers. The antihypertensive activity of beta-adrenergic blockers in these patients correlates well with the degree of inhibition of plasma renin activity [16]. This mechanism, by no means, explains the antihypertensive effects of all beta-receptor blocking agents since those which selectively block beta-1 receptors will also lower blood pressure without decreasing, and sometimes actually increasing, plasma renin activity [17]; moreover, patients with low-renin hypertension respond to beta-blockade by a reduction of blood pressure [18]. Thus, in the majority of hypertensive patients, inhibition of renin release is probably not the primary mechanism through which blood pressure is lowered.

c. Effects on central mechanisms. Some beta-receptor blocking agents readily cross the blood–brain barrier and a central site for their antihypertensive activity has been suggested [19]. Since isoproterenol was shown to increase blood pressure and propranolol to decrease blood pressure when given directly into the central nervous system, the existence of central beta-receptors was postulated. It has been suggested that blockade of these central beta-receptors results in unopposed central alpha-adrenergic stimulation leading to decreased efferent sympathetic traffic. However, this hypothesis does not explain the time-lag between the reduction in cardiac output and the lowering of blood pressure following administration of these compounds for there is apparently no accumulation of beta-receptor blocking agents in the brain with time. Moreover, this hypothesis does not explain the antihypertensive activity of agents such as timolol which do not cross the blood–brain barrier [20]. Others have suggested that beta-receptor blocking agents affect afferent mechanisms to inhibit efferent sympathetic discharge; i.e., the 'set-point' of the baroreceptors is altered. The evidence for this proposed mechanism is not yet convincing [21].

d. Effects on sympathetic nerves. The possibility that beta receptors were present at presynaptic sites was suggested by the work of Adler-Graschinsky and Langer [22] who reported that norepinephrine release in response to sympathetic nerve stimulation was enhanced by isoproterenol and inhibited by propranolol. Langer [23] has, therefore, formulated a hypothesis to explain the participation of presynaptic alpha- and beta-receptors in neurotransmitter release. According to this hypothesis, during low frequency sympathetic stimulation, norepinephrine release is facilitated from the postganglionic sympathetic nerve through beta-receptor stimulation; whereas, at higher frequencies, release is inhibited by presynaptic alpha-receptor stimulation. Hence inhibition of the presynaptic beta-receptors would lead to unopposed stimulation of presynaptic alpha-receptors with resultant reduction of norepinephrine release. This hypothesis, although attractive, awaits further evaluation. It, too, is difficult to reconcile with the delay in the antihypertensive response which is seen after administration of these agents.

e. Effects on catecholamine synthesis. Several beta-receptor blocking agents, when administered chronically to rabbits, were shown to reduce the activity of both tyrosine hydroxylase and dopamine-beta-hydroxylase in superior cervical ganglia [24]. Since both of these enzymes are involved in the synthesis of norepinephrine by the postganglionic sympathetic nerve, their reduced activity would be expected to reduce the amount of neurotransmitter available for release. It is not clear, however, whether this reduction in enzyme activity occurs because of a direct effect on the two enzymes, because of a reduction in preganglionic activity, or because of increased end-product accumulation consequent to inhibition of its release. Thus, although reductions in the activity of these two enzymes may contribute to the blood pressure lowering effect of beta-adrenergic blocking agents, it does not necessarily represent the primary mechanism of action.

4. Pharmacokinetic considerations

Propranolol and most of the other beta-receptor blocking agents are almost completely absorbed following oral administration; however, several of these compounds, such as propranol and metoprolol, are metabolized by the liver during its first passage through the portal circulation ('first-pass elimination') and only about one-third of the administered dose reaches the systemic circulation. In addition, there is considerable interindividual variation in the degree of hepatic elimination of these compounds. Thus, there is not a good correlation between the size of the oral dose and the blood level of compounds which undergo 'first-pass elimination.' Nadolol, on the other hand, is not metabolized by the liver and is excreted unchanged in the urine; thus, the size of the oral dose *does* correlate with the blood level. Since the elimination of nadolol is dependent on renal function, dose adjustments must be made in patients with renal disease to avoid toxic blood levels. Although the degree of beta-receptor blockade is related directly to the blood level of the beta-blocker, there is no such correlation with blood pressure reduction. Frequently, the blood levels required to reduce pressure are considerably larger than those required to effect beta blockade. Thus, the consequences of beta blockade will be seen at the lower doses. Since the major dangers of therapy with beta-adrenergic blocking agents are related to receptor blockade per se, most untoward effects are seen at lower doses.

5. Untoward effects

Blockade of beta-2 receptors in bronchial smooth muscle will consistently increase airway resistance. This effect is of no consequence in individuals without lung disease; however, in patients with chronic lung disease, particularly in those with bronchospastic disease, the increase in airway resistance can be marked and extremely dangerous. Moreover, these agents will block the bronchodilation induced by epinephrine and other sympathomimetic amines, so that therapeutic attempts to reverse the brochoconstriction will be hampered. Thus, if a beta-receptor blocking agent is to be used in a patient with chronic lung disease, only those which exhibit cardioselectivity may be tried at low (less than 100 mg/day) doses for cardioselectivity is progressively lost with increasing doses.

The inhibition of glycogenolysis because of blockade of beta-2 receptors when nonselective beta-blockade is used is of particular importance in patients with diabetes mellitus who are being treated with insulin. Thus, in the presence of hypoglycemia, compensatory increases in blood sugar mediated by catecholamine induced glycogenolysis will be blocked. The hypoglycemia, therefore, will be more severe and of longer duration. The situation is made potentially more dangerous because several of the warning signs of hypoglycemia, such as tachycardia and muscular tremor, may be blocked in the presence of beta-blockade.

The relationship between beta-receptor blockers and blood glucose levels has become even more complex with the observations that some patients develop hyperglycemia when treated with these agents. This phenomenon, which occurs in patients who exhibit no glucose intolerance when the medication is removed, has been attributed to blockade of beta-2 receptors which participate in insulin release from the pancreas.

Since cardiac contractility is, in part, dependent on beta-receptor stimulation, patients with compromised myocardial function may develop heart failure when treated with beta-receptor blocking agents. The inotropic action of digitalis is not prevented by beta-receptor blocking agents, although both drugs depress A-V conduction and, when used together, may cause A-V dissociation and cardiac arrest.

Beta-adrenergic blocking agents should not be discontinued abruptly for this may produce a withdrawal syndrome characterized by either angina pectoris or frank myocardial infarction.

B. Alpha-adrenergic blocking agents

1. Introduction

The clinical usefulness of alpha-receptor blocking agents has been extremely limited because of problems with orthostatic hypotension and reflex tachycardia. Hence, they have been used as diagnostic tests for pheochromocytoma, in the preoperative or intraoperative management of patients with pheochromocytoma or for long-term management of patients with that disease when inoperable. However, with the advent of beta-adrenergic blocking agents and the development of selective alpha-1 receptor antagonists, these compounds may become more important in the management of the patient with essential hypertension.

2. Properties

Although all of these agents possess the capacity to block alpha-adrenergic receptors, they do not exhibit identical pharmacologic properties because of other distinguishing characteristics. Thus, the blockade of the alpha-receptor may be either irreversible (noncompetitive), such as is produced by phenoxybenzamine and dibenamine, or reversible (competitive), such as that produced by phentolamine, tolazoline and prazosin. Moreover, the capacity to block alpha receptors may be nonselective, i.e., the compound may exhibit similar affinities for both alpha-1 and alpha-2 receptor, such as phentolamine or selective for alpha-1 receptor blockade, such as prazosin and phenoxybenzamine. Yohimbine, which is a selective alpha-2 receptor inhibitor, has no clinical indication at the present time.

3. Clinical considerations

Phenoxybenzamine effectively inhibits the responses that are mediated by alpha-adrenergic agonists. Its half-life is approximately 24 hr. In normal subjects, in a supine position, phenoxybenzamine causes little change in systemic blood pressure. Decreases in blood pressure are appreciated only with assumption of upright posture or with a reduction in intravascular volume. The chronotropic and inotropic effects of catecholamines or sympathetic nerve stimulation on the heart are not inhibited by alpha-adrenergic blocking drugs, since the myocardium contains beta-adrenergic receptors exclusively. Excessive reduction of blood pressure, postural hypotension and reflex tachycardia are common occurrences when phenoxybenzamine is used alone. Inhibition of compensatory vasoconstriction also exaggerates the reductions in blood pressure observed with other agents when used simultaneously such as those which relax vascular smooth muscle directly. Other untoward effects include miosis, nasal stuffiness and inhibition of ejaculation.

Phentolamine exhibits a wide spectrum of pharmacological actions including alpha-adrenergic blockade, antihistaminic properties, as well as sympathomimetic, cholinomimetic and histamine-like effects. The competitive alpha-adrenergic blockade is relatively transient. Therapeutic doses of phentolamine cause cardiac stimulation that is out of proportion to the degree of blood pressure reduction. This is frequently associated with cardiac arrhythmias and angina pain. This is most likely related to the fact that phentolamine blocks both alpha-1 and alpha-2 adrenergic receptors; hence, norepinephrine secretion at the level of the myocardium would not be modulated because of alpha-2 adrenergic inhibition as well as unopposed action of the norepinephrine on the beta-receptors of the myocardium. Because of the severe side effects, phentolamine has not been used in the routine management of the hypertensive patient. Its clinical uses have been as a diagnostic tool for pheochromocytoma and for the intraoperative management of pheochromocytoma.

Although originally thought to be a direct vasodilator, prazosin is now thought to lower blood pressure because of selective blockade of post-synaptic alpha-adrenergic receptors [24]. Thus, prazosin reverses the pressor response to epinephrine and inhibits the vasoconstrictor action of norepinephrine. Although prazosin inhibits the vasoconstriction produced by norepinephrine that is released from the sympathetic nerve endings, its relative lack of effect on alpha-2 receptors allows norepinephrine to exert negative feedback control of its own release, thus, reducing the cardiac stimulation that follows nonselective alpha-adrenergic blockade. Thus, the tachycardia observed with the use of phentolamine is not seen with prazosin and the side effects are usually well tolerated. The untoward effects include drowsiness, dizziness, palpitations, headaches and easy fatigability. Sexual dysfunction is uncommon. The most puzzling effect is postural hypotension and syncope that can occur with the first dose [25]. The likelihood of syncope is related to the size of the dose, and it occurs more readily in patients who are already salt depleted.

C. *Agents which block adrenergic neurons*

1. *Guanethidine*

Although guanethidine exhibits local anesthetic effects, its antihypertensive properties are related to its ability to impair the release and to deplete stores of norepinephrine from peripheral adrenergic nerves. It does not cross the blood–brain barrier. To be effective, guanethidine must enter post ganglionic sympathetic nerves via the amine transport system. This mechanism of entrance into the nerve is shared by norepinephrine as well as many drugs, such as the phenothiazines and the tricyclic antidepressants. Hence, any of these agents can inhibit the uptake and, consequently, the effects of guanethidine. When given acutely, guanethidine may, as an initial response, cause the release of sufficient amounts of norepinephrine to produce an increase in blood pressure. Moreover, when guanethidine is given on a chronic basis, sensitivity of effector organs to norepinephrine is greatly enhanced in a manner similar to that observed with denervation. In spite of increased effector organ sensitivity, rebound hypertension does not occur when the drug is abruptly discontinued.

Postural hypotension is the most common side effect of chronic guanethidine administration. Frequently the hypotension is severe enough to produce syncope. Guanethidine should not be used in patients with pheochromocytoma because of the possibility of severe hypertensive reactions, most likely related to the development of effector supersensitivity and the failure of guanethidine to deplete catecholamines from either the adrenal gland or tumors of the adrenal gland.

2. *Reserpine*

A considerable portion of the antihypertensive effects of reserpine is related to its depletion of catecholamines in peripheral adrenergic nerves. Because of its large central action, reserpine is discussed below under 'Agents Which Affect Central Mechanisms.'

3. *Alpha-methyltyrosine*

Alpha-methyltyrosine inhibits tyrosine hydroxylase which is the rate-limiting enzyme in the synthesis of norepinephrine. It has little effect on the blood pressure of patients with essential hypertension, but is effective in patients with pheochromocytoma reducing not only total catecholamine excretion, but also the frequency and severity of hypertensive attacks, headache, sweating and palpitations. It is used in the preoperative preparation of patients with pheochromocytoma and for the management of inoperable patients with pheochromocytoma [26].

4. Monoamine oxidase inhibitors

Originally introduced as antidepressants, the monoamine oxidase (MAO) inhibitors were soon found to possess antihypertensive properties. These findings were unanticipated in view of the fact that the monoamine oxidases are enzymes which degrade norepinephrine. It was soon recognized, however, that MAO inhibitors also blocked the catabolism of tyramine, which was then transported into the adrenergic nerve and converted to octopamine. Octopamine then served as a false neurotransmitter for it has little ability to stimulate adrenergic receptors. Because of their toxicity, the MAO inhibitors are no longer used in the treatment of the hypertensive patients.

D. Agents which block autonomic ganglia

1. Introduction

There are a number of compounds with diverse chemical structures which are capable of blocking neurochemical transmission in autonomic ganglia. These compounds inhibit ganglionic transmission by functioning as receptor inhibitors of acetylcholine and by stabilizing the post synaptic membrane against acetylcholine-induced stimulation.

2. Properties

Hexamethonium served as the prototype of the bis-quaternary ammonium compounds which were found to block transmission through autonomic ganglia. Pentolinium, with a longer duration of action, was the most extensively used of this group. Later triethylsulfonium salts were found to exhibit similar pharmacological properties. This eventually led to the development of trimethaphan. Agents, such as mecamylamine, a secondary amine, were introduced later. Its blockade of acetylcholine has both a competitive and noncompetitive aspect. Since ganglionic blocking agents inhibit transmission through *all* autonomic ganglia, i.e., sympathetic as well as parasympathetic, the physiological consequences of their use are large. Thus, in addition to a reduction of blood pressure, generalized ganglionic blockade may produce cycloplegia, bladder and gastrointestinal tract atony and impaired sexual function. Moreover, the greatest reductions in blood pressure are observed with the assumption of upright posture so that postural hypotension is a major untoward effect of these agents.

3. Therapeutic uses

The untoward effects of these agents preclude their use in the management of chronic hypertension. Trimethaphan by intravenous drip is used in the treatment of hypertensive emergencies since it has a rapid onset of action, a short duration of action and its use is not associated with a reflex tachycardia.

E. Agents which affect central mechanism

1. Clonidine
Clonidine is an antihypertensive agent which lowers blood pressure by reducing sympathetic tone. Although clonidine stimulates alpha-adrenergic receptors, it exerts an antihypertensive effect most likely because its primary site of action is within the central nervous system, probably in the region of the *nucleus tractus solitarius*, where stimulation of central alpha-receptors is thought to produce a decrease in the sympathetic outflow from the brain [27]. The major pharmacological actions of clonidine appear to be related to its capacity to stimulate central as well as peripheral alpha-1 and alpha-2 adrenergic receptors. Clonidine is a potent stimulator of alpha-2 (presynaptic) receptors. As a consequence, release of norepinephrine from postganglionic sympathetic fibers is inhibited by the drug. The hemodynamic consequences of clonidine administration are a reduced blood pressure and a reduced cardiac output and heart rate. The most common, and frequently severe, side effects of clonidine in man are dry mouth and sedation. Impotence occurs occasionally and orthostatic hypotension, rarely. Other adverse affects include nausea and vomiting, Raynaud's phenomenon, depression, insomnia and nightmares. When clonidine is the sole drug used to control hypertension, its sudden withdrawal can result in a hypertensive crisis within 12–48 hr which may be life threatening [28]. The withdrawal syndrome has occurred most commonly in patients receiving doses larger than 1.2 mg daily. Patients with this syndrome often first develop symptoms of restlessness, insomnia, irritability, tremors, tachycardia and sweating. This is followed by a rebound increase in blood pressure associated with headache, abdominal pain and a hypertensive crisis which may be fatal. This reaction can be controlled by reinstituting clonidine.

2. Alpha-methyldopa
Alpha-methyldopa is a commonly used antihypertensive agent. The present evidence suggests that alpha-methyldopa acts through central mechanisms to interfere with sympathetic function. Initially it was thought to exert its antihypertensive action by interfering with norepinephrine synthesis through inhibition of aromatic amino acid decarboxylase. Later, it was suggested that alpha-methyldopa was decarboxylated to form alpha-methylnorepinephrine in peripheral adrenergic nerves. This false neurotransmitter, alpha-methyl norepinephrine, was suggested to have reduced potency compared with norepinephrine. Later studies, however, failed to confirm that the metabolite was a less potent vasoconstrictor than norepinephrine. At the present time it is generally accepted that the major antihypertensive effect of methyldopa is on the central nervous system [29]. Within the central nervous system it forms alpha-methyl norepinephrine which, when released, stimulates central alpha-adrenergic re-

ceptors thereby inhibiting sympathetic outflow. Many of the side effects of methyldopa are related to the fact that it has large central nervous system effects and causes sedation, with persistent lassitude and drowsiness. In addition, vertigo, extrapyramidal signs, nightmares and psychic depression are not uncommon. Dry mouth and nasal stuffiness may also be central in origin. Sexual dysfunction, primarily impotence, occurs in an appreciable number of males. Drug fever can be severe and may mimic sepsis with shaking chills and high spiking temperature. Hepatic dysfunction, reflected by elevation of hepatic enzymes in plasma and occasionally by the appearance of jaundice can progress to hepatic necrosis. A positive Coombs test develops in 25% of patients taking 1000 mg of methyldopa daily for six months or more. However, hemolytic anemia occurs in less than 5% of those with a positive Coombs test. Methyldopa-induced lactation can appear in either sex.

3. Reserpine

Reserpine depletes catecholamines in adrenergic nerve endings as well as in the brain and adrenal medulla; similarly, it depletes 5-hydroxy-tryptamine from several organs. Most of its pharmacological effects have been attributed to these actions. Untoward responses to reserpine are predominantly referable to the central nervous system and the gastrointestinal tract and have resulted in a progressive reduction in the doses employed in the treatment of hypertension. However, doses as small as 0.25 mg/day can produce a considerable incidence of nightmares and psychic depression, sometimes severe enough to require hospitalization. Hence, this drug should probably not be used in the routine treatment of the hypertensive patient.

F. Agents which affect afferent mechanisms – the veratrum alkaloids

Many naturally occurring veratrum alkaloids have been identified and many have been synthesized by substitution. The cardiovascular effects of the veratrum alkaloids include decreases in heart rate, blood pressure and cardiac output. The repetitive firing in the baroreceptor induced by the veratrum alkaloids accounts for their blood pressure lowering properties.

The clinical usefulness of the veratrum alkaloids is limited by the narrow range between the hypotensive and the emetic doses. The emesis is now known to be a central effect due to stimulation at the level of the nodose ganglion.

References

1. Veterans Administration Cooperative Study Group on Anti-hypertensive Agents: Effects of treatment on morbidity in hypertension: results in patients with diastolic blood pressure averaging 115 through 129 mmHg. JAMA 202:1028–1034, 1967.
2. Veterans Administration Cooperative Study Group on Anti-hypertensive Agents: Effects of treatment on morbidity in hypertension. II. Results in patients with diastolic blood pressure averaging 90 through 114 mmHg. JAMA 213:1143–1152, 1970.
3. Langley JN: The autonomic nervous system. Brain 26:1–26, 1903.
4. Gaskell WH: The involuntary nervous system. London, Longman, Green, 1916.
5. Loewi O: Über humorale Ubertragbarkeit der Herznervenwirkung. Pfluegers Arch 189:239–242, 1921.
6. Langley JN: On the reaction of cells and of nerve-endings to certain poisons, chiefly as regards the reaction of striated muscle to nicotine and to curari. J Physiol (Lond) 33:374–413, 1905.
7. Clark AJ: Handbuch der experimentellen Pharmakologie. In: Heffter A, Heubner H (eds) General pharmacology, Vol 4. Berlin, Springer, 1937.
8. Ahlquist RP: A study of the adrenotropic receptors. Am J Physiol 153:586–600, 1948.
9. Lands AM, Arnold A, McAuliff JP, Luduena FP, Brown TG: Differentiation of receptor systems activated sympathomimetic amines. Nature 214:597–598, 1967.
10. Westfall TC: Local regulation of adrenergic neurotransmission. Physiol Rev 57:659–728, 1977.
11. Prichard BNC: Hypotensive action of prenethalol. Br Med J 1:1227–1228, 1964.
12. Prichard BNC: β-adrenergic receptor blockade in hypertension, past, present and future. Br J Clin Pharmacol 5:379–399, 1978.
13. Fitzgerald JD: Perspectives in adrenergic beta-receptor blockage. Clin Pharmacol Ther 10: 292–306, 1969.
14. Tarazi RC, Dustan HP: Beta adrenergic blockade in hypertension. Am J Cardiol 29:633–640, 1972.
15. Struyker-Boudier HAJ, Smits JF, van Essen H: The role of the baroreceptor reflex in the cardiovascular effects of propranolol in the conscious spontaneously hypertensive rat. Clin Sci 56:163–167, 1979.
16. Buhler FR, Laragh JH, Baer L, Vaughan ED, Brunner HR: Propranolol inhibition of renin secretion. A specific approach to diagnosis and treatment of renin dependent hypertensive diseases. N Engl J Med 287:1209–1214, 1972.
17. Stokes GS, Weber MA, Thornell IR: Beta-blockers and plasma renin activity in hypertension. Br Med J 1:60–62, 1974.
18. Hollifield JW, Sherman K, Zwagg RV, Shand DG: Proposed mechanisms of propranolol's anti-hypertensive effect in essential hypertension. N Engl J Med 295:68–73, 1976.
19. Day MD, Roach AG: The brain as a possible site for the cardiovascular effects of β-adreno-ceptor blocking agents in cats. Clin Sci Mol Med 48:2695–2725, 1975.
20. Lohmollers G, Frohlich ED: A comparison of timolol and propranolol in essential hypertension. Am Heart J 89:437–442, 1975.
21. Tuttle RS, McCleary M: A mechanism to explain the anti-hypertensive action of propranolol. J Pharmacol Exp Ther 207:56–63, 1978.
22. Adler-Graschinsky E, Langer SZ: Possible role of β-adrenoceptors in the regulation of nor-adrenaline release by nerve stimulation through a positive feed-back mechanism. Br J Pharmacol 53:43–50, 1975.
23. Langer SZ, Cavero I, Massingham R: Recent developments in noradrenergic neurotrans-mission and its relevance to the mechanism of action of certain anti-hypertensive agents. Hypertension 2:372–382, 1980.

24. Oates HF, Graham RM, Stokes GS: Mechanism of the hypotensive action of prazosin. Arch Int Pharmacodyn Ther 227:41–48, 1977.
25. Stokes GS, Oates HF: Prazosin: new alpha-adrenergic blocking agent in treatment of hypertension. Cardiovasc Med 3:41–57, 1978.
26. Engelman K, Horwitz D, Jequier E, Sjoerdsma A: Biochemical and pharmacologic effects of alpha-methyltyrosine in man. J Clin Invest 47:577–594, 1968.
27. Kobinger W: Central alpha-adrenergic systems as targets for hypotensive drugs. Rev Physiol Biochem Pharmacol 81:39–100, 1978.
28. Hansson L, Hunyor SN, Julius S, Hoobler SW: Blood pressure crisis following withdrawal of clonidine (Catapres, Catapresan), with special reference to arterial and urinary catecholamine levels, and suggestions for acute management. Am Heart J 85:605–610, 1973.
29. Heise A, Kroneberg G: Central nervous alpha-adrenergic receptors and the mode of action of alpha-methyldopa. Naunyn Schmiedebergs Arch Pharmacol 279:285–300, 1973.

6. Vasodilators and their association with remission

H. MITCHELL PERRY, JR.

A. Vasodilators

Vasodilators represent the third and last class of antihypertensive drugs, and their discussion is appropriate here. I would like to extend my comments to include a very important but often neglected topic, *remission*. The extension is logical since one type of remission, at least, is specifically related to hydralazine, the most commonly used vasodilator. Hydralazine is considered in some detail since there is much more information regarding it than other vasodilators. The section on remission, which relies very heavily on data from our own clinic, is designed to demonstrate that remission can and does occur and therefore warrants further study.

Blood pressure is the product of cardiac output and peripheral resistance. Thus, to lower blood pressure, one must lower one or both of these variables. Obviously, the vasodilators lower peripheral resistance. A vasodilator is the recommended third step in the step-care regimen of the Joint National Committee on Detection, Evaluation, and Treatment of High Blood Pressure [1]. In the United States, hydralazine is the only drug of this class which is effective by mouth and recommended for general use. A second more potent antihypertensive vasodilator, minoxidil, has recently been made available for treatment of severe hypertension that cannot be otherwise controlled. These drugs have a direct relaxant effect on arteriolar smooth muscle. Alone, however, they are seldom effective in long-term control of hypertension because they have no sympatholytic action and hence do not block the compensatory reflex increase in myocardial contractility and cardiac output which is triggered by the decreased peripheral resistance. Even more recently, a third drug, captopril, which is probably most appropriately classed as a vasodilator, has been made available. It was devised as an inhibitor of the converting enzyme of the renin-angiotensin system, and it does that and more. It too is currently recommended only for seriously hypertensive patients whose blood pressure cannot be otherwise controlled. Finally, the adrenergic blocking agent, prasozin, has a peripheral vasodilatory action (Table 1).

Table 1. Antihypertensive peripheral vasodilators

Drug	Use in United States	Route of administration	Usual starting dose (mg/da)	Usual maximum dose (mg/da)	Untoward effects and comments
Hydralazine	general	By mouth	50	300	Palpitations and headache; 'LE' with >400 mg/da for >6 mos
Minoxidil	restricted	By mouth	10	40	Fluid retention (must use loop diuretic) and hair growth
Captopril	restricted	By mouth	12.5	50	Proteinuria, granulocytopenia, rash, hypoguesia
Prazosin	general	By mouth	1	20	Syncope, usually early (note: postsynaptic adrenergic-blocking agent)
Indapamide	experimental	By mouth	2.5	2.5	Hypokalemia
Diazoxide	emergency	Intravenous	300 mg in bolus	'prn'	Decreased carbohydrate tolerance
Nitroprusside	emergency	Intravenous	0.025– 0.25 mg per min by drip	'prn'	Most potent antihypertensive available

Hydralazine

Hydralazine is the oldest antihypertensive agent that is still in clinical use. It is a substituted hydrazine, like the antituberculous agent isoniazid, and it was originally studied for activity against the tubercle bacillis. Its use as an antihypertensive agent began in 1949 [2]. In 1951 the Hypertension Division at Washington University initiated the use of hydralazine in combination with the other available antihypertensive agent of the time, hexamethonium, a ganglioplegic agent which decreased venomotor tone and allowed blood to pool in the great veins, thereby diminishing the amount returned to the heart. Use of these two drugs in combination produced a dramatic change in the treatment of hypertension. Although either drug used alone would lower elevated blood pressure for a short period, the antihypertensive effect quickly wore off, whereas the combination of hydralazine with a ganglion blocking agent provided the first effective long-term control of 'malignant' hypertension [3]. The four patients with malignant hypertension whom our group treated during August of 1951 immediately showed dramatic improvement in both blood pressure and cardiovascular status. One of them survived for more than 20 years, a previously unheard of survival time for a patient with malignant hypertension.

Hydralazine or 1-hydrazinophthalazine, contains the extremely reactive hydrazino group. As has been pointed out, hydrazines are used as rocket fuel. The hydrazino group is the business end of the molecule; it apparently has its effect directly on vascular smooth muscle, although its precise mode of action has still not been elucidated. It is very effective and may lower the peripheral resistance as much as 75%. Unfortunately, except in the elderly where the reflexes in question are markedly blunted or absent, even a 75% fall in peripheral resistance has little effect on blood pressure since there is a compensatory increase in cardiac output if hydralazine is used alone.

The orally and parenterally effective doses of hydralazine are approximately equal. In man, the half life of the drug is 6–12 hr. Only a few percent of the administered drug appear in the urine. The rest is metabolized by an hepatic acetyl transferase, the level of which is genetically controlled. For both black and white populations, there are about equal numbers of slow and fast 'acetylators.' The latter metabolize the drug much more rapidly and, hence, need higher doses for the same effect. In contrast, Oriental populations have about 90% rapid acetylators.

Oral hydralazine is available in 10, 25, 50 and 100-mg sizes. In a patient who is receiving 'Step 1 and 2' drugs, i.e., a diuretic and adrenergic-blocking agent without controlling his blood pressure, it is reasonable to add, as a 'Step 3' drug, 25 mg of hydralazine twice or thrice a day. This starting dose can be increased stepwise to 50, then 75 and finally 100 mg two or three times daily. For the usual hospitalized patient, increases in dosage can be made every two days, but for outpatients, with their generally less severe hypertension, it is usually preferable to have their doses increased at weekly or biweekly intervals. Although the usual dose required, (in combination with both a diuretic and an adrenergic-blocking agent) for effective control of moderate or severe hypertension is 200 or 300 mg daily, we do not hesitate to use 400 mg or even larger doses if they are necessary for adequate control of the blood pressure since such control is vital to effective treatment. When we do use more than 400 mg of hydralazine daily, we measure the patient's acetylation rate.

It is worth emphasizing that in elderly people with pure or primarily systolic hypertension, hydralazine can often be used as a 'Step 2' drug since the usual reflex increase in cardiac output is ordinarily absent or markedly blunted in such patients. The advantage of using hydralazine as a 'Step 2' drug is that, unlike the adrenergic-blocking agents, hydralazine does not slow the patient down mentally or make him somnolent; this is a real advantage since one certainly does not want to decrease the mental function of an elderly patient in any way.

The major side effects of hydralazine are tachycardia and headache. If one starts with sufficiently small doses, these are rarely problems in patients who are already taking 'Step 1 and 2' drugs. When side effects do occur, they ordinarily disappear within a relatively short period of time. When the drug is used alone, however, the side effects are frequently significant and patients may refuse to take the drug.

In the light of today's interest in cholesterol, it may be worth noting that hydralazine lowers circulating cholesterol. Our average hydralazine-treated patient had a decrease of 25 mg/100 ml of plasma, starting within a few days of his first dose of hydralazine and continuing with no visible change for over ten years (Figure 1) [4]. In confirmation of these data on patients receiving several drugs,

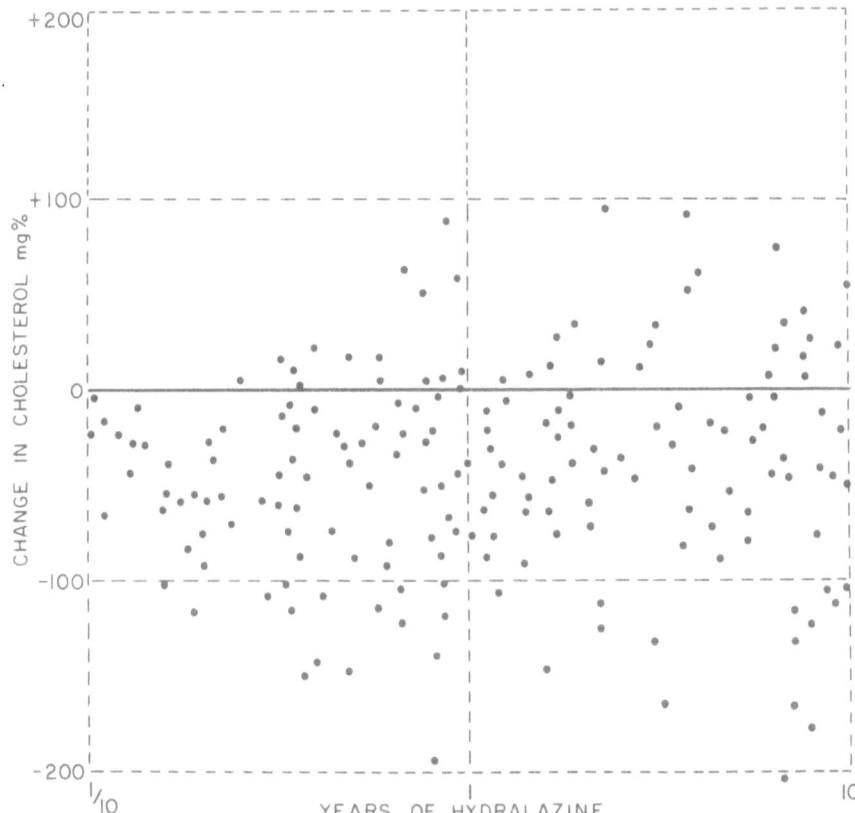

Figure 1. Tendency of total circulating extracellular cholesterol to decrease in patients with high initial concentrations during effective antihypertensive therapy with hydralazine and ganglionic blockade: changes in cholesterol for 93 patients with initial concentrations greater than 215 mg per 100 ml of plasma are plotted against time. One value from the first year and one from the next nine are indicated for each patient. Most of the points fall well below the solid 'zero line' indicating that the cholesterol concentration usually decreased during therapy. For the group of patients with high cholesterol levels the decrease during the first year averaged 46 mg/100 ml and for the next nine years, averaged 41 mg/100 ml of plasma.

the data in Figure 2 refer to ten normotensive women who were given hydralazine alone. With small doses, there was no significant change. With moderate doses, there was a statistically significant fall of about 20 mg/100 ml. With large doses, there was a larger fall in circulating cholesterol amounting to some 40 mg/100 ml. Return to pretreatment levels required more than two months. I should hasten to add that there is no indication that the cholesterol lowering effect of hydralazine is beneficial. The change is in the 'right' direction, and it may be beneficial; it certainly makes both physician and patient happy, but it must be remembered that lowering cholesterol by other therapeutic modalities has not been shown to lower the risk associated with a naturally high level of cholesterol.

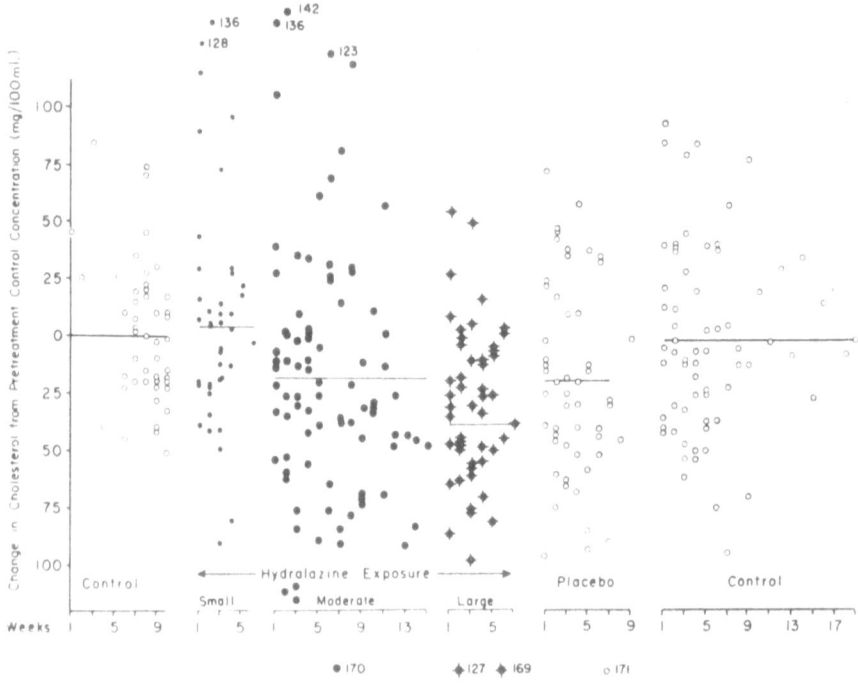

Figure 2. Decrease of total circulating extracellular cholesterol in normotensive hypercholesterolemic women during hydralazine administration: differences between individual concentrations and the appropriate patient's mean pretreatment concentration are plotted. For each of ten patients 16–40 weekly values are cited. These are divided into a pretreatment control period (open circles), three periods of increasing hydralazine exposure (increasingly accentuated solid dots), and two posttreatment control periods (open circles). The average for each period is indicated by a horizontal line. Of the 173 values obtained during hydralazine exposure, 8.1% differed from their mean pretreatment concentrations by more than 100 mg of cholesterol per 100 ml of plasma, whereas only 0.74% of the 136 values obtained without hydralazine differed by this much from their pretreatment values.

Hydralazine toxicity

A peculiar late autoimmune reaction to hydralazine was recognized after the drug had been used for several years. This was reported from our clinic in late 1953 [5], about 20 months after the observation that hydralazine in combination with hexamethonium could control malignant hypertension [3]. Over the next several years, it became obvious that hydralazine had the dubious distinction of being the first drug to regularly induce a syndrome that resembled idiopathic lupus erythematosus or rheumatoid arthritis. By 1956, it was evident that such a reaction, which had prior to the advent of hydralazine been observed only sporadically and very rarely, was occurring in over 10% of hydralazine-treated patients [6–9]. An obvious result was that, as other antihypertensive drugs became available, they replaced hydralazine which became much less popular.

This is not the entire story, however. This reaction to hydralazine deserves further comment. First, this reaction has an unusual pattern of occurrence: it rarely occurs in anybody until he has been exposed to 400 mg of hydralazine daily for six months [10]. Second, it rarely occurs in blacks; and among whites it is limited to the 50% of the population, who are slow acetylators of hydralazine [10]. This syndrome has been reported in a few blacks, but it is much rarer than in whites, and it is atypical when it does occur [10]. Third, the reaction differs in several significant ways from idiopathic lupus erythematosus and rheumatoid arthritis: all evidence of its presence eventually disappears following withdrawal of the drug, although regression of symptoms sometimes requires considerable time. Moreover, even if the drug is continued, the kidney and the brain, the most worrisome target organs of the idiopathic disease, do not become involved in the iatrogenic process, and deforming arthritis does not occur [11].

Minoxidil

Minoxidil is a very potent, orally effective antihypertensive vasodilator [12]. Its action is therefore similar to that of hydralazine. Its usual dose ranges from 10 to 40 mg daily in either single or divided doses. In the United States, it is recommended that its use be reserved for those whose serious hypertension cannot be otherwise controlled. Based on very few cases, its use in patients with significant azotemia has been reported to be associated with some increase in renal function [13]. Its major untoward effect is fluid retention which usually requires the use of a concomitant 'loop' diuretic such as furosemide. This excessive fluid retention makes it undesirable to prescribe this drug for patients who cannot be closely supervised. Minoxidil apparently increases the incidence of pericardial effusion with resultant life-threatening cardiac tamponade in patients on dialysis [14] and perhaps in patients with normal or nearly normal renal function as well. Minoxidil also promotes growth of hair, a particularly undersirable side effect in women.

Captopril

Captopril is the most recent orally effective antihypertensive agent to become available [15]. It was designed to be a vasodepressor by virtue of inhibiting 'converting enzyme' which is responsible for the conversion of the inert deca-peptide Angiotensin I to the extremely pressor octapeptide Angiotensin II. It would therefore be expected to be effective in controlling hypertension related to excess renin. It seems, however, to lower the blood pressure of most hypertensive patients, regardless of whether the renin-angiotensin system can be implicated. Moreover, it is known to have effects other than its inhibition of converting enzyme. Specifically it prevents the metabolic degradation of bradykinin, a naturally occurring nonapeptide which produces vasodilatation; one of the kininases which inactivates bradykinin is identical with the angiotensin-con-verting enzyme and hence is inactivated by captopril [15]. Like minoxodil, captopril is also recommended only for serious hypertension that cannot other-wise be controlled. Its usual daily dose range is 12.5–50 mg, and it is usually given three times daily. The major untoward effects of captopril are agranulo-cytosis and proteinuria [15]. The first is thought to be lifethreatening when other major disease complications are present. The second may be extreme with as much as 15 gm of urinary protein per day, and it may reach its maximum after the drug has been withdrawn, although eventually it apparently disappears without residual. Rashes and loss of taste may also be sufficient to require discontinua-tion of the drug [15].

Prazosin

Prazosin is a postsynaptic alpha-adrenergic blocking agent, and as such it has already been discussed. Here it is enough to say that because its site of action is so close to the vascular smooth muscle its effect is similar to that of the direct peripheral vasodilator, hydralazine. It is reported not to produce the reflex increase in cardiac output that counteracts the efficacy of hydralazine when it is used alone, but it may well be that much of this apparent difference is simply that prazosin is a less potent peripheral vasodilator. The major untoward effect of prazosin is syncope which usually, but not always, occurs with the first dose or soon after an increase in dose [16].

Diazoxide

Diazoxide, a close chemical relative of the thiazides, is not available for oral use in the United States because of the very high incidence of significantly decreased carbohydrate tolerance. When used systemically it is not a diuretic, but parenterally administered diazoxide produces a dramatic lowering of blood pressure, apparently by a direct effect on resistance arterioles [17].

Nitroprusside

Nitroprusside is also a very effective antihypertensive vasodilator, but only when given parenterally. By intravenous injection, it is probably the most effective antihypertensive agent available [18].

Indapamide

Indapamide is a long-acting, orally effective vasodilator, which apparently acts by inhibiting the net inward flow of calcium into vascular smooth muscle and thereby reducing its contraction [19]. It is also a diuretic; as such, it can induce hypokalemia. It is not yet available in the United States.

B. Remission

Although seldom discussed, remission of the hypertensive process, either partial or complete, has obvious great potential significance. Remission of hypertension is not merely a remote theoretical possibility. It occurs, and Table 2 lists some complete remissions that have been reported. Our experience suggests that there are two basic types of remission. First, there is the spontaneous remission which occurs in some patients whose hypertension has been well controlled. Thurm and Smith [20] and a VA Study [21] have reported such remissions in 22 and 15% of patients with mild hypertension. Because of the mildness of the original hypertension in these two studies, some of the alleged remissions probably represented relatively trivial changes. Thus, the percentage incidence may be inflated by patients who did not originally have the fixed hypertension that was ascribed to them and by hypertensive patients who did not have the subsequent normotension that was ascribed to them. Apparently belonging to the same category of spontaneous remission were the less frequent (3.3%) – and apparently temporary – remissions reported by Dustan et al. [22] and the equally frequent (3.3%) – and apparently permanent – remissions observed by us [23] in patients

Table 2. Complete remission of hypertension

Authors	Number of patients[a]	Severity of hypertension	% with remission	Reference
Perry et al.	272	Moderate & severe	3.3	Circ 33:958, 1966
Perry et al.[b]	42	Moderate & severe	17	Am J Med 54:58, 1973
Perry et al.[b]	13	Moderate & severe	54	J Chron Dis 30:519, 1977
Dustan et al	60	Moderate & severe	3.3	Circ 37:370, 1968
VA Study 3	60	Mild & moderate	15	Circ 51:1107, 1975
Thurm et al.	69	Mild	23	JAMA 201:301, 1967

[a] Total patient population from which the remittant patients were taken.
[b] These reports involve subpopulations of the population of the first report.

with more severe hypertension. All of these remissions occurred in patients whose blood pressures had been maintained at or near normotensive levels. This type of spontaneous remission seems to be the extreme case of the general lessening in the severity of the hypertensive process that we reported in an entire population of patients whose blood pressure had been controlled by treatment [24]. The second type of remission is associated with the late reaction to hydralazine described above [23]. It is therefore limited to the relatively small population of white patients who develop this syndrome. In our experience, one-sixth of all patients with this peculiar autoimmune reaction have developed a complete remission [25], and in one small but well-defined subgroup the incidence has actually exceeded 50% [11]. This type of remission is obviously related to hydralazine and hence is peculiarly appropriate to this presentation.

Spontaneous partial remission

A general lessening in the severity of hypertension which has been effectively treated was reported in 1956 [24], just five years after long-term control of elevated blood pressure by orally administered antihypertensive agents had first been effected. The decrease in severity was not limited to a few unusual patients; rather it was a general phenomenon characteristic of the entire population with adequately controlled diastolic pressures. This observation seems to be of sufficient importance to warrant a detailed look at the data to see how convincing they are and to note their limitations.

Every hypertensive patient discharged from Barnes Hospital between August of 1951 and May of 1954 after treatment with the combination of oral hexamethonium chloride and hydralazine was included in the population considered below, provided he met three criteria: (1) Adequate daily follow-up blood pressure and drug intake data, obtained and reported by the patient or his family, were available for at least one year. (2) No antihypertensive drugs other than hexamethonium chloride or hydralazine had been used. (Data on patients who had had only a single antihypertensive regimen were easier to obtain in 1955 when there were only a few antihypertensive agents available and therefore the tendency to switch from one regimen to another was much less marked than it is in 1981, when a great many agents are available; however, even then some severely hypertensive patients had to be removed from the series because penta-pyrrolidinium was substituted for hexamethonium and/or reserpine was added to their regimens.) (3) There was no evidence of the late reaction to hydralazine which has been discussed above. A total of 114 patients fulfilled these criteria: 59 were white males, 42 were white females and 13 were black. Their average age was 46, with a range of 24–65 years. Before treatment, 40 had diastolic pressures of 100–115 mmHg, 41 had pressures of 115–130 mmHg, and 33 had pressures of 130 mmHg or higher, all pressures being taken at 'hospital rest.'

The 114 patients were arbitrarily divided into two subgroups on the basis of their diastolic pressures during treatment. Those with mean pressures below 100 mmHg with the patient seated were considered 'controlled,' and those with mean pressures of 100 mmHg or higher were considered 'uncontrolled.' The mean pressure for each patient was calculated by averaging 28 or 35 diastolic pressures obtained and recorded at home immediately before each dose of medicine during the week which began exactly one month after hospital discharge. Each patient's mean intakes of hexamethonium and hydralazine were obtained for the same period and from the patients' own records. Comparable calculations were made for the week which began precisely a year later. This process was repeated at two and three years for those patients whose home pressure and drug data continued to be available.

According to these criteria, 79 patients were controlled one month after hospital discharge and 35 were uncontrolled. A year later, the mean diastolic pressure of the controlled patients had decreased slightly, and their intakes of hexamethonium and hydralazine had decreased to 74% and 89%, respectively, of their one-month intakes. For the uncontrolled patients, the result was different. Their mean diastolic pressure had increased slightly, and they were ingesting 97% and 98% of their initial doses of the drugs. At two and particularly at three years, the decrease in drug requirement for the controlled patients, and hence the difference between the groups, was more marked. *After three years of treatment, the controlled group needed an average of about 50% of their one-month doses*, while the uncontrolled group was taking almost 80% of their one-month doses. The diastolic pressures of the former had decreased 3 mmHg while those of the latter had increased (Table 3).

The decrease in medication for the controlled group represented a real change. Initially, the required dose for these patients had been carefully titrated, particu-

Table 3. Decrease in severity of treated hypertension with time

	One year		Three years	
	Hexa-methonium*	Hydralazine*	Hexa-methonium*	Hydralazine*
79 controlled	74%	89%	42%	55%
35 uncontrolled	97%	99%	84%	77%

* Percent of original effective doses still required after one and three years.

Legend: A group of 114 consecutive patients is included. For the 79 controlled patients, the original effective dose, i.e., the one month intake of hexamethonium and hydralazine averaged 2.01 and 0.50 gm/day; for the 35 uncontrolled patients, the corresponding averages were 2.36 and 0.59 gm/day.

larly in the case of the hexamethonium. If they took 10% less than their prescribed doses, their hypertension became uncontrolled; whereas, if they took a 10% excess, they became hypotensive and had to remain flat in bed. Thus, the decrease of 50% within three years appeared to be meaningful. In contrast, the drop to 80% for the uncontrolled group may well represent frustration with failure to achieve control rather than any real decrease in requirement. Unfortunately we could not predict with any certainty which patients were going to become controlled, although those with mild hypertension and those requiring smaller than average doses of drug were the most likely candidates. To illustrate the first of differences, four-fifths in the mild hypertensives followed for three years and just over half of the severe hypertensives belonged to the controlled group.

It should be noted that for a patient with good control, the decrease of hexamethonium intake was an automatic process, since it depended on the patient's dosage instructions, which generally were to take a full dose for a 'sitting' systolic pressure over 140 mmHg, half that dose for a presssure between 140 and 130 mmHg, a quarter of that dose for a pressure between 130 and 120 mmHg and nothing for a pressure below 120 mmHg. The decrease in hydralazine was not similarly automatic; it depended on the physician's decreasing the dose of that drug when the intake of hexamethonium had decreased. Great attention, however, was paid to decreasing the hydralazine as rapidly as possible, since we had observed that only by such decreases could we avoid the late reaction to hydralazine which involved our best therapeutic results [26].

Follow-up of partial remission

A long-term follow-up of partial remission was completed for 101 of the original 114 patients [25] who were followed for a minimum of 18 years or to death. Sixty-eight had originally been listed as controlled. Of that group, 54% were still alive in mid-1972. Thirty-three had originally been listed as uncontrolled, and only 27% of them were still alive in mid-1972. The difference between 54% and 27% was highly statistically significant with p < 0.001. Moreover, the average survival time for the controlled group was 172 months; for the partly controlled group, it was 108 months (25).

Length of survival was not related to the initial dose of hydralazine, i.e., whether or not the patient's initial (one month after hospital discharge) intake of hydralazine was more than 400 mg/day. Survival time, however, was related to whether the dose of hydralazine increased or decreased significantly during the first year. Twenty-one of the 101 had a decrease in hydralazine to less than two-thirds of what it was initially, whereas ten had an increase to more than $1\frac{1}{2}$ of the initial daily dose. In mid-1972, 57% of the former (those with a decrease) but only 10% of the latter (those with an increase) were still alive. This difference in percentage survival was reflected by an average survival time of 175 months for the former and 94 months for the latter. The difference in survival time is now presumably larger since many of the former but only a few of the latter were alive in mid-1972 when the last follow-up was completed [25].

Spontaneous complete remission

Some of the 79 controlled patients considered above had far more than the average decrease in their drug requirement. This is illustrated by Figure 3 which provides monthly mean pressures and intakes for a 34-year-old white male with a malignant stage of hypertension; for both drugs the 34-month intake was less than 10% of the one-month intake [24]. A total of 19 patients were able to completely discontinue hexamethonium, and ten of them were able to discontinue hydralazine as well [24]. The ten apparently represented the decreasing requirement for medication described above, carried to its ultimate limit, namely discontinuation of all drug with persistent normotension.

A follow-up report on the six of these 'remittant' patients who initially had moderate and severe hypertension plus ten additional patients who were subsequently able to entirely discontinue their antihypertensive medications was made ten years later [23]. These 16 patients constituted 5.1% of the entire group of 316 patients with pretreatment diastolic pressures of 110 mmHg or more who were treated by the Hypertension Division at Washington University during the six years beginning in August of 1951. The 16 had complete remissions which lasted 29 to 112 months. All remissions that lasted two years were apparently permanent over the observation period which averaged 6.25 years. Since there was no recrudescent hypertension, there was no further need for antihypertensive drugs. There was no change in life style to which the normotension could be ascribed.

J.C. ♂ 34

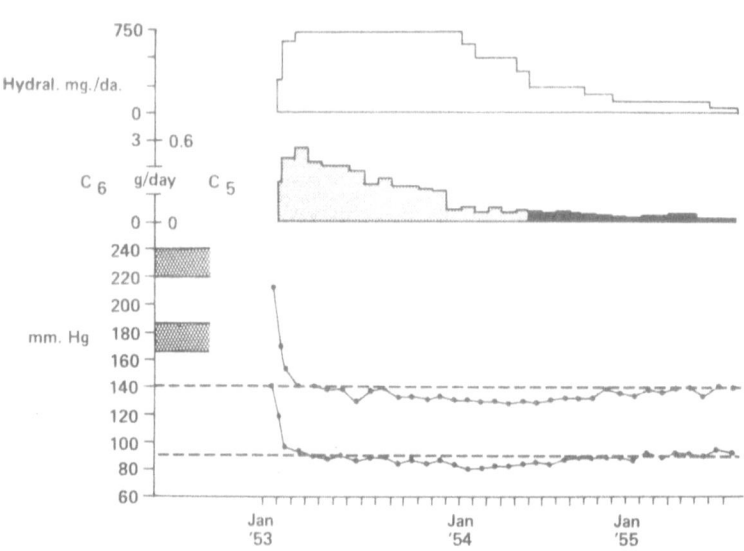

Figure 3. Blood pressure and oral medication for a 34-year-old white male with a malignant stage of hypertension. The range of pretreatment blood pressure is indicated by crosshatching. The bar graphs indicate the drug intake, the open area representing hydralazine, the dotted hexamethonium (C6) and the solid pentolinium (C5). Note that the scale is different for the two methonium compounds since the second is approximately five times more potent than the first [24].

Seven of these 16 remittant patients had the late hydralazine reaction which resembled lupus erythematosus and/or rheumatoid arthritis [11]; their remissions will be discussed later. The remaining nine who had no such reaction constituted 3.3% of the 272 patients without late hydralazine reactions. Before their remissions, the nine had little to distinguish them. Six had had non-accelerated hypertension, and three had had accelerated hypertension. All seemed to have had a real change in the severity of their underlying hypertension. Finally, all nine were white, although blacks constituted one-fifth of the 316 patients at risk. Unfortunately we do not know how many were slow acetylators of hydralazine, although all of the seven with 'hydralazine toxicity' were necessarily slow acetylators.

Complete remission with hydralazine toxicity

Of our 308 white patients who began antihypertensive treatment between mid-1951 and mid-1957, 42 developed late toxicity to hydralazine, giving an incidence of 13.6% [26]. Those destined for toxicity had significantly higher baseline diastolic pressures than the rest of the group; moreover, 50% of them had accelerated hypertension, while less than 25% of the nontoxic population did [26]. Among our patients, however, toxicity was a disease of normotension. It ordinarily did not occur until the diastolic pressure was strictly normal.

When late toxicity to hydralazine was first recognized, we noted that it involved only those with good therapeutic results; patients with poor control of their pressures seemed immune. Later, when more than 10% of our treated patients were developing toxicity and some warning of impending difficulty was desperately needed, normotension provided such a warning. We found that by cutting the hydralazine intake back as soon as the average 'home diastolic pressure' fell below 90 mmHg – and cutting it as rapidly as possible without compromising the new 'normotension' – the incidence of toxicity was dramatically decreased. Thus, we noted 33 new cases in the two years before August of 1954 when this algorithm was adopted; and only five new cases were seen in the next two years [11].

Our previously mentioned 308 white patients, all of whom were treated according to the same algorithms, provide the data to document the reciprocal relationship between toxicity and blood pressure. Toxicity developed in 42 after an average daily intake of just over 0.5 gm hydralazine for an average of 17 months, whereas the remaining 266, who never developed any evidence of toxicity, ingested only 10% less hydralazine and for considerably longer than 17 months on the average. Table 4 compares the 42 toxic patients not only to the

Table 4. Average diastolic pressure as taken by the patient at home several times daily

	Before therapy	After one month of therapy at home	One month before first toxic symptom	At time of maximum toxic symptoms	Most recent
42 toxic patients	130	93	88	80	94
42 matched nontoxic patients	126	99*	97**	98**	101*
All 266 nontoxic patients	120*	99*	98**	99**	101*

Legend: Tabulated values are average diastolic pressures in mmHg. Their standard deviations ranged from 15 to 18 mmHg for the first and last columns and from 8 to 12 mmHg for the middle three columns. One and two asterisks indicate values which differed significantly from the comparable value for the toxic patients, with $p < 0.05$ and < 0.001, respectively.

For each patient, the diastolic pressure 'before therapy' was the average of values in hospital before antihypertensive drugs were administered. Diastolic pressures during therapy were averages of 3–5 readings taken and recorded per day by the patient or a family member during a week at home. *Note:* For the two nontoxic groups, 'one month before first toxic symptom' and 'at time of maximum toxic symptoms' were averages at 18 and 30 months, respectively. Most recent pressure is averaged only for patients who survived at least ten years after beginning treatment. In this group there were 26 toxic and 183 nontoxic patients, of whom 17 were 'matched' non-toxic patients.

entire 266 nontoxic patients, but also to 42 who were matched with respect to sex, age (within three years), and the presence of accelerated hypertension [25]. Despite their higher average pretreatment pressure, once treatment had begun the 42 patients who were destined to develop toxicity, but who had not yet done so, had consistently and significantly lower average diastolic pressures than nontoxic patients – lower than the entire group of 266 and lower than the matched group of 42 nontoxic patients. The difference in pressure between the groups was evident, although small, at the end of the first month of treatment at home, i.e., one month after hospital discharge. It was larger a month *before* the first toxic symptoms appeared, and it became maximal when the toxic symptoms were maximal, at which time it averaged almost 20 mmHg. As symptoms regressed, this difference decreased to its initial value of 6 or 7 mmHg.

The lower average pressure of the toxic patients was reflected in longer survival. The entire group of 42 toxic patients survived an average of 141 months after begining therapy, while the 42 matched nontoxic patients survived an average of 108 months. The number of both 10- and 15-year survivors in the toxic group was significantly larger than in the matched nontoxic group, with $p < 0.05$. The survival curves in Figure 4 suggest that the difference in favor of the toxic patients began about the sixth year of therapy for those with accelerated hypertension and somewhat earlier for those with less severe hypertension [25].

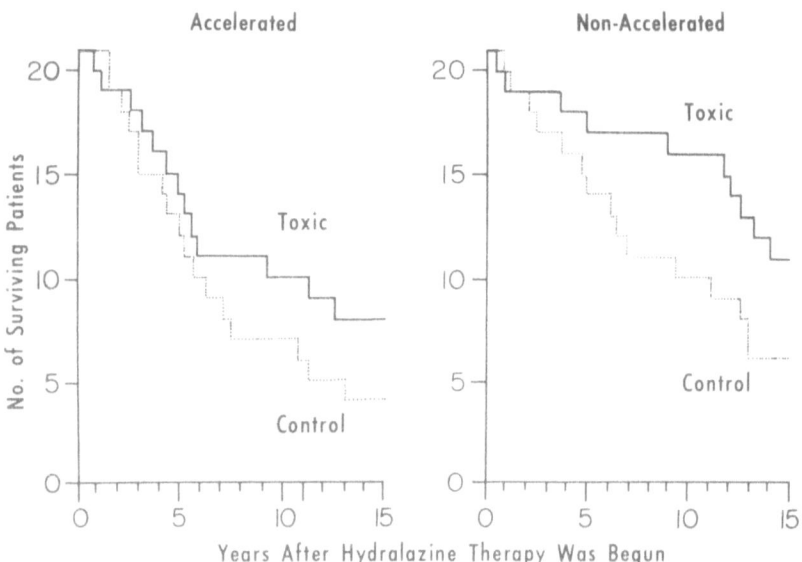

Figure 4. Fifteen-year survival for 42 toxic and 42 matched nontoxic patients. There happened to be 21 toxic patients with accelerated and 21 with less severe hypertension. The difference in both 10 and 15 year survival (after therapy began) was significant, with $p < 0.05$, when all 42 toxic patients were compared to the 42 matched nontoxic patients.

A patient's course after he developed toxic symptoms depended on his subsequent hydralazine intake. Eleven toxic patients discontinued hydralazine completely and promptly, i.e., within two months of their first symptom; in general, their pretreatment hypertension quickly returned, and their average survival was only 87 months after beginning therapy. In contrast, 13 continued much-reduced doses of hydralazine (20–25% of their maximum dose) for more than 18 months after toxic symptoms began; in general, the normotension characteristic of toxicity persisted, and they survived an average of 191 months (Table 5). This difference in survival was significant, with $p < 0.005$ [25]. To further emphasize the differences in survival, six of the 11 patients who discontinued taking hydralazine promptly were dead within a year; whereas all of the 13 who reduced their doses but continued some exposure lived longer than a year after their toxic symptoms began [11]. The shortened mean survival of those who 'discontinued promptly' was usually related to severe recrudescent hypertension.

Of the 13 patients with long-term, low-level exposure to hydralazine after their initial toxic symptoms, seven, including two with accelerated hypertension and three others with severe nonaccelerated hypertension, had prolonged remissions of their hypertension. Their total length of exposure to hydralazine averaged 50 months. Once their hypertension had disappeared and toxic symptoms appeared, their antihypertensive drugs were gradually discontinued; for them no recrudescence of hypertension occurred during a followup period of 29–112

Table 5. Survival of toxic patients as a function of how long hydralazine was ingested after toxic symptoms appeared

	Recrudescent hypertension (%)	Persistent symptoms (%)	Months survived (Mean ± SD)
40 toxic patients	54*	63*	138±78
11 continuing <2 months	89*	30*	87±90
16 continuing 2–11 months	56	63	129±64
13 continuing >18 months	25*	92*	191±46

* Data not available for 1–3 patients.
Legend: With the onset of toxicity, hydralazine was quickly discontinued entirely (i.e., in <2 months), temporarily continued (i.e., for 2–12 months) at about half of the prior dose, or prolongedly continued (i.e., for >18 months) at 1/4–1/8 of the prior dose. 'Recrudescent hypertension' indicates that one year after the onset of toxicity the diastolic pressure, as taken by the seated patient at home during a two week period, averaged more than 100 mmHg. 'Persistent symptoms' indicates that toxic symptoms persisted for more than three months after the last dose of hydralazine. Survival is in months (mean ± standard deviation) after the beginning of therapy. *Note:* Forty, rather than 42, patients are considered; a pair of living patients (they had survived 217 and 222 months by mid-1972) were excluded because they temporarily discontinued but subsequently restarted hydralazine. Including them as 'continuing >18 months' would have made survival time of that group even higher.

months during which no antihypertensive drugs were ingested. It should be emphasized that these patients were not sick or infirm when they were normotensive. They felt good, they were healthy, and they worked and led normal lives [26].

In summary, hydralazine toxicity was associated with better control, longer survival and prolonged remission. Before treatment, toxic patients had higher pressures than nontoxic patients; however, chronic hydralazine exposure had a more marked effect for them so that their pressures during treatment were lower. Moreover, these lower pressures led to increased survival, with half of an extended exposure group having apparent complete remissions of their originally severe hypertension.

Conclusion

The very large numbers of hypertensive patients who are currently being treated with drugs make *remission*, either complete or partial, of tremendous potential significance. The current efforts to 'stepdown' antihypertensive therapy are predicated on the reality of *remission*. To some, remission brings to mind decreasing sodium and perhaps increasing potassium intake, but it is uncertain whether this is really remission or simply the establishment of a new steady-state equilibrium. In any case, it proves very difficult for many patients to change their dietary habits to the required extent. The data just reported suggest, however, that true remission does occur. Partial remission would seem to be the general rule for effectively treated patients, with a small part of the treated population progressing to complete remission. In addition, complete remission would seem to be common among the small group of patients who become normotensive and develop hydralazine toxicity but continue low level exposure to the drug – and hence remain normotensive for significant periods of time.

The fact that there is little confirmation of our reports of general partial remission and of complete remission with hydralazine toxicity is somewhat disturbing, although it seems to be relatively easily explained. The amount of effort required to demonstrate partial remission was very large and could only be relatively easily done when the number of antihypertensive drugs and therapists were few. Hydralazine-related remission, of course, depends on the availability of relatively large numbers of toxic patients. If remission can be achieved, its importance in the treatment of millions of patients who otherwise will be forced to take full doses of medication for decades is obvious.

Acknowledgment

This research was supported by the Veterans Administration.

References

1. The 1980 Report of the Joint National Committee on Detection, Evaluation, and Treatment of High Blood Pressure. Arch Intern Med 140:1280, 1980.
2. Schroeder HA: The effect of 1-hydrazinophthalazine in hypertension. Circulation 1:28, 1952.
3. Schroeder HA, Morrow JD, Perry HM Jr: Studies on the control of hypertension by Hyphex. I. Effects on blood pressure. Circulation 8:672, 1953.
4. Perry HM Jr, Mills EJ: The effect of oral hydralazine on circulating human cholesterol. Am J Med Sci 243:72, 1962.
5. Morrow JD, Schroeder HA, Perry HM Jr: Studies on the control of hypertension by Hyphex. II. Toxic reactions and side effects. Circulation 8:829, 1953.
6. Dustan HP, Taylor RD, Corcoran AC, Page IH: Rheumatic and febrile syndrome during prolonged hydralazine treatment. JAMA 154:23, 1954.
7. Perry HM Jr, Schroeder HA: Syndrome simulating collagen disease caused by 1-hydrazinoph-thalazine (Apresoline). JAMA 14:670, 1954.
8. Muller JC, Rast DL, Pryor WW, Orgain ES: Late systemic complications of hydralazine (Apresoline) therapy. JAMA 157:894, 1955.
9. Erickson JC, Hines EA, Pease GL, Brunsting LA: Rheumatoid and lupus-erythematosus-like syndromes. Arch Dermatol 74:640, 1956.
10. Perry HM Jr, Tan EM, Carmody S, Sakamoto A: Relationship of acetyl transferase activity to antinuclear antibodies and toxic symptoms in hypertensive patients treated with hydralazine. J Lab Clin Med 76:114, 1970.
11. Perry HM Jr: Late toxicity to hydralazine resembling systemic lupus erythematosus or rheumatoid arthritis. Am J Med 54:54, 1973.
12. Lowenthal DT, Onesti G, Mutterperl R et al: Long-term clinical effects, bioavailability, and kinetics of minoxidil in relation to renal function. J Clin Pharmacol 18:500, 1978.
13. Mitchel HC, Graham RM, Pettinger WA: Renal function during long-term treatment of hypertension with minoxidil. Ann Intern Med 93:676, 1980.
14. Marquez-Julio A, Uldall PR: Pericardial effusions associated with minoxidil. Lancet 2:816, 1977 (Letter to Editor).
15. Heel RC, Brogden RN, Speight TM, Avery CS: Captopril: a preliminary review of its pharmacological properties and therapeutic efficacy. Drugs 20:409, 1980.
16. Graham RM, Thornell IR, Gain JM et al: Prazosin: the first-dose phenomenon. Br Med J 27:1293, 1976.
17. Olgilvie RI, Mikulic E: Effects of diazoxide and ethacrynic acid on sequential vascular segments in the canine gracilis muscle. J Pharmacol Exp Ther 180:368, 1972.
18. Page UH, Corcoran AC, Dustan HP, Koppanyi T: Cardiovascular actions of sodium nitro-prusside in animals and hypertensive patients. Circulation 11:188, 1955.
19. Campbell DB: Chemistry, pharmacology and pharmacokinetics of indapamide. In: Velasco M (ed) Arterial hypertension, International Congress Series 496. Excerpta Medica, Amsterdam, Exford, Princeton, 1980, p 151.
20. Thurm RH, Smith WM: On resetting of 'barostats' in hypertensive patients. JAMA 201:35, 1967.

21. Veterans Administration Cooperative Study Group on Antihypertensive Agents: Return of elevated blood pressure after withdrawal of antihypertensive drugs. Circulation 51:1107, 1975.
22. Dustan HP, Page IH, Tarazi RC, Frohlich ED: Arterial pressure responses to discontinuing antihypertensive drugs. Circulation 38:370, 1968.
23. Perry HM Jr, Schroeder HA, Catanzaro FJ, Moore-Jones D, Camel GH: Studies on the control of hypertension. VIII. Mortality, morbidity and remissions during twelve years of intensive therapy. Circulation 33:958, 1966.
24. Perry HM Jr, Schroeder HA: Studies on the control of hypertension. VI. Some evidence for reversal of the process during hexamathonium and hydralazine therapy. Circulation 13:528, 1956.
25. Perry HM Jr, Camel GH, Carmody SE, Ahmed KS, Perry EF: Survival in hydralazine-treated hypertensive patients with and without late toxicity. J Chron Dis 30:519, 1977.
26. Perry HM Jr: Possible mechanisms of the hydralazine-related lupus-like syndrome. Arthritis Rheum 24:1093, 1981.

7. Nonpharmacologic treatment of hypertension

GEORGE N. AAGAARD

The thesis to be proposed and supported here is that the hygienic measures of treatment should be utilized in all hypertensive patients, mild to severe. They should also be used in normotensives who are at risk of developing persistent hypertension: those with a family history of hypertension, and those with a history of even a single transitory elevation of blood pressure. Hygienic measures include: (1) reduction of body weight, (2) restriction of dietary salt, (3) recreational exercise and (4) relaxation and psychological methods.

Hygienic measures should be widely applied because they are effective and because they do not have adverse effects. Patients feel better and function more effectively. Drug therapy, in contrast, may cause distressing symptoms in previously asymptomatic patients. Physicians who treat patients should read the poignant letter written by a physician-patient to the editor of 'Lancet' describing how he felt and functioned while receiving antihypertensive drugs [1].

The treatment of hypertension, hygienic or with drugs, begins with the education of the patient. In order to gain patient acceptance and to maintain cooperation over time, it is important that patients understand and accept four concepts:

1. Borderline and occasionally hypertensive patients carry a greater risk of developing persistent hypertension later in life, but statistical chances are good that sustained hypertension will not develop if hygienic measures are followed.
2. Hypertension and secondary damage may develop without any symptoms.
3. Blood pressure should be monitored periodically, with the frequency depending on its level.
4. Treatment must be individualized and adjusted according to the need of the individual.

Reduction of body weight

There has been much misunderstanding about body weight and many writers have denigrated the importance of obesity in hypertension. Good evidence is available to support the idea that populations with increased body weight have an associated increase in blood pressure. Of course, this is not true for everyone, and there is considerable individual variation within a population, with many subjects having perfectly normal blood pressures. Unfortunately, many physicians have loose standards of acceptable body weight when dealing with hypertensive patients. Little attention is paid to the loss of muscle mass with aging. This effect was demonstrated by studies from the University of Rochester which showed that the average sedentary male in the United States loses 12 kg or 26 lbs of lean body mass between ages 25 and 65. Thus the individual who weighs exactly the same at 65 as he did at 25 is actually 26 lbs fatter because he has replaced that much muscle with fat [2]. Unfortunately, most American males actually gain in weight while losing muscle mass. Therefore, the amount of obesity is even greater than this.

Because of the prognostic implications of a hypertensive patient being overweight, our standard for desirable weight should be more stringent for hypertensive patients, and for those normotensive patients who are at increased risk of developing hypertension, than for other patients. Individual weight history is important. Weight at the time an individual played a varsity sport, or weight for a woman prior to her first pregnancy, would help to suggest a weight goal. Measurement of the subcutaneous fat layer is also helpful. A Lang caliper is not necessary for routine patient care. A good estimate can be attained by pinching the subcutaneous fat layer between one's fingers and estimating thickness at three sites: the anterior abdominal wall, one inch lateral to the umbilicus; the posterior chest wall at the angle of the scapula; and the triceps area at the back of the arm. These three estimates should total no more than 25 mm (1 in). Values in excess of that, in a hypertensive person, are regarded as overweight.

Excellent laboratory and clinical studies support the concept that weight reduction will lower blood pressure. In laboratory animals, fasting caused a decrease in sympathetic nervous system activity as estimated by norepinephrine turnover rate of cardiac muscle [3]. Forced feeding caused an increase [4]. Studies in human beings have shown a decrease in urinary catecholamines and metabolites in patients who lost weight [5]. Reisin et al. reported a substantial blood pressure decrease in hypertensive patients who reduced weight. They reported an average weight loss of 10 kg [6], a remarkable result.

Restriction of dietary salt

Population studies have shown a correlation between salt intake and blood pressure [7]. The United States and Japan, countries with high salt intakes, have a high incidence of hypertension. The Yanomamo Indians, who live on the border of Venezuela and Brazil, have never had salt introduced into their culture.

Average systolic and diastolic pressure for males and females does not change after the second decade of life. For females over fifty years of age, average systolic blood pressure was 106 and diastolic blood pressure 64 mmHg [8]. Studies done at the University of Iowa demonstrated that after an oral salt load, men with borderline hypertension reacted differently than normotensive young men. Those with borderline hypertension had a decrease in blood flow to the forearm and an increase in peripheral resistance, whereas those with normotension did not show this type of response [9].

Dietary salt restriction is an important aspect of treatment for patients who require drug therapy, because excess salt can negate the hypotensive response of drug therapy, particularly diuretic therapy [10]. Salt restriction will also decrease the likelihood of hypokalemia in patients who are receiving a thiazide-type diuretic [11]. A daily sodium intake of 1000 mg (43mEq) is the goal for patients. This is difficult to achieve for anyone who must frequently eat away from home, because many chefs use salt as an inexpensive way to make food tasty. Patients who eat meals prepared at home can maintain a sodium intake less than or equal to 1000 mg without undue difficulty if processed meats, canned vegetables and grossly salty foods are avoided, while still enjoying a balanced diet and pleasant tasting dishes. The sodium contents of foods which might be included in a daily basic diet are shown in Table 1. These are the foods of highest sodium content. Fruits contain negligible amounts of sodium. Fresh and properly processed frozen vegetables will not add a great deal of sodium to the diet. Large amounts of sodium are added and potassium leeched out in canning of vegetables. Unfortunately, this reverses the natural favorable potassium/sodium ratio.

Table 1.

	Na (mg)
Whole milk (two glasses)	260
Bread (two slices, not salt-free)	250
Butter (2 pats)	100
Fresh meat (six ounces)	150
Egg	60

Exercise

Exercise contributes in several ways to the care of the hypertensive patient. First, it helps to control body weight. Exercise is often minimized in weight reduction programs, and reduced caloric intake emphasized. However, a constant caloric intake coupled with an increase in physical activity to the extent of one mile of walking per day will result in a weight reduction of 1 lb per month or 12 lbs in a year. Second, exercise causes a small but significant reduction in blood pressure. A recent report from St. Louis showed a blood pressure decrease from exercise in hypertensive adolescents [12]. Third, exercise gives most patients a sense of wellbeing and relaxation. In modern urban society, nervous energy is generated constantly at home, at work and in social activities. There is little or no vigorous physical activity which might release tension. Sustained physical activity each day is helpful and healthful. Therefore, in our clinic we try to get all patients to walk for thirty minutes daily, starting slowly with sedentary patients and increasing gradually to thirty minutes.

An exercise program which the patient will enjoy is important. Games such as tennis are excellent, but few can play tennis daily. A walk is a good alternative for days when tennis is impossible. Rope jumping is a good, albeit vigorous, exercise which is suggested for people when they are traveling and other exercise is impractical. A good workout is possible in a hotel room with a jump rope. Our patients are urged to jump rope until their breathing quickens, then walk around the room until their breathing returns to normal and then resume rope jumping. Thus, rope jumping and walking is alternated in the same fashion that jogging and walking can be alternated. For individuals who find it impractical or inconvenient to leave home for their daily exercise, dancing at home has sometimes proven very satisfactory. Picture, if you will, a little 75-year-old lady, who didn't like walking in rainy winter weather. It was suggested that she might try dancing. On her return visit one month later, she was all aglow! She had started dancing in her living room for 45 min a day on the days when she couldn't get outside to walk. Most important, she was enjoying this exercise – it was great fun!

Relaxation techniques

Physicians who care for hypertensive patients frequently observe the powerful influence of psychological and emotional factors on blood pressure. In college and university students, blood pressure may rise just before and during examination week. Conflict at home between husband and wife or between parent and child may cause a blood pressure increase. Tension in the employment environment may be equally potent and adverse.

Two concepts are emphasized in efforts to use relaxation and psychological methods. First, stress is not the cause of hypertension, but stress causes a greater and more prolonged elevation of blood pressure in hypertensive than in normotensive persons. Second, it is not true that hypertensive individuals are more angry, anxious or hurried than normotensive persons. However, since situations which cause these emotions cause increased blood pressure, it is desirable that patients are helped to prevent stress, if possible, or to cope more effectively when stress cannot be avoided. To help a patient change life style to prevent stress or to handle it more effectively, it is efficacious for the physician to have continuing contact with him or her. Time and sensitive supportive care on the part of the physician are needed to help patients with the psychological aspects of hypertension.

It is important that hypertensive patients become aware of their feelings of anger, anxiety and time pressure and of the situations which cause them. Techniques of muscular relaxation, meditation and biofeedback may be useful for lowering blood pressure because of the passive quietness achieved during their. practice. A daily quiet period can make the patient more readily aware of anger, anxiety or time pressure. With recognition comes the opportunity to prevent or deal more effectively with the causal noxious situation.

It is especially beneficial to help patients plan their activities to avoid a sense of hurry and time constraint. In work, recreation and social activities the watchword is 'enjoy.' Patients are urged to schedule their work so that they can do a good job and enjoy it – even the most difficult tasks.

It is important and encouraging for patients to recognize that sources of stress are not perpetual. Some sources of stress may be resolved. Children mature and leave home. Relationships improve. The work environment may improve. An unreasonable supervisor may retire or move on to another job. As patients are being encouraged to improve their sence of self-esteem, special effort is made to avoid any sense of guilt over lack of success in weight control and other aspects of the program. A supportive and helpful attitude is shown, rather than one which is critical or judgmental.

Follow-up care

In continuing to provide care for hypertensive patients, a specific inquiry is made into their progress on each element of hygienic care at each return visit. Body weight is carefully measured. The extent and regularity of the exercise program is evaluated; and finally the use of salt and sodium-rich foods, including processed meats, like ham, bacon and sausage, at the table and in the preparation of meals is questioned. If blood pressure readings, both at home and in the office, are higher than desired, a particular effort is made to find a cause, rather than to simply increase the antihypertensive medications. If there is a possibility that dietary salt has been incre:sed because of meals in restaurants and hotels, a 24-hr urine specimen is checked for sodium. There is concern about emotional problems, and the patient is always invited to comment on changes in his life situation which might have been stressful. The point to be emphasized is that each visit serves to increase understanding of the patient and to stimulate him or her to closer observance of hygienic measures.

For many patients, the blood pressure readings make it apparent that a reduction of antihypertensive drug therapy is appropriate. In these circumstances, an attempt is made to reduce the dose of drugs very slowly. For patients who are receiving two or more antihypertensive drugs, the daily dose of one drug at a time is reduced. For example, if a patient is receiving a diuretic and a beta-blocker, the diuretic is maintained at the same level and the daily dose of the beta-blocker is reduced. The daily dose of the beta-blocker is reduced by 10–25% every two weeks as long as home blood pressure readings are satisfactory. When the daily intake has been reduced to a low level and the drug is taken only once a day, the patient omits the drug every third day and then every other day, until finally it is being taken once a week. At this time we can usually discontinue it completely.

It should be emphasized that these gradual reductions in drug dosage are accomplished in patients whose blood pressure is being observed at home and is known to be in a satisfactory range. With carefully followed hygienic measures, many patients can enjoy good blood pressure control with a significant reduction in their antihypertensive medications.

As an example of the effectiveness of hygienic measures in the management of hypertension, let me cite the experience of a physician who came to our clinic one morning after visiting his ophthalmolagist the day before, at which time a screening blood pressure reading had been recorded at 240/140 mmHg; this was the first time he had been told of any elevation in blood pressure. A brief examination revealed blood pressures of 210–230/108–120 mmHg supine, and 200/106 mmHg sitting. Funduscopic examination was normal. These findings suggested that his blood pressure was not as high as it had been the previous day in the ophthalmolagist's office. There was confidence that he was moving in the right direction, and he was asked to return in two days. Then, his blood pressure was recorded at 195/105 mmHg sitting. Asked if he would like to be started on drug therapy or if he wished to follow a hygienic program without drug therapy for a time, he chose to postpone drug therapy. He was seen again one week later, at which time he had already lost $2\frac{1}{2}$ lbs, and his blood pressure was 165–170/96–100 sitting. He and his wife had become interested in the sodium content of his diet, and estimated that he was ingesting approximately 500 mg of sodium a day. Six weeks after his initial visit, he had lost approximately 19 lbs. His blood pressure was 155–175/85 mmHg supine, and 124–15–124–150/84 mmHg sitting. None of the readings on that visit was over 85 mmHg diastolic.

It is possible that in the future significant hypertension may be prevented and that the majority of patients with established hypertension may be treated with hygienic measures and without drug therapy. The report of the Hypertension Detection and Follow-up Study provides some hopeful information concerning the severity of the hypertension found in a widespread screening program [13]. Approximately 158,000 people were initially screened at home. Those with blood pressures of 95 mmHg diastolic and above were invited to a clinic evaluation where a diastolic pressure of 90 mmHg or higher was considered to indicate hypertension. Of 10,000 patients so classified, approximately 72% were in the range of 90–104 mmHg diastolic. This is very encouraging because many of these patients can be effectively managed with hygienic measures, without drug therapy. Obviously, it is essential that their blood pressure level be monitored at appropriate intervals throughout life. The important point, however, is that a significant number of hypertensive patients are being recognized at a time when hygienic measures may be effective in preventing the development of established hypertension and thereby preventing the morbidity and mortality which is related to this important health problem.

References

1. Trials and tribulations of a symptom-free hypertensive physician receiving the best of care. Lancet 2(8032):291–292, 1977.
2. Forbes GB, Reino Julio C: Adult lean body mass declines with age: some longitudinal observations. Metabolism 19:653–663, 1970.
3. Young JB, Landsberg L: Suppression of sympathetic nervous system during fasting. Science 196:1473–1475, 1977.
4. Young JB, Landsberg L: Stimulation of the sympathetic nervous system during sucrose feeding. Nature 269:615–617, 1977.
5. Jung RT, Shetty PS, Barrand M, Callingham BA, James WPT: Role of catecholamines in hypotensive response to dieting. Br Med J 1:12–13, 1979.
6. Reisin E, Abel R, Modan M, et al: Effect of weight loss without salt restriction on the reduction of blood pressure in overweight hypertensive patients. N Engl J Med 298:1–6, 1978.
7. Page LB, Damon A, Moellering RC: Antecedents of cardiovascular disease in six Solomon Islands societies. Circulation 49:1132–1154, 1974.
8. Oliver WJ, Cohen EL, Neel JV: Blood pressure, sodium intake, and sodium-related hormones in the Yanomamo Indians, a 'no-salt' culture. Circulation 52:146–151, 1975.
9. Mark AL, Lawton WJ, Abboud FM et al: Effects of high and low sodium intake on arterial pressure and forearm vascular resistance in borderline hypertension. Circ Res 36, 37 (Suppl. 1): I(194)–I(198), 1975.
10. Parijs J, Joossens JV, Van der Linden L et al: Moderate sodium restriction and diuretics in the treatment of hypertension. Am Heart J 85:22–34, 1973.
11. Fallis N, Ford RV: Electrolyte excretion and hypotensive response. JAMA 176:581–584, 1961.
12. Haberg JM: Beneficial effects of endurance exercise training in adolescent hypertension. Am J Cardiol 45:489A, 1980.
13. Hypertension Detection and Follow-Up Program Group: Five-year findings of the Hypertension Detection and Follow-Up Program. JAMA 242:2562–2578, 1979.

8. The enigma of mild hypertension: how much treatment?

H. MITCHELL PERRY, JR.

A. Introduction

Currently, the major question with respect to the treatment of hypertension is when and how to treat mild hypertension. There is no general consensus as to the most effective method of managing this entity. Mild hypertension, an unfortunate term but the only one in common use, is characterized by a *usual* diastolic blood pressure of from 90 through 104 mmHg. In the United States, its overall incidence is almost 15% of the population, as defined by a single diastolic pressure – and single diastolic pressure data constitute the only available prevalence information. Its incidence is a function of age, increasing rapidly from a rather constant average approximating 5% in young adults to about 15% at age 40 and more than 20% at age 60 [1].

Complications of hypertension are directly related to the level of diastolic blood pressure. Framingham-type data, which are the basis for much of our information, indicate that even an isolated elevation in pressure is accompanied by an increase in morbidity and mortality [2]. National Pooling Project data indicate that with diastolic pressures of 95–105 mmHg, total deaths increase 50% and coronary deaths more than 100%, when compared with the death rates associated with pressures in the 75–85 mmHg range [3].

While the associated risks of serious cardiovascular complications of untreated mild hypertension are well documented, the benefits of treatment are not! Despite the recent suggestive data from the Hypertension Detection and Followup Program (HDFP) [4, 5], there are no definitive data on the benefits of treating mild hypertension or on the risks of such treatment. The first step then in considering how to manage mild hypertension is to examine carefully the available information on benefits and risks of drug therapy – there are no data at all on nonpharmacological therapy – in order to determine whether therapy is justified and if so, when and how enthusiastically it should be pursued. A summary of the available information follows:

B. The benefits of treating mild hypertension

When the first effective antihypertensive agents became available in the early 1950s, their ability to prolong life for patients with the most severe kinds of hypertension was quickly appreciated. Since these first dramatic results, the benefit of drug therapy has been successively demonstrated for less and less severe hypertension. By demonstrating decreased morbidity and mortality for patients with moderate hypertension (diastolic pressures 105 through 114 mmHg), the well-known Veterans Administration Study of Antihypertensive Agents III (VA Study 3) made a major contribution to this progressive extension of the range of blood pressures benefited by treatment [6]. This study proved to be a turning point in the general attitude toward hypertension, both in the United States and throughout the world; before its publication, there was widespread apathy regarding effective antihypertensive treatment; after it, there was universal enthusiasm.

From the time the VA Study III data [6, 7] became available, there has been a tendency to extrapolate the results to patients with mild hypertension (diastolic pressures 90 through 104 mmHg). There are difficulties with such extrapolation, however. Not only were the morbid events of moderate hypertension quantitatively different from those of severe hypertension, but they were qualitatively different as well. Thus, with untreated hypertension, the total event rate decreased as the severity of the disease decreased. In addition, so-called *hypertensive events*, progressively rising pressure, congestive heart failure, hemorrhagic stroke and renal damage were increasingly replaced by *atherosclerotic events*, primarily myocardial infarction, including 'sudden death', and thrombotic stroke. The VA Study III demonstrated this change in the pattern of events for a single population of untreated (i.e., placebo) veterans whose hypertension ran almost the entire gamut of severity, with diastolic pressures ranging from 90–130 mmHg. The frequency of all events per patient per year decreased from 0.23 in severe hypertension to 0.11 in moderate hypertension. At the same time, the ratio of hypertensive to other arteriosclerotic events also decreased from 2.14 to 1.08 (Table 1). This study indicated that antihypertensive treatment was far more effective in preventing hypertensive events than in preventing atherosclerotic events. Keeping in mind that the number of patients involved was very small, treatment seemed to prevent most hypertensive events in all patients, regardless of the severity of their underlying hypertension, whereas it markedly diminished atherosclerotic events in severely hypertensive patients, but prevented only half of them in moderately and mildly hypertensive patients.

The overall results of six major studies of mild hypertension are summarized in Table 2 and discussed below. The first three studies are double-blind, placebo-controlled trials. The fourth and fifth – and by far the largest – were unblinded and had no placebo controls. They also differed from the others in that different

118

Table 1. Morbid and mortal events for placebo patients (VA Study III)

Severity of hypertension and no. of patients	Hypertensive events (BP & CHF)	Atherosclerotic events (MI & CVA)	Hypertensive to atherosclerotic ratio	Total events per patient per year
73 Severe	15	7	2.14	0.23
110 Moderate	25	21	1.19	0.13
84 Mild	13	12	1.08	0.093

Legend: Pattern of Events in VA Study III: Numbers of hypertensive events (significant rise in blood pressure and congestive heart failure) and atherosclerotic events (myocardial infarction and thrombotic stroke), their ratio, and the incidence of all events are listed for severe, moderate and mild hypertension.

Table 2. Mild hypertension: benefits of drug treatment

Study	Patients	Mean years followed	Summary results	References
VA-III*	170	3.3	4 times as many placebo as treatment events in moderate hypertension but only 1.5 times as many in mild hypertension	JAMA 213:1143, 1970
PHS*	389	7	Twice as many hypertensive events in placebo as in treated patients but equal numbers of artherosclerotic events.	Circ Res 40 (Suppl 1):98, 1977
VA-NIH*	1012	1.5	Increased heart block and increased plasma cholesterol in *treated* patients. A third of placebo patients were normotensive.	Circ Res 40 (Suppl 1):180, 1977
HDFP	7825	5	20% lower mortality in 'special care' than in 'referred care' patients.	JAMA 242:2562, 1979
MRFIT	8011	6	No significant difference between 'special intervention and 'usual care'	JAMA 248:1465, 1982
Austra-lian**	3251	4	Twice as many CVAs and more fatal MIs in placebo patients but no differences for those with diastolic pressures less than 95 mmHg	Lancet 1:1261, 1980

* These studies were double-blind and placebo-controlled.
** This study was single-blind and placebo-controlled.

groups of physicians, using different regimens, and with differing amounts of time and ancillary resources, treated the two groups of patients studied. Finally, the first was interpreted as showing marked benefit from aggressive treatment while the other failed to confirm this benefit. The sixth study was single-blind and placebo-controlled; it suggested that maximum benefit of treatment was associated with a diastolic pressure in the 90s.

VA Study III included 170 patients with mild hypertension. For them, no definitive benefit of treatment was demonstrated, in part because the absolute event rates were very low and in part because of the relatively small difference between 'treated' and 'placebo' event rates. The data are as follows: for the entire 380 patients of the second report, i.e., those with baseline diastolic pressures of 90–115 mmHg, the ratio of the percentage of placebo patients with morbid events divided by the percentage of treated patients with morbid events, i.e., the 'therapeutic efficacy ratio,' approximated 2.5. Patients with moderate hypertension at baseline, however, benefitted more from treatment than the whole group, and those with mild hypertension less. Thus, for those with diastolic pressures of 105–115 mmHg, the therapeutic efficacy ratio approximated 4, whereas, for those with pressures of 90–105 mmHg, the ratio was only about 1.5 (Table 3) [8]. It must be emphasized that even a ratio of 1.5, if it proves to be sufficiently different from unity, could represent a major benefit for society, since there are millions of people with mild hypertension in the United States, and 60% of the excess mortality attributable to high blood pressure occurs in those with mild hypertension [9]. There is, however, a very large uncertainty in the ratio of 1.5, and it could be that 'treated' and 'placebo' event rates are the same.

This study also demonstrated how difficult it is to evaluate the side and toxic effects of therapy. Out of the total study population of 380 patients, 29 were dropped from the study because of effects that both patient and physician

Table 3. Efficacy of antihypertensive treatment (VA Study III)

Number of patients	Pretreatment diastolic range (mmHg)	Placebo patients (% with events)	Treated patients (% with events)	Therapeutic efficacy ratio*
170	90–105 (mild)	25	16	1.5
210	105–115 (mod)	32	8	4.0
380	90–115 (total)	29	12	2.5

* Percentage of placebo patients with morbid events divided by the percentage of treated patients with morbid events.

Legend: The percentages of placebo and treated patients with moderate and mild hypertension in VA Study III who developed morbid events during the average follow-up period of 39 months and the therapeutic efficacy ratio for each group.

ascribed to 'active drug' treatment. When the 'double-blind' was broken, two-thirds of the dropped patients were indeed found to have been on active drug; however, one-third were on placebo and hence could hardly have had any drug-related effect (Table 4) [6]. Thus, without a double-blind study, it is probably not possible to determine which complaints are due to drugs; likewise it is probably impossible to quantitate drug-induced effects in any meaningful way.

Although there are few data dealing with the goal level to which diastolic pressure should be lowered in order to obtain the maximum benefit of therapy, the same study suggests that lowering the diastolic pressure to strictly normal levels is no more protective than partial lowering. When the actively treated patients of the VA Study III were divided on the basis of how far therapy lowered their diastolic pressures, the third with the lowest pressures (treated diastolic pressure below 80 mmHg) and the third with the highest pressures (treated diastolic pressure above 90 mmHg) had the same event rates despite the fact that the pressure in the 'high third' had been lowered an average of only 8 mmHg and in the 'low third' an average of 28 mmHg (Table 5) [10]. Thus, lowering the pressure into the 90s may be as effective as lowering it into the 70s.

Finally, an extension of this study apparently demonstrated 'remission' of mild hypertension. After the efficacy of treatment had been proven by a significant decrease in morbidity and mortality, those patients (with either moderate or mild hypertension) whose diastolic pressure had been well controlled (less then 90 mmHg) for two years on 'active drugs' were offered an extension of the study to determine whether they had a continuing need for treatment. Eighty-six of them agreed to be rerandomized in double-blind fashion. Some were continued on active drug, but the majority were switched to placebo. Figure 1 indicates that most of these new placebo patients had a relatively rapid return of their hypertension and required reinstitution of treatment within six months. At least 15%

Table 4. Toxic and side effects (VA Study III): patients dropped from study because of toxic or side effects

Toxic or side effect	Active	Placebo	Total
Depression	7	5	12
Peptic ulcer	6	4	10
Impotence	1	1	2
Lupus erythematosus	6	5	1
	20	11	29*

* The 20 and 11 effects occurred in 29 patients, because two patients had two events each.
Legend: Analysis of the 29 patients (out of a total study population of 380 moderately and mildly hypertensive patients) who were dropped from the study because of presumed 'drug-induced' effects. Two-thirds were receiving antihypertensive drugs, and one-third were not!

Table 5. Similar benefit from paritial or complete control (VA Study 3)

Patient group	'Treated' diastolic pressure (mean, mmHg)	Patients with events	Percent of patients with events
194 Placebo	106	56	28.9%
186 Treated	86	22	11.8%
66 Treated	98	8	12.1%
61 Treated	76	7	11.5%

Legend: Comparison of placebo and active drug patients and then of partially controlled and well-controlled active drug patients (out of the total study population of 380 moderately and mildly hypertensive patients): Treatment with active drug abolished (or delayed) 60% of the events that placebo patients had, but active treatment that lowered the average diastolic pressure to 98 mmHg was no better than active treatment that lowered it to 76 mmHg!

of them, however, remained normotensive without active drugs for a year, with no additional patients developing recrudescent hypertension after six months [11]. The 15% remission rate is actually a minimum figure; the rate may have been twice this high since another 15% were removed from the study while they were still normotensive because they dropped out or because of the appearance of symptoms, such as angina pectoris. In confirmation of this observation, a similar study with mildly hypertensive patients reported a similar 22% remission rate [12]. Thus, a fifth to a sixth of the patients with effectively treated mild hyper-

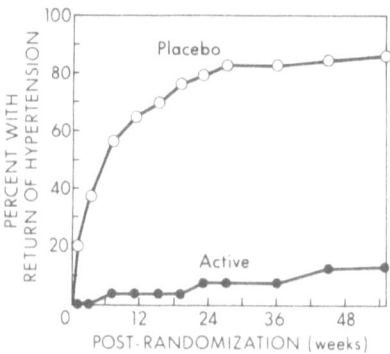

Figure 1. Apparent remission of hypertension in VA Study III patients whose diastolic pressures were controlled below 90 mmHg for two years by active drug treatment: After completion of the original trial and breaking of the 'double-blind,' consenting controlled patients who had been on active drug were rerandomized in double-blind fashion to active or placebo drug. Vertical scale represents recrudescent hypertension for active patients, but it represents removal from the trial for 'placebo' patients. Of the latter, 85% were removed from the trial, but only 70% actually became hypertensive; the other 15% dropped out or were again begun on antihypertensive treatment because of symptoms, such as angina pectoris, while still normotensive.

tension have been able to discontinue treatment and remain normotensive for a significant period.

Public Health Service Hospital Study (PHS Study) followed 389 men and women (20%) for seven to ten years [13]. These patients were 21–55 years old at entry and had average baseline diastolic pressures (taken at home during six weeks by patient or family) of 90–115 mmHg. Sixteen percent of them had 'hypervoltage,' but none had other evidence of target organ damage. Thus, not all of these patients had mild hypertension and not all of them had completely uncomplicated hypertension. After three months of 'single-blind' placebo, the patients were randomly assigned in double-blind fashion to placebo or drug treatment, the latter consisting of 500 mg of chlorothiazide and 100 mg of rauwolfia serpentina root twice daily. Blood pressure fell promptly in the treated group by an average of 16/10 mmHg, and the new lower level was maintained without change for the remainder of the study. There never was anything more than a trivial fall in blood pressure for the placebo group.

Major morbid events were myocardial infarction, including sudden death, and stroke. These occurred with equal frequency in the two groups, with eight myocardial infarctions in the treated and seven in the placebo groups; there were also two strokes in the placebo group [13]. Less serious *hypertensive* events, almost exclusively the appearance of cardiomegaly, were twice as frequent in the placebo as in the treated group, and progression to more severe hypertension was seen only in the placebo group. Thus, treatment provided no benefit recognizable to the patient, although it prevented changes that placed him in a higher risk group and therefore many have protected him from eventual complications.

VA-NIH Mild Hypertension Feasibility Trial (VA-NIH Trial) randomized a total of 1012 men and women (19%) from 21 to 50 years old with mild hypertension and no evidence of target organ damage; they were treated for an average of 18 months with a three-step regimen, consisting either of 50 mg of chlorthalidone, 100 mg of chlorthalidone, or that plus 0.25 mg of reserpine or with a matched three-step placebo regimen [14, 15]. Unlike the prior two studies, this one included only patients with mild uncomplicated hypertension. It is worth noting that during screening the diastolic pressures became normal without any treatment for half of the subjects, who were otherwise suitable and whose initial diastolic pressures ranged from 90 to 120 mmHg; this half was excluded from the study by the requirement that average diastolic pressure remain above 90 mmHg on four successive screening visits.

Following randomization, the average baseline diastolic pressure of 93.2 mmHg fell 5.3 mmHg for the placebo group and 10.9 mmHg for the treated group. A detailed distribution of pressures during the first six months after randomization is shown in Figure 2 for both placebo and treated cohorts; after six months there was little further change in the distribution. The figure shows that a significant fraction of patients with mild hypertension, as rigorously

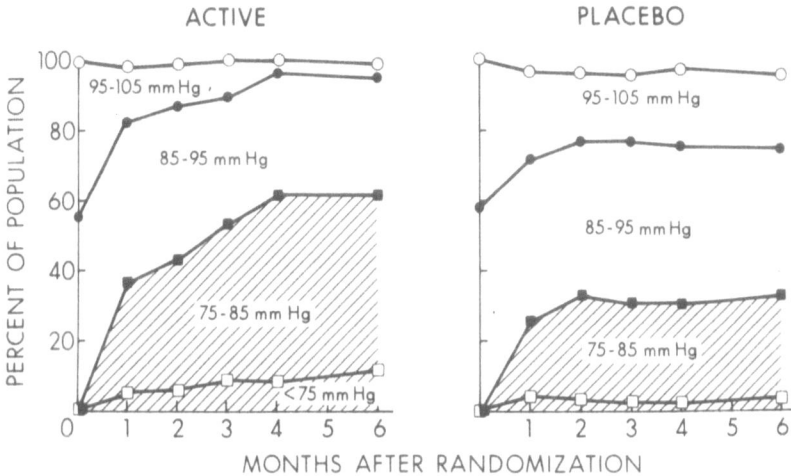

Figure 2. Distribution of diastolic pressures for subjects with consistent mild hypertension during the first six months of treatment in the VA-NHLBI Trial: the shaded areas represent the percentage of active drug and placebo subjects with diastolic pressures below 85 mmHg. The areas 85–95 mmHg and 95–105 mmHg indicate the percentage of subjects with treated diastolic pressures in these ranges. Note: to be randomized, all subjects had had four successive screening pressures above 90 mmHg.

defined by diastolic pressures greater than 90 mmHg on four consecutive visits, became and remained well controlled without antihypertensive drugs. Thus, one third of *placebo* patients maintained diastolic pressures less than 85 mmHg. For treated patients, the fraction under control increased for the first four months after randomization as the intensity of treatment increased. At that time, three-fifths of the treated patients had diastolic pressures below 85 mmHg. Thus, aggressive treatment brought an additional fourth of the patients under control. Although the data are not presented here, this was true irrespective of whether their pretreatment diastolic pressure was in the high or low part of the mildly hypertensive range.

Increased severity of hypertension requiring the institution of treatment occurred in 2% of placebo patients but in no treated patients. There were no significant differences in morbid events between the two groups. Thus, among placebo patients, there were five nonfatal myocardial infarctions; among the treated patients, there were six, plus two sudden deaths. There was, however, one statistically significant difference in the incidence of a predetermined morbid event: first-degree heart block appeared in 27 treated patients and in only seven placebo patients. Not surprisingly, asymptomatic chemical abnormalities were more common in the treated than in the placebo group. Thus, more than 20% of treated patients and less than 1% of placebo patients developed a potassium level below 3.0 mEq/l of plasma; 20% of the treated patients also developed uric acid levels above 9.0 mg/100ml. Treatment was also associated with average increases in plasma cholesterol of about 10 mg/100ml and in plasma glucose of about 3.5 mg/100ml. A total of 1642 side effects were recorded for the treated patients versus 920 for placebo patients (Table 6). Based on their distribution between placebo patients, side effects belonged in one of two categories. Either they occurred equally often in the two groups (rash, diarrhea and headache) and were of the type which would not be expected to be associated with the antihypertensive drugs used in this study, or they were two to three times as frequent in treated as in placebo patients (asthenia, muscle aches, nasal stuffiness, impotence and somnolence) and could reasonably be expected as side effects of chlorthalidone and reserpine. The events recorded in this study are summarized in Table 6.

Hypertension Detection and Follow-up Program (HDFP) was not double-blind or placebo-controlled; instead it randomized patients into one of two tracks, either referring them to the *usual community health care provider*, i.e., referred care (RC); or giving them *intensive antihypertensive treatment by a special clinic*, i.e., special care (SC) [4, 5]. Thus, this is the first large scale cooperative study which compared patients who were treated by entirely different types of health care providers – on the one hand investigators for whom money and time were no object, on the other whatever health care providers the community offered – and several of these communities were in the ghetto. Of a total of 10,940 hypertensive men and women from 30 to 70 years old who were randomized, 7825 had mild hypertension, as manifested by a diastolic pressure

Table 6. All predefined events during treatment (VA-NIH Trial)

	504 Placebo subjects	508 Active subjects
Treatment failures*	12	0
Major morbid events	5	8
Minor electrocardiographic events**	12	38
Subjects with chemical abnormalities***	8	176
Side effects	920	1642

* Treatment failures were defined before the start of the trial as diastolic pressures above 110 mmHg on four consecutive clinic visits or above 120 mmHg on two.

** Only first-degree heat block is considered here, since the other predefined minor morbid events' were rare and equally distributed between the active and placebo groups.

*** Only potassium levels below 3.0 mg and uric acid levels above 9.0 mg/dl of plasma are considered here, since only they met the requirements for predefined chemical events.

Legend: Summary of all events for mildly hypertensive subjects without target organ damage who were treated with either 50 mg chlorthalidone, 100 mg of chlorthalidone, or that plus 0.25 mg reserpine daily, or placebos for these agents during an average of 18 months of follow-up.

of more than 95 mmHg at home and more than 90 mmHg at a follow-up clinic visit but less than 105 mmHg at both times. Patients were included regardless of whether or not they had target organ damage.

The trial was designed to detect whether aggressive treatment, as opposed to usual community care, produced any significant difference in total mortality between the two groups, and indeed, for the mildly (but not for severely) hypertensive patients, there was such a difference. Unfortunately it was not designed to determine whether antihypertensive therapy was beneficial. After five years of follow-up, the mildly hypertensive patients in the SC group had 20% fewer deaths than the initially comparable RC group, but there was no difference for the subpopulation of patients below 50 years of age – and none for white women. At the end of the trial the diastolic pressures of the SC group averaged 83.4 mmHg and those of the RC group 87.8 mmHg. (The average diastolic pressure of the SC group is similar to but about 1 mmHg *above* the level achieved by the treated patients in the VA-NIH Trial; the RC value was about 1 mmHg *lower* than the placebo patients in the VA-NIH Trial. Thus, the difference in pressures between treated and placebo patients in the VA-NIH Trial was about 2 mmHg greater than the difference between SC and RC in HDFP [4, 8, 15].) Moreover, 64% of the SC group was controlled at 'goal diastolic pressure' versus 43% of the RC group. *Unfortunately, however, the relationship between an individual patient's level of treated diastolic pressure and his mortality has not yet been published;* however data presented at the 1982 American Heart Association meeting suggested that about two-thirds of the lower mortality among SC patients was related to lower pressure.

Although the 20% lower mortality of the SC group is probably due in part at least to the more intensive antihypertensive treatment provided to these patients, it may also be partly due to more frequent, complete and sympathetic attention, i.e., closer and better overall therapy, which this group very probably received. A necessarily tentative assignment of 'cause of death' suggested that for the mildly hypertensive patients there was a 26% drop in cardiovascular-renal mortality and a 13% drop in *noncardiovascular* mortality; the latter, of course, cannot be directly ascribed to antihypertensive treatment, but it might be related to generally improved cardiovascular status. The same tentative analysis of cause of death suggested that both stroke and myocardial infarction were diminished by almost half in the SC group; the effect on stroke but not on myocardial infarction is consistent with findings in other studies. Unfortunately, no valid comparision of morbid events can be made since differences in visit frequency might well have caused transient events to be differentially missed. In addition, the absence of a placebo group, which would serve as a control, effectively precludes quantitation of any undesirable effects of therapy.

Australian Therapeutic Trial in Mild Hypertension (Australian Study) was a randomized, single-blind, placebo-controlled study of 3251 patients with mild hypertension (diastolic pressures 95–110 mmHg), who were followed for an average of four years [16]. It demonstrated a halving of cerebrovascular events in the actively treated group. There was no significant difference in the incidence of myocardial infarction; however, the infarcts proved fatal for eight patients in the placebo but for only two in the actively treated group. Active therapy was not associated with significantly fewer trial endpoints than placebo for those less than 50 years old or for white women, although the trends in both groups favored treatment.

Finally and perhaps most important, all of those with treated diastolic pressures below 95 mmHg, whether receiving placebo or active drug, had the same total event rates (Table 7). Even trends were nonexistent. This is in sharp contrast to the interpretation of HDFP which holds that the difference in average diastolic pressure between 83 and 87 mmHg was associated with a 20% difference in mortality. It agrees, however, with the VA Study, which found that essentially the same event rates were associated with average diastolic pressures in the 90s and in the 70s. Thus, the Australian Study suggests that a diastolic pressure below 95 mmHg, whether achieved by active treatment or occurring in placebo patients, provides maximum protection.

Multiple Risk Factor Intervention Trial (MRFIT), like HDFP was not 'blinded' or 'controlled'. Although MRFIT was limited to high risk men and was seeking the effects of reducing other risk factors as well as blood pressure, the two trials were otherwise similar in design. Of a total *12,866* men between *35* and *57* who were randomized, *8011* were hypertensive. Unlike HDFP, 'special intervention,' including intensive antihypertensive treatment, did not decrease mortality in MRFIT. In fact, there were no statistically significant differences between 'Special Intervention' and 'Usual Care.' The general trend was reminiscent of the Australian Study in seeming to suggest that treatment was not helpful for subjects with diastolic pressures less than 95 mmHg.

Table 7. Event rate by treated diastolic pressure (Australian Study)

Treated diastolic pressures	Numbers of patients		Trial end points rates*		Total
	Active	Placebo	Active	Placebo	
90 mmHg	1044	407	14	17	15
90–94 mmHg	373	482	20	16	18
95–99 mmHg	143	412	55	23	31
100 mmHg	77	316	36	59	54

* Incidence rates given in end points (i.e., morbid events) per 1000 patient-years of risk.
Legend: Incidence of trial end points in active drug and placebo patients as a function of treated diastolic pressure. There seem to be no meaningful differences in 'end point rates' of 14–20 events per 1000 patient-years. Thus, active drug and placebo patients with treated diastolic pressures below 95 mmHg have apparently achieved 'maximum benefit', and the primary effect of active treatment seems to be to increase the percentage of patients with diastolic pressures less than 95 mmHg.

C. Summary of advantages and disadvantages of treating mild hypertension

(1) Because of the relatively low stroke and myocardial infarction rates associated with mild hypertension, one can only expect small benefits from treatment; however, because of very large numbers involved, even a small decrease could be significant. (2) Until HDFP was interpreted by some as demonstrating that treating mild hypertension lowered mortality by 20%, there was no suggestion that treatment decreased the incidence of any major morbid event. The critical HDFP data suggest that the observed benefit depends on a difference in treated average diastolic pressures of 83 and 87 mmHg: intuitively this seems unlikely; thus, the interpretation of benefit may be overly optimistic. (3) The upper limit of the goal diastolic pressure has been traditionally, but arbitrarily, set at 90 mmHg. Since HDFP, some have felt it should be in the low 80s; however, both the VA Study and the Australian Study suggest that lowering the diastolic pressure to 95 mmHg may provide many benefits. (4) The price of treatment in terms of such things as toxicity, inconvenience and expense are real but difficult to evaluate, particularly since there are no useful data on lifelong treatment of mild hypertension, i.e., for 30 or 40 years. (5) For as many as a third of mildly hypertensive patients, a concerned physician using placebos may be able to lower the pressure to normal and keep it there for a significant period of time. (6) One patient in five or six whose mild hypertension has been treated and controlled at normal levels with antihypertensive drugs may be able to discontinue those drugs and maintain normotension for significant periods.

D. Management of mild hypertension

What, then, are reasonable goals in managing mild hypertension? As indicated in the Introduction, the risk associated with mild hypertension is unquestioned; although perhaps not very high for a specific individual. There is, however, a major uncertainty as to whether drug therapy lowers the risk and what price, in terms of undesired effects, is associated with such therapy. As indicated by the studies discussed above, myocardial infarction is probably little influenced by drug therapy. HDFP is alone in suggesting that treatment lessens coronary events, and this interpretation must be considered problematic since that study was designed to provide data on mortal events as a whole, rather than various types of events, and there could be significant biases in the morbid event data from that study. Other studies may have been too small or too short to show an effect on coronary artery disease, but it seems more likely that the apparent HDFP effect will prove to be considerably smaller than current estimates. Cerebrovascular accidents, in contrast, seem very likely to be lessened by treatment, although treatment did not alter the incidence of a second stroke in mildly hypertensive patients with a prior stroke [17]. Progression to more severe hypertension and development of electrocardiographic changes (hypervoltage and cardiomegaly) are prevented by treatment. Although the mildly hypertensive patient may have no symptomatic improvement, these complications, which are highly correlated with serious trouble, are almost eliminated by treatment. Cardiac failure is very probably lessened in the mildly hypertensive subjects older than 60 years of age. Retinopathy and renal failure are also often listed as being diminished by treatment; however, since they are seldom if ever caused by mild hypertension, the benefit of treatment cannot be great.

Young patients, i.e., less than 50 years old, with mild diastolic hypertension, particularly those who are asymptomatic and without target organ damage or other major risk factors, continue to pose a major unresolved therapeutic question: to treat or not to treat. For them, even HDFP did not suggest benefit, and the VA-NIH Trial documented undesired effects in the form of side effects, induced chemical abnormalities, and first-degree heart block. The usual question is whether prophylactic antihypertensive treatment will give better eventual

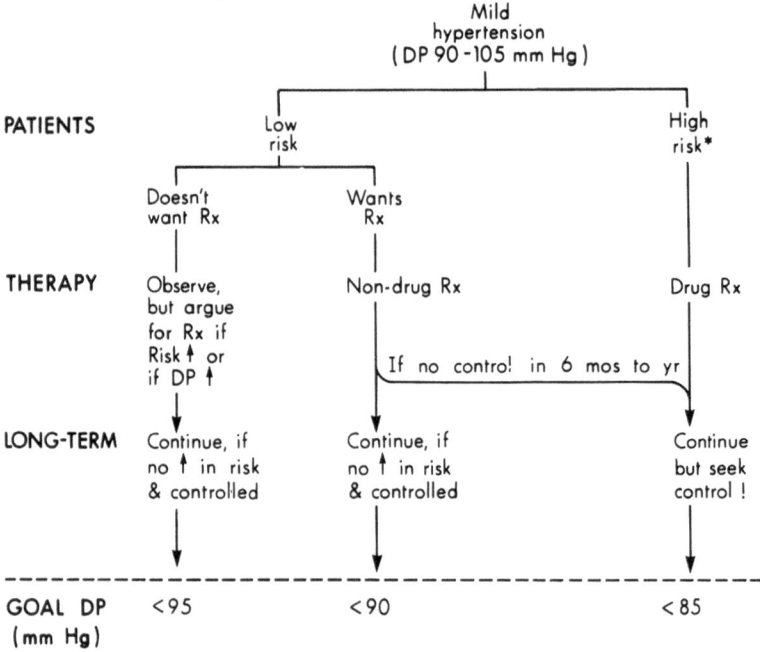

Figure 3. A general plan for managing mild hypertension which permits observation in low-risk patients who do not want treatment.
* 'High risk' is present if there is target organ damage, family history of trouble *before* age 50, or high cholesterol; or if the patient is a smoker; or if the patient is young, black, or male (two of three); or if the patient has a usual diastolic pressure (DP) above 95–100 mmHg (with cutoff depending on other risk factors).

results than careful observation coupled with intervention only when certain specific criteria are surpassed, and there are no data on this point. If prophylaxis is indeed beneficial to a group as a whole, there is the question of whether it is sufficiently beneficial to justify treating the whole group – and therefore subjecting everyone to undesirable side effects. Even if antihypertensive treatment is beneficial to the entire mildly hypertensive population or to specific subpopulations, a great many patients in the group would never have developed any complications and therefore could presumably not benefit from therapy. Are the many to be treated in order to benefit the relatively few who will eventually develop hypertensive complications which treatment might have aborted, mitigated or delayed?

As suggested in the foregoing, for the moment there would seem to be two reasonable ways to manage mild hypertension: (1) careful follow-up with definitive treatment only when the process progresses; (2) immediate but limited definitive nonpharmacologic or pharmacologic treatment designed to do minimal harm (Figure 3). It seems logical to base the decision about how to manage the condition on the perceived risk-benefit ratio for the individual patient. In order to assess risk, one needs an evaluation of the severity of the hypertensive process and the amount of existing cardiovascular compromise.

E. Initial evaluation

The work-up of a patient with mild hypertension need not include extensive diagnostic procedures designed primarily to discover rare secondary causes of hypertension. It should begin with careful blood pressure measurements made under conditions which are not unusually stressful. The finding of an elevated blood pressure at first screening categorizes an individual as hypertensive in the 'Framingham epidemiologic context' [18], since such epidemiologic data are essentially based on a single blood pressure measurement. Obviously, however, all patients with a single elevated blood pressure are not at similar risk since risk depends on many variables. One of these is the subsequent blood pressure course. Many patients will remain mildly hypertensive, but for a large fraction most subsequent blood pressures will be normal.

Usual pressure, rather than first pressure – or lowest pressure – is needed to determine whether treatment is appropriate for a given individual, and how aggressive it should be. A first approximation of the usual pressure can be obtained by taking and recording the pressure of the seated patient twice – or, if practical, thrice – at each of three visits, and then using the average value. These measurements are often less stressful when made by an adequately trained nurse or physician's assistant than when made by a physician. In general, blood pressures taken in various positions are done primarily in a search for secondary hypertension and are not necessary for evaluation of mild hypertension; however, it is appropriate to check the 'standing pressure' to be certain that there is no unusual postural response.

Because of the importance of usual pressure to the decision about lifelong treatment, it should be based on as many measurements as possible. The most convincing usual pressure is obtained if the patient or a member of his family takes and records his blood pressure at home at least twice daily for whatever period is required to obtain a stable value. Ordinarily the weekly average of home pressures will trend slowly downward for at least the first two to four weeks; eventually it will reach a relatively constant level which can be taken as a reasonable approximation of the usual pressure. If home blood pressure readings are to be used, detailed instruction on the technique of taking blood pressure and a subsequent check for accuracy of home measurements are mandatory. In addition, adequate counseling regarding isolated high or low readings must be provided so that single observations will not be overinterpreted.

History pertinent to the decision of how mild hypertension should be managed includes: (1) age, race and sex because of their relationship to incidence of cardiovascular disease; (2) family history of hypertension or its complications, with emphasis on heart attack, stroke or kidney failure before age 50; (3) past medical history of any of these three or other cardiovascular-renal problems, including transient ischemic attacks, congestive heart failure, angina pectoris, arryhthmia, or renal disease; (4) 'risk factors' for hypertensive complications, specifically for coronary artery disease, i.e., cigarette smoking, hypercholesterolemia, diabetes mellitus and obesity.

Physical examination should pay particular attention to: (1) Ocular fundi – where tortuosity and spasm, either localized or generalized, are the best indications of the extent of the hypertensive process. Mild hypertension is not associated with hemorrhages, exudates or papilledema. (2) Chest – where arrhythmia, cardiomegaly without anatomic cause or pulmonary edema suggest a compromised myocardium. Even though such compromise is not likely to result from mild hypertension alone, it represents a very real 'risk factor' for the patient. (3) Extremities – where edema again suggests compromised cardiac function, neurologic deficits may represent residua of a stroke (if localized and motor) or diabetic neuropathy (if symmetric and sensory) and peripheral vascular disease can be recognized by poor pulses.

Laboratory data should include: (1) electrocardiogram as the best index of cardiac arrhythmias, hypertrophy and coronary artery disease; (2) urinalysis with a check for proteinuria and glycosuria; (3) creatinine clearance to demonstrate and quantitate renal dysfunction which has not progressed to azotemia. Proteinuria, depressed creatinine clearance or azotemia is likely to be caused by underlying renal disease, since mild hypertension does not ordinarily have a demonstrable effect on the kidney; nonetheless, any of these indicates greatly increased risk of eventual renal failure.

F. Subsequent follow-up

When a patient has been evaluated and found to have mild hypertension, and his other significant risk factors have been assessed, the situation must be explained to him in understandable form, and then a decision as to how to manage the hypertension should be made jointly by the patient and his physician. Two approaches are possible: (1) careful observation with a view to intervention when the risk of hypertensive complications is felt to have reached some predetermined threshold value at which treatment becomes definitively indicated; (2) prompt treatment with a view to lowering the pressure to some predetermined goal, perhaps with some specified limit on the number and extent of the therapeutic modalities to be used.

Obviously, the greater the number and magnitude of risk factors, the greater the incentive to treat rather than merely observe. Since antihypertensive drugs have not been clearly shown to benefit patients with mild hypertension, a period of observation does not seem inappropriate, particularly in young patients with no target organ damage or other risk factors. Such patients are asymptomatic, at least with respect to their hypertension, and it seems very important not to induce side effects or a significant decrease in the quality of life. The physician is certainly indispensable for the evaluation of the risks involved and then to explain the situation to the patient; however the patient is the key factor in making the final decision about treatment, which he must presume will be lifelong with all that this implies. If the patient indicates that he will not comply, attempting treatment will almost surely be an exercise in futility. If the risk of complications appears sufficiently great, however, the physician is obligated to make a maximum effort to persuade his patient to accept therapy.

Observation requires careful monitoring of the patient's pressure at relatively frequent intervals, at least until its stability has been demonstrated. Home blood pressures have the double advantage of providing the best in monitoring at the same time that they involve the patient in his own care and so enhance his compliance. When monitoring is done in the physician's office, visits must be frequent enough that the patient does not feel abandoned, and yet not so frequent that neither patient nor physician can tolerate them over the long term. Observation also requires monitoring of target organ damage – the risk factor that is most likely to progress significantly with time – primarily by periodic electrocardiograms. If the physician feels that treatment is indicated, but the patient declines it, the physican may reasonably accept temporary observation in order to maintain or improve his rapport with the patient until the latter can be cajoled into accepting therapy.

Nonpharmacologic antihypertensive treatment is often espoused because it is thought to be less likely to do harm than pharmacologic treatment; however, this may simply mean that it has little effect – for either good or bad – because by and large most patients pay relatively little attention to it. Although it has great appeal to some patients and to the community, it has never been shown to lower morbidity or mortality. Currently nonpharmacologic therapy generally consists of encouraging the patient to do one or more of the following: lose weight, limit salt intake, exercise regularly, stop smoking and eat a diet low in saturated fat. Losing weight will lower blood pressure, but weight loss is difficult to maintain. There is remarkably little evidence that a limited but attainable restriction of salt intake is beneficial, and even less that exercise induces any chronic decrease in blood pressure. Discontinuation of smoking lowers the risk of cardiovascular complications even though it may have little effect on blood pressure; in contrast, lowering plasma cholesterol seems to have little effect on morbidity or mortality. The most important parameter to follow is probably the level of diastolic pressure, since it can be affected and, at least in the high part of the mildly hypertensive range, such alterations probably affect survival and health. If nonpharmacological therapy – or any other harmless procedure – induces a reduction in pressure to the 'goal' level, it should be continued. If it does not bring the pressure to some specified goal within some specified period, e.g., six months to a year, the choices are to proceed to pharmacologic treatment or to return to careful observation, and again the patient must be involved in the decision.

Drug treatment, as recommended by the Joint National Committee on Detection, Evaluation and Treatment of Hypertension [19], usually begins with a thiazide diuretic. There are few data comparing the relative benefits of long-acting and short-acting diuretics, although administration once daily is obviously desirable. Furosemide and the loop diuretics in general are more potent natriuretic agents, but less potent antihypertensive drugs, perhaps because the thiazides have a weak peripheral vasodilatory effect which becomes significant during long-term use. Potassium-sparing diuretics have no advantages over thiazides except to prevent hypokalemia, e.g., levels below 3 mEq potassium/l plasma. Triampterine, in particular, is much less effective in lowering blood pressure and can lead to hyperkalemia; ameloride may be more effective and less dangerous. For patients without contraindications, beta-blockade is reasonable initial therapy in individuals with recent myocardial infarction [20] or in whom there seems a high risk of imminent myocardial infarction. There is also a basis for using it as the first step drug in patients with 'high renin hypertension' or in young patients with so-called 'hyperdynamic hearts.' To identify high renin hypertension, however, would require 'renin profiling'; although this has sometimes been advocated, it is very expensive and hence generally considered not worthwhile. It should be remembered that beta-blockade is relatively ineffective in blacks and in the elderly.

As a second drug, reserpine offers maximum efficacy at minimum cost; no other drug, when combined with a thiazide, has been shown to be more effective. Quite possibly the efficacy of reserpine depends on its uniquely long biological half-life and the fact that the usual dose of 0.25 mg daily is far more than is needed. A recent VA Cooperative Study reveals that a daily dose of 0.05 mg provides 80% of the antihypertensive effect of the usual maximum dose of 0.25 mg [21]. Thus, the patient who takes only two or three pills weekly may still get maximum benefit. Because both reserpine and thiazide offer once-a-day dosage and because both have very flat dose–response curves, so that titration is unnecessary, combination pills are both logical and available. If a beta-blocking agent has not been used as the first drug, it may be added to thiazide as the second drug. Beta-blocking agents may provide primary protection against recurrent myocardial infarction in high-risk patients [20], and they could have value in preventing first infarctions. If there is an effect on first infarction which involves the general population, the use of beta-blocking agents will be greatly increased, but this will be hard to prove. Other adrenergic-blocking drugs may be used according to the preference of the physician.

A third step drug is rarely, if ever needed for the treatment of mild hypertension. In the United States hydralazine is the only available vasodilator recommended for general use. Minoxidil is similar in action but more potent; the major difficulty with it is fluid retention. It should therefore be used with a 'loop diuretic.' Captopril is the final step three drug; it has a different mechanism of action and is associated with disturbing effects: agranulocytosis and proteinuria.

Compliance is a major problem in mild, asymptomatic and uncomplicated hypertension, particularly for the patient in the younger age group which is mobile and busy and generally considers itself far removed from disease and death. The most effective ways of increasing long-term compliance are genuine concern for the patient by the physician and selfinvolvement in his own treatment by the patient. The value of 'tender loving care' is obvious. In addition, by informing the patient of his goal blood pressure and encouraging him to monitor his pressure, the physician can usually obtain a dedicated ally who will insist on this goal. Almost all hypertension can be controlled by three antihypertensive drugs, and mild hypertension can usually be controlled by one or at the most two. Simple and convenient treatment regimens are very helpful in increasing compliance. Unnecessary drugs, like sedatives and vitamins, and secondary drugs, like potassium and allopurinol, should not be prescribed promiscuously but used only when there are real and sufficient indications. Compliance is improved by drugs that are effective on a once-a-day schedule, by combination in a single pill of drugs that do not require titration, and by using exactly the same pill year in and year out, rather than using generic pills which may vary over a wide range of color, size and shape.

Goal diastolic pressure should traditionally be a value of 90 mmHg or below. HDFP has been used as evidence that the goal diastolic pressure should be in the low 80s, but this is questionable, and it is certainly not indicated unless there are no undesirable side effects. On the other hand, the data from VA Study III [8] make it reasonable to accept a goal above 90 mmHg, choosing the lowest level between 90 and 100 mmHg that can be attained without undesirable effects.

Step-down should always be considered in patients who have had well-controlled blood pressures for some time. About 20% of mildly hypertensive patients may be able to 'step-down' their antihypertensive drugs and discontinue therapy completely; others may be able to decrease but not discontinue therapy. An attempt at step-down should be seriously considered for patients who have been well controlled for two or more years *whenever careful monitoring of the pressure is available*, e.g., if the patient is taking reliable home pressures or if he can obtain frequent blood pressure measurements at his place of work or anywhere else. Without frequent monitoring, stepdown may not be a feasible or safe alternative, despite its obvious appeal.

Basically, the step-down procedure is the reverse of the 'step-care' approach to therapy, with a stepwise decrease in drug intake beginning with the drug at the highest 'step,' which is decreased and finally discontinued. This process is continued until the pressure begins to rise. At that point, the procedure is temporarily discontinued – or, if necessary, therapy is stepped back up to where goal diastolic pressure is again achieved. Step-down is more likely to succeed in warm weather, perhaps due to general vasodilation.

G. Summary

Mild hypertension, defined by a *usual* diastolic pressure of 90–105 mmHg, becomes common after age 35 when it is found in one of six Americans. There is no question that even mild elevations of diastolic pressures are associated with an increased morbidity and mortality, although the increase may not be evident for decades. There are, however, serious unresolved questions about who, when and how to treat. The currently available data suggest that those with *usual* diastolic pressures greater than 95 mmHg deserve pharmacologic therapy unless other measures have established control. There is no convincing evidence to support prompt agressive drug treatment for mild hypertension. Similarly there is no convincing evidence to support the concept of thiazide toxicity. Under the circumstances, it therefore seems appropriate to individualize the decision of whether to treat, basing that decision on the degree of risk and its immediacy, but most importantly on the patient's desires. For the young, uncomplicated, mildly hypertensive patient who is not likely to get into trouble for many years, there is no evidence that prompt treatment is more effective than delayed treatment. Age, target organ damage or other significant risk factors increase the morbidity and mortality rates, and so decrease the margin for error, but there still is no evidence of benefit from treating mild hypertension.

The choices for managng mild hypertension include (1) initial observation with subsequent treatment if needed, or (2) immediate treatment, with the informed patient being the final arbiter. In general he should be treated only if he wants to be treated – and if the thinks he can and will comply. He should not be coaxed or coerced if he is unwilling. Either nonpharmacologic or pharmacologic treatment can be tried. If a treatment is effective, i.e., lowers diastolic pressure to goal without causing changes that the patient does not want to tolerate, it should be continued. If it is ineffective, it ought to be discontinued or increased to the point where it is effective. For treatment, the bottom line is adequate blood pressure control without significant untoward effects.

References

1. Gordon J: Blood pressure of addults by age and sex, United States, 1960–1962. National Center for Health Statistics, Public Health Service (Publication No 1000 – Series 11, No 4), Washington, DC, 1964.
2. Kannel WB, Sarlie P: Hypertension in Framingham. In: Paul O (ed) Epidemiology and control of hypertension. New York, Stratton Intercontinental Medical Book Corp, 1975, p 533.
3. Pooling Project Research Group: Relationship of blood pressure, serum cholesterol, smoking habit, relative weight and ECG abnormalities to incidence of major coronary events: final report of the Pooling Project. J Chronic Dis 31:201, 1978.
4. Hypertension Detection and Follow-up Program Group: Five-year findings of the Hypertension Detection and Follow-up Program. JAMA 242:2562, 1979.
5. Hypertension Detection and Follow-up Program Cooperative Group: Five-year findings of the Hypertension Detection and Follow-up Program. II. Mortality by race-sex and age. JAMA 242:2572, 1979.
6. Veterans Administration Cooperative Study Group on Antihypertensive Agents: Effects of treatment on morbidity in hypertension: results in patients with diastolic blood pressure averaging 90 through 114 mmHg. JAMA 312:1143, 1970.
7. Veterans Administration Cooperative Study Group on Antihypertensive Agents: Effects of treatment on morbidity in hypertension. I. Results in patients with diastolic blood pressures averaging 115 through 129 mmHg. JAMA 202:1028, 1967.
8. Perry HM Jr: Veterans Administration cooperative studies of hypertension. Angiology 29:804, 1978.
9. Labarthe DR: Problems in definition of mild hypertension. In: Perry HM Jr, Smith WM (eds) Mild hypertension: to treat or not to treat. Ann NY Acad Sci 304:3–14, 1978.
10. Taguchi J, Freis E: Partial reduction of blood pressure and prevention of complications in hypertension. N Engl J Med 291:329, 1974.
11. Veterans Administration Cooperative Study Group on Antihypertensive Agents: Return of elevated blood pressure after withdrawal of antihypertensive drugs. Circulation 51:1107, 1975.
12. Thurm RH, Smith WM: On resetting of 'barostats' in hypertensive patients. JAMA 201:301, 1967.
13. Smith WM (for the VA-NHLBI Study Group for Cooperative Studies on Antihypertensive Therapy): Mild hypertension. Treatment of mild hypertension: results of a ten-year intervention trial. Circ Res 40 (Suppl 1):180, 1977.
14. Veterans Administration National Heart, Lung, and Blood Institute Study Group for Cooperative Studies on Antihypertensive Therapy: Mild hypertension, treatment of mild hypertension, preliminary results of a two-year feasibility trial. Circ Res (Suppl 1) 40:180, 1977.

136

15. Perry HM Jr, Schnaper HW, Lavin MA, Goldman AI, Fitz AE, Frohlich ED: Evaluation of drug treatment in mild hypertension. In: Perry HM Jr, Smith WM (eds) Mild hypertension: to treat or not to treat. Ann NY Acad Sci 304:267, 1978.
16. The Australian Therapeutic Trial in Mild Hypertension: Report by the Management Committee. Lancet 1:1261, 1980.
17. Hypertension-Stroke Cooperative Study Group: Effect of antihypertensive treatment on stroke recurrence. JAMA 229:409, 1974.
18. Shurtleff D: Some characteristics related to the incidence of cardiovascular disease and death: Framingham Study, 18-year Follow-up. In: The Framingham Study: an epidemiological investigation of cardiovascular disease. Publication No (NIH) 74-599, Section 30, Washington, DC, US Dept of Health, Education, and Welfare, February 1974.
19. The 1980 Report of the Joint National Committee on Detection, Evaluation, and Treatment of High Blood Pressure. Arch Intern Med 140:1280, 1980.
20. The Norwegian Multicenter Study Group: Timolol-induced reduction in mortality and reinfarction in patients surviving acute myocardial infarction. N Engl J Med 304(14):801–807, 1981.
21. Veterans Administration Cooperative Study Group on Antihypertensive Agents: Low doses of reserpine versus standard doses of reserpine: a randomized double-blind multi-clinic trial in hypertensive patients taking chlorthalidone. JAMA 248:2471–2477, 1982.

9. Antihypertensive drug interactions

ANDREW J. LONIGRO

I. Introduction

The administration of more than one drug to a patient always raises the possibility that the efficacy and/or toxicity of one drug might be altered by the simultaneous or prior administration of the other. When such an event occurs, it is termed a 'drug interaction'. Not unexpectedly, the incidence of drug interactions is directly related to the number of drugs administered; hence, the treatment of the hypertensive patient, which often requires a multiple drug regimen, would be predicted to be associated with a significant number of drug interactions. It should be clearly recognized, however, that not all drug interactions are deleterious; indeed, in the development of therapeutic objectives, advantage can be taken of known drug interactions to provide the patient with the greatest efficacy at the lowest toxicity. In general, when efficacy is improved and toxicity diminished, the drug interaction can be beneficial, whereas, when efficacy is diminished and toxicity enhanced, the interaction is harmful and is referred to as an 'adverse drug interaction' [1].

The question of the overall clinical significance of drug interactions is crucial; the answer to this question is, unfortunately, elusive [2]. In the patient drug interactions may not be recognized, for it may be difficult to distinguish toxic interactions from the primary disease [3–5]. A drug interaction defined in animal studies cannot be simply extrapolated to the clinical situation; considerations relative to species variation in terms of drug metabolism, as well as to the doses used in such animal studies, may render the results difficult to translate into clinical applicability. In addition, all-too-many reports of drug interactions are based on single case reports or on studies of 'normal' volunteers. Often this has resulted in the practitioner being presented with ponderous lists of drug interactions which go mostly unread, let alone remembered. In the initial portion of this chapter, those pharmacological principles considered prerequisite to an understanding of drug interactions will be described in detail. Comprehension of these principles, not only obviates, to a large extent, the need to commit lists of drug interactions to memory, but, in addition, permits many such interactions to be predicted with a reasonable degree of accuracy [6]. The latter portion of this chapter will describe those interactions of antihypertensive agents considered to be of clinical import.

II. Principles of drug interactions

Drugs are usually administered repetitively at regular intervals to achieve and to maintain a constant concentration of the drug in plasma and, hence, in tissues where the drug receptors are located. The *minimum effective concentration* of a drug in plasma is that concentration which produces a large enough tissue concentration such that a desired response is detectable. The intensity of the response will increase as the plasma concentration of the drug increases until a maximum response or toxicity is produced. Hence, maintenance of a *steady-state plasma concentration* above the minimum effective concentration and below the *minimum toxic concentration* is a fundamental goal of applied therapeutics. Most drug interactions are produced by one drug altering the steady-state plasma concentration of another drug such that enhanced toxicity or reduced efficacy results. These interactions have been termed *pharmacokinetic interactions*, viz., those produced by alterations in the absorption, distribution or elimination of one drug by another.

A. Pharmacokinetic interactions

When a drug is administered repetitively at regular intervals, the drug accumulates until the amount of drug absorbed is equal to the amount of drug being eliminated, at which time there is a *steady-state plasma concentration* (C_{ss}). The *time* required to reach C_{ss} for any drug given repetitively is estimated to be four or five half-lives ($t_{\frac{1}{2}}$) of that drug. To determine the actual steady-state concentration requires a more complicated formula:

$$C_{ss} = \frac{(F)\,(D)}{(K_{el})\,(V_d)\,(\Delta t)}$$

where; C_{ss} = steady-state plasma concentration; F = fraction of the dose reaching the general circulation (bioavailability); D = dose; K_{el} = the rate constant of elimination; V_d = the apparent volume of distribution; Δt = dosage interval.

From the above equation, it is clear that with repetitive administration of a drug, the steady-state plasma concentration is a function of (1) the dose, (2) the fraction of the dose reaching the general circulation, (3) the elimination half-life, (4) the apparent volume of distribution and (5) the dosage interval.

1. Drug absorption interactions

Several mechanisms have been described whereby one drug alters the absorption of another [7]. In any consideration of drug absorption, one must distinguish between *extent* and *rate* of drug absorption. A change in the rate of absorption is usually of little consequence during chronic drug therapy. In contrast, a change in the fraction of a dose of a drug reaching the general circulation can be of major importance because of the resultant change in the steady-state plasma concentration of the drug. Drug interactions which alter absorption generally result in decreased efficacy rather than increased toxicity. Thus, most of these interactions produce a decrease in the extent of drug absorption; i.e., a decrease in the fraction of the dose reaching the general circulation, and, thereby, a reduction in the steady-state plasma concentration.

2. Distribution interactions

After absorption into the blood stream, a drug is distributed throughout the body, the degree of distribution being dependent upon several factors including (1) the blood/tissue partition coefficient for the particular drug which is generally a function of lipid solubility and, hence, its ability to pass through membranes, (2) the degree of binding to plasma proteins and to tissue macromolecules, (3) regional blood flows and (4) active transport and storage mechanisms. Although most drugs exhibit a nonuniform distribution, determined largely by their lipid solubility and their ability to pass through membranes, the range of distribution may vary from confinement to the vascular system (those drugs avidly bound to plasma proteins) to uniform distribution (those drugs of low molecular weight which are water soluble) to sequestration within a particular cell, tissue or organ (active transport and storage).

a. Protein binding. A drug may bind tightly or loosely to a plasma protein such as albumin by means of electrostatic attraction (ionic binding), hydrogen binding or van der Waals forces [8]. The albumin-bound fraction of a drug is pharmacologically inactive, but that fraction is usually protected from biotransformation and from glomerular filtration. When appreciable protein binding occurs, the biological half-life and, hence, the duration of action are prolonged. Mathematically, this relationship, which obeys the law of mass action, is described as:

$$[D] + [P] \rightleftharpoons [D - P]$$

where: $[D]$ = the concentration of 'free' or 'unbound' drug; $[P]$ = the concentration of protein; $[D - P]$ = the concentration of drug-protein complex.

Thus, as the plasma concentration (free *plus* bound drug) rises, the concentration of free drug will increase slowly initially and then more sharply as the proteins become saturated. It is important to recognize that only free drug can diffuse into tissues, the drug-protein complex being too large to cross membranes. Hence, only free drug can gain access to and interact with drug receptors. It is the free drug, therefore, which may be considered the active form of the drug. Hence, the concentration of a free drug will determine whether no effects, desired therapeutic effects or toxic effects occur. It would be predicted that drugs with the same protein binding sites would compete, one with the other, for those sites. Whether one agent would be able to displace the other is determined by their concentrations and relative affinities for the sites. In order for competitive interactions at protein binding sites to alter the concentration of free drug in plasma, certain criteria must be met. First, the bound fraction should constitute the major fraction of the drug in the blood [9]. Secondly, the volume of distribution should be small so that the drug displaced from the protein will add enough to the free fraction such that its concentrations are significantly altered. Thirdly, drug levels in the blood should approach saturation of the available binding sites. Relatively few drugs satisfy these criteria in normal therapeutic usage.

When free drug diffuses across membranes, it may or may not bind to tissue macromolecules. When drugs are bound to tissue proteins, a new factor is introduced into the equilibrium reaction, shown above; that is, free drug (D) can now interact with tissue macromolecules (M) to form drug-macromolecule complexes (D − M) such that:

tissue	membrane	plasma
$[D - M] \rightleftharpoons [M] + [D]$	$\rightleftharpoons$	$[D] + [P] \rightleftharpoons [D - P]$

Thus, the amount of free drug in plasma will now be influenced by its avidity for the tissue macromolecule; indeed, the plasma can be effectively cleared of drug if the binding to tissue macromolecules is great enough.

b. Active transport and drug storage. Most drugs traverse cellular membranes passively, i.e., the process does not require the expenditure of energy and occurs because of a concentration gradient across the membrane [10]. With passive diffusion the intracellular concentrations of free drug can never exceed the plasma concentration. Some drugs are, however, transported into tissues by energy-requiring processes [11]. Active transport can be inhibited by reduced temperature and by drugs, it is saturable and may occur against a concentration gradient, leading to intracellular levels of the drug greater than the plasma concentration and, most importantly, the process is subject to competitive inhibition by related compounds. Although active transport and storage does not occur for most drugs, such mechanisms are of paramount importance in the discussion of antihypertensive drugs. Most of these active transport processes occur in the neurones of the peripheral sympathetic nervous system or in the central nervous system. Hence, many of those antihypertensive agents which must gain access to the nervous system do so through active transport. There are numerous examples of drugs used to treat hypertensive patients which are affected by concomitant administration of other agents which prevent their active uptake into the nervous system.

c. Apparent volume of distribution. Estimates of the apparent volume of distribution (V_d) of a drug describe the amount of drug in the total body relative to that in plasma at any one time and give us an indication of its distribution within the body [12]. Thus, if the apparent volume of distribution were small, e.g., 2–3 liters for an adult, this would suggest that the drug was confined to the vascular compartment; whereas a large volume of distribution, e.g., 30–50 liters would indicate concentration of the drug at some storage site. Mathematically, the volume of distribution is described by the equation:

$$V_d = \frac{D}{C_0}$$

where: V_d = apparent volume of distribution; D = the dose; C_0 = the concentration of the drug in plasma at zero time (obtained by extrapolation of the plasma concentration vs. time curve after intravenous administration or rapid oral administration of a drug).

3. Elimination interactions

Drugs are eliminated from the body, in large part, by renal, biliary, intestinal and pulmonary mechanisms [13]. Water soluble drugs are excreted mainly unchanged through the kidney and will reach toxic concentrations when renal function is impaired. Lipid soluble drugs, on the other hand, must be metabolized to water soluble compounds before they can be excreted in the urine. The metabolites formed are usually less active than the parent compound. Although drugs are metabolized in the lung, the kidneys and the intestine, the primary site of drug metabolism is the liver. A variety of biochemical transformations occur to render a drug inactive and to produce water soluble metabolites. For example, polar groups may be introduced into the drug molecule by oxidation, reduction or hydrolysis. In addition, drugs may be conjugated with glucuronic acid, sulphate, glycine or other groups. Drug-metabolizing enzymes are chiefly associated with the smooth endoplasmic reticulum. Oxidation is the most important metabolic pathway and is catalyzed by enzymes present in the endoplasmic reticulum. These reactions include aliphatic oxidation, aromatic hydroxylation, N- and O-dealkylation, S-demethylation, deamination, sulfoxide formation, desulfuration, N-oxidation and N-hydroxylation. Cytochrome P_{450}, a hemoprotein, serves as a terminal oxidase in a complex chain of events and is directly involved in the binding of the drug to the microsomes. There are three clinically important features of cytochrome P_{450}-mediated oxidation [14]: (1) nonspecificity, (2) large potential for drug interactions, particularly induction of metabolism, and (3) marked inter- and intra-species variation.

There are many other factors which affect the rate of drug metabolism such as genetic influences, age, sex, pregnancy, liver disease, environment, diet, alcohol ingestion and other drugs. Since the hepatic microsomal enzyme has a relatively low degree of substrate specificity, many drugs can compete with one another for oxidation. A number of other drugs can bring about an increase in the activity of the hepatic microsomal drug metabolizing system. Increased enzyme activity can only be produced by treatment in vivo and not by exposure of microsomes to drugs in vitro.

The rate of change in concentration of a drug is, in most instances, described mathematically as:

$$dC/dt = -K_{el} C$$

Where: C = concentration; K_{el} = the rate constant of elimination; t = time; and $K_{el} = 0.693/t_{\frac{1}{2}}$.

The elimination of a drug is best described by its *clearance*, which is defined as the volume of plasma cleared of drug by elimination per unit time. Total clearance is the sum of clearances by renal and hepatic mechanisms (and other minor mechanisms).

$$\text{Clearance} = (K_{el})\,(V_d) = \frac{0.693\,V_d}{t_{\frac{1}{2}}}$$

b. Pharmacodynamic interactions

Drug receptors are molecular structures at or near cellular membranes and represent the chemical entity of the cell with which drugs interact. A single receptor can be occupied by only one molecule of a drug at one time. When a drug contacts a receptor, the resulting drug-receptor complex may be very short-lived, dissociating rapidly to form unoccupied receptor and free drug; on the other hand, the relationship of drug to receptor may be prolonged if there is chemical binding between them, resulting in irreversible interactions. To produce an effect, a drug must first have an 'affinity' for the receptor; secondly, the drug must have 'intrinsic' activity, viz., it must produce a response. The greater the intrinsic activity, the fewer the number of receptors will have to be occupied to produce a given response. Two drugs may act on the same receptor to produce enhanced or inhibited effects. The magnitude of the observed effects is dependent on the relative intrinsic activities, affinities and doses of the two drugs. Two drugs may act on different receptors to produce either enhanced or blunted effects. Such an interaction often results in an effect which is greater (potentiation) or less (inhibition) than the sum of the component effects.

III. Antihypertensive drug interactions

In the formulation of a therapeutic regimen to treat the hypertensive patient, advantage is taken of one or more drug interactions in order to enhance efficacy and/or to reduce toxicity. When blood pressure is altered in the hypertensive patient through the administration of antihypertensive drugs, compensatory mechanisms, effected through alterations in cardiac output and total peripheral resistance, will be set into motion to return blood pressure to its abnormally high value. Successful management of the hypertensive patient must address not only blood pressure reduction, but also control of the pathophysiological processes which are operative or set into motion by the application of therapy. In the remainder of this chapter, those drug interactions which are beneficial as well as those which are detrimental will be discussed.

A. Diuretic agents

1. The benzothiadiazides (thiazides)

Although thiazide diuretics have been used extensively in the management of the hypertensive patient, considerable debate regarding their mechanism of action persists. The antihypertensive effects of thiazide diuretics most likely reside in their capacity to affect movement of sodium ion across membranes resulting in either a reduced cardiac output secondary to natriuresis and diuresis (reduction of intravascular volume) and/or changes in disposition of sodium ion at the level of the arteriolar smooth muscle membrane to produce vasodilation and reduced sensitivity to vasoconstrictor stimuli. The mechanism notwithstanding, thiazide diuretics potentiate the hypotensive action of the other antihypertensive drugs [15] permitting lower doses of the latter agents and, thereby, avoiding many of their side effects which are dose-dependent. The thiazides, when given together with other agents to reduce blood pressure, represent a prime example of a drug interaction characterized by enhanced efficacy with reduced toxicity, i.e., a beneficial drug interaction.

The thiazide diuretics produce a predictable increase in potassium excretion because of activation of a renin-angiotensin-aldosterone system and increased delivery of sodium to the distal tubule. This mechanism may, on occasion, lead to frank hypokalemia. When a patient is on concomitant cardiac glycoside therapy, the potential exists for enhanced digitalis intoxication. An increased incidence of digitalis toxicity in patients receiving potassium-depleting diuretics has been often documented [16, 17]. Digitalis and potassium compete for myocardial Na^+, K^+-ATPase. In the presence of hypokalemia, exaggerated effects of digitalis may be seen resulting in cardiac arrhythmias.

In order to be effective as a diuretic agent, the thiazide diuretics must gain entrance to the renal tubule which they do through the organic acid transport mechanism located in the proximal tubule. This secretory mechanism is blocked by probenecid; hence, the diuretic and natriuretic actions of thiazide diuretics may be inhibited when probenecid is given simultaneously, an event which probably occurs all too frequently since thiazides may produce hyperuricemia. It must be remembered that any agent which uses this active tubular transport mechanism, of which there are many [18], might interfere with the actions of thiazide diuretics.

2. Potassium-sparing diuretics

The competitive receptor antagonist of aldosterone, spironolactone, which is frequently used in conjunction with other diuretic agents and less frequently as a sole agent in the management of cirrhosis with ascites and as a diagnostic tool for evaluation of possible primary aldosteronism, when used together with potassium supplementation, will almost always result in dangerous elevations of serum potassium levels. Similarly, toxic levels of potassium will result when either spironolactone or potassium supplementation are given together with other potassium-sparing-diuretics such as triamterene or amiloride.

B. Agents which block adrenergic receptors

1. Alpha-receptor blocking agents

The inhibitors of alpha-receptors have had limited clinical applicability in the past largely because of the attendant reflex tachycardia which was out of proportion to the degree of blood pressure lowering. It is now recognized that there are two alpha-receptors, namely, the $alpha_1$-receptor, which is postjunctional (postsynaptic) in location and which, when stimulated, produces vasoconstriction and the $alpha_2$-receptor which is prejunctional (presynaptic) in location and which when stimulated. inhibits the release of the neurotransmitter [19]. Thus, under physiological conditions, when norepinephrine is released from postganglionic sympathetic nerves, $alpha_1$-receptors are stimulated on the effector organ to produce vasoconstriction and $alpha_2$-receptors are stimulated at the prejunctional site to inhibit release of norepinephrine; hence, under normal conditions norepinephrine modulates its own release from the nerve ending. In the presence of an agent which blocked both $alpha_1$ and $alpha_2$-receptors, such as phenoxybenzamine or phentolamine, excessive amounts of norepinephrine were released because of the $alpha_2$ blockade. In spite of the excessive amounts of norepinephrine present, blood pressure fell because of $alpha_1$ blockade; however, the beta-receptors of the myocardium which when stimulated, produce positive inotropic and chronotropic response, were subjected to the excessive release of norepinephrine from the nerve ending; hence, tachycardia and palpitation ensued. With the advent of beta-receptor blocking agents, these reflex cardiac effects of alpha-receptor blockade can be controlled. The clinical use of alpha and beta receptor blocking agents together is an example of two drugs acting on different receptors to produce a highly desirable therapeutic effect; i.e., the antihypertensive properties of alpha-receptor blockade will be enhanced and the undesirable side effects will be diminished.

Two other agents which interfere with alpha-adrenergic mechanisms should be mentioned at this points; prazosin is a selective inhibitor of alpha$_1$-adrenergic receptors and because of its relative lack of effects on alpha$_2$-receptors, reflex tachycardia is not a major problem with the clinical use of this drug. The drug, labetalol, which has been used extensively in Europe for the treatment of hypertension possesses both alpha- and beta-receptor inhibiting properties; hence, reflex tachycardia does not occur [21].

2. Beta-receptor blocking agents

Beta-receptor blocking agents are used extensively in the treatment of the hypertensive patient. Most of the interactions with other therapeutic agents have been beneficial; thus, when used in conjunction with alpha-receptor blockers (vide supra) or with direct vasodilators (vide infra), antihypertensive efficacy has been enhanced and toxicity diminished.

Care must be taken when beta-receptor blocking agents are used in patients who are being treated with hypoglycemic agents. Glycogenolysis is, in part, stimulated by catecholamines via beta$_2$-receptors. Thus, in the presence of hypoglycemia, compensatory increases in blood sugar mediated by catecholamine-induced glycogenolysis will be blocked in the patient on beta-receptor blocking agents. The hypoglycemia will be more severe and of longer duration. The situation is made potentially more dangerous because several of the warning signs of hypoglycemia, such as tachycardia and muscular tremor, may be blocked in the presence of beta-blockade.

As described later in this section, both clonidine and alpha-methyldopa, the latter through formation of alpha-methyl norepinephrine, lower blood pressure through stimulation of alpha-receptors, their effects being most predominant on alpha$_2$-receptors located either within the central nervous system or on peripheral nerves to inhibit efferent sympathetic mechanism. In the presence of beta-receptor blockade, the possibility exists that stimulation of the alpha$_1$-receptors by clonidine or alpha-methyl norepinephrine, will result in vasoconstriction and hypertension. Indeed one such case has been reported [22]. Whether this interaction occurs more frequently than the literature would suggest is unknown.

Finally since cardiac contractility is, in part, dependent on beta-receptor stimulation, patients with compromised myocardial function may develop heart failure when treated with beta-receptor blocking agents. If digitalis is given and

A-V dissociation should occur, the beta-blocker may depress the ventricular rhythm leading to cardiac arrest.

C. Vasodilating agents

The arteriolar vasodilating drugs, namely, hydralazine, diazoxide, nitroprusside and minoxidil act directly on vascular smooth muscle to reduce vascular resistance and, thereby, to lower blood pressure. Since these agents do not interfere with nervous mechanisms of blood pressure control (cardiovascular reflexes) when they are used alone to lower blood pressure, mechanisms are set into motion to return blood pressure to its abnormally high values. Thus, reflex tachycardia, increased myocardial contractility, increased plasma renin activity and retention of salt and water are all predictable side effects of these agents. These may result in coronary insufficiency becoming symptomatic, i.e., development of angina pectoris or frank myocardial infarction; increasing refractoriness to their antihypertensive effects; and even heart failure [23]. Hence, these agents should never be used alone in the management of the hypertensive patient; rather, advantage should be taken of known beneficial drug interactions to prevent the unwanted and sometime dangerous untoward effects. A rational therapeutic regimen would include agents which block the reflex responses, such as methyldopa, clonidine or beta-receptor blocking agents [24]. Hydralazine, an effective antihypertensive agent, was almost discarded until it was recognized that it is a highly effective antihypertensive agent when used in conjunction with other drugs to block its unwanted side effects. Diazoxide, the use of which is generally limited to the hypertensive emergency, is a nondiuretic thiazide. Its side effects include excessive hypotension, reflex sympathetic stimulation, hyperglycemia and marked salt and water retention [25]. Because of its salt and water retention, it is often recommended that the drug be given with a diuretic agent such as furosemide. The drug will displace Warfarin from albumin-binding sites [26] thus increasing anticoagulation. Moreover, diazoxide antagonizes the hypoglycemic actions of sulfonylureas and increases the hyperglycemic actions of thiazide diuretics primarily because it inhibits insulin release from the pancreas. In addition, diazoxide has been reported to decrease plasma levels of phenytoin in man presumably because of increased metabolism of the latter agent.

Minoxidil, recently released for clinical use, is a potent antihypertensive agent, which in addition to the side effects described above for all vasodilators, produces exaggerated fluid retention and hypertrichosis. Adverse drug interactions have not yet been reported.

Sodium nitroprusside is a potent antihypertensive agent which is available only for intravenous use. It has a rapid onset of action and an extremely short biological half-life. The major side effects include hypotension and, on rare occasion, thiocyanate toxicity. Patients receiving other antihypertensive therapy may exhibit enhanced sensitivity to the action of nitroprusside.

D. Other antiadrenergic drugs

1. Guanethidine

The antihypertensive agent guanethidine, which lowers blood pressure by impairing release of transmitter from postganglionic sympathetic nerves, must gain access to the neuron via the amine transport mechanism before it can deplete the vesicles of norepinephrine and thereby reduce blood pressure. Several substances, such as sympathomimetic amines, phenoxybenzamine, phenothiazines, tricyclic antidepressants and cocaine, interfere with the amine transport process, thereby preventing entrance of guanethidine into the postganglionic sympathetic nerve and reducing its antihypertensive effects. In addition, patients treated chronically with guanethidine develop a functional denervation hypersensitivity and may demonstrate an enhanced hypertensive response to ephedrine and epinephrine [27].

2. Monoamine oxidase inhibitors

In the past, monoamine oxidase (MAO) inhibitors were commonly used in the treatment of hypertensive patients, although use of these agents for that purpose is no longer recommended. When MAO inhibitors are given not only will MAO be inhibited, but many other enzymes as well [28]. Hence, not only will the biological activities of sympathomimetic amines be prolonged, but, in addition, the hepatic metabolism of many drugs will be impaired. Indirect acting sympathomimetic amines such as tyramine and amphetamine will exhibit potentiated effects following the use of MAO inhibitors.

When foods rich in tyramine, such as cheese or wine, are ingested by a patient being treated with a MAO inhibitor, the possibility exists for a most serious drug interaction leading to a hypertensive crisis. Thus, the ingested tyramine will not be metabolized by the liver, but will enter into the general circulation and, since it is an indirect-acting sympathomimetic amine, will promote release of the supranormal amounts of catecholamines contained in the postganglionic sympathetic nerves and, thereby, produce marked elevations of blood pressure [29]. Similar syndromes may occur when MAO inhibitors are used with sympathomimetic amines, methyldopa, dopamine, reserpine and guanethidine.

3. Clonidine

Clonidine is an antihypertensive agent which lowers blood pressure by reducing sympathetic tone. Although clonidine stimulates alpha-adrenergic receptors, it exerts an antihypertensive effect most likely because its primary site of action is within the central nervous system. The tricyclic antidepressant, desipramine, abolishes the hypotensive effect of clonidine [30].

4. Alpha-methyldopa

Alpha-methyldopa, which lowers blood pressure by affecting central mechanisms, is remarkably free of reported drug interactions, the most important potential one being that reported with beta-receptor blocking agents [22]. In addition, alpha-methyldopa competes with the renal tubular reabsorption of amino acids, which may lead to aminoaciduria.

In summary, most of the drug interactions known to exist for antihypertensive agents are of benefit in planning a therapeutic regimen. Other drug interactions, if not appreciated, could have disasterous consequences. An understanding of the pharmacology of the individual agent, as well as an appreciation of the principles of drug interaction will, on most occasions, allow a prediction of a possible drug interaction.

References

1. Boston Collaborative Drug Surveillance Program: Adverse drug interactions. JAMA 220:1238, 1972.
2. Crooks J, Stevenson IH, Shepherd AMM, Moir DC: The clinical significance and importance of drug interactions. In: Grahame-Smith DG (ed) Drug interactions. Baltimore, University Park Press, 1977, p 3.
3. Melmon KL: Preventable drug reactions – causes and cures. N Engl J Med 284:1361, 1971.
4. Karch FE, Lasagna L: Adverse drug reactions. A critical review. JAMA 234:1236, 1975.
5. Brater DC, Morrelli HF: Cardiovascular drug interactions. Annu Rev Pharmacol Toxicol 17:293, 1977.
6. Prescott LF: Clinically important drug interactions. In: Avery GS (ed) Drug treatment. Principles and practice of clinical pharmacology and therapeutics. New York, Adis Press, 1980, p 236.
7. Koch-Weser J: Bioavailability of drugs. N Engl J Med 291:233; 503, 1974.
8. Ma JKH, Jun HW, Luzzi LA: Determination of equilibrium constants and binding capacities using a modified Scatchard method in drug-protein binding studies. J Pharm Sci 62:2038, 1973.
9. Koch-Weser J, Sellers EM: Binding of drugs to serum albumin. N Engl J Med 294:311, 1976.
10. Brodie BB: Physico-chemical factors in drug absorption. In: Burns TB (ed) Absorption and metabolism of drugs. Baltimore, Williams & Wilkins, 1964, p 16.
11. Boullin DJ: Drug interactions involving cellular transport and storage mechanisms. In: Grahame-Smith DG (ed) Drug interactions. Baltimore, University Park Press, 1977, p 57.
12. Sjogvist F, Borga O, L'E Orme M: Fundamentals of clinical pharmacology. In: Avery GS (ed) Drug treatment. Principles and practice of clinical pharmacology and therapeutics. New York, Adis Press, 1980, p 1.
13. Creasey WA: Drug disposition in humans. The basis of clinical pharmacology. New York, Oxford University Press, 1979.
14. Burns JJ, Conney AH: Enzyme stimulation and inhibition in the metabolism of drugs. Proc R Soc Med 58:955, 1965.
15. Dustan HP, Tarazi RC, Bravo EL: Dependence of arterial pressure on intravascular volume in

treated hypertensive patients. N Engl J Med 288:861, 1972.

16. Hurwitz N, Wade OL: Intensive hospital monitoring of adverse reactions to drugs. Br Med J 1:531, 1969.

17. Shapiro S, Slone D, Lewis GP, Jick H: The epidemiology of digoxin. J Chronic Dis 22:361, 1969.

18. Prescott LF: Mechanisms of renal excretion of drugs. Br J Anaesth 44:246, 1972.

19. Westfall TC: Local regulation of adrenergic neurotransmission. Physiol Rev 57:659, 1977.

20. Oates HF, Graham RM, Stokes GS: Mechanism of the hypotensive action of prazosin. Arch Int Pharmacodyn Ther 227:41, 1977.

21. Levy GP, Richards DA: Labetalol. In: Scriabine A (ed) Pharmacology of antihypertensive drugs. New York, Raven Press, 1980.

22. Nies AS, Shand DG: Hypertensive response to propranolol in a patient treated with methyldopa – a proposed mechanism. Clin Pharmacol Ther 14:823, 1973.

23. Ablad B: A study of the mechanism of the hemodynamic effects of hydralazine in man. Acta Pharmacol Toxicol (Copenh) 20 (Suppl 1):1–53, 1963.

24. Gilmore E, Weil J, Chidsey C: Treatment of essential hypertension with a new vasodilator in combination with beta-adrenergic blockade. N Engl J Med 282:521, 1970.

25. Thomson AE, Nickerson M, Gaskell PI, Grahame GR: Clinical observations on an anti-hypertensive chlorothiazide analogue devoid of diuretic activity. Can Med Assoc J 87:1306, 1962.

26. Sellers EM, Koch-Weser J: Influence of intravenous injection rate on protein binding and vascular activity of diazoxide. Ann NY Acad Sci 226:319, 1973.

27. Mitchell JR, Oates JA: Guanethidine and related agents. I. Mechanism of the selective blockade of adrenergic neurons and its antagonism by drugs. J Pharmacol Exp Ther 172:100–107, 1970.

28. Costa E, Sandler M: Monoamine oxidases – New vistas, advances in biochemical psycho-pharmacology, Vol 5. New York, Raven Press, 1972.

29. Ayd FJ Jr, Blackwell B: Discoveries in biological psychiatry. Philadelphia, J.B. Lippincott Co, 1970.

30. Pettinger WA: Clonidine, a new anti-hypertensive drug. N Engl J Med 293:1179, 1975.

10. Complications of hypertension and their relation to therapy

H. MITCHELL PERRY, JR. and WILLIAM H. NEAL

I. Introduction

In general people do not die of high blood pressure itself but of its complications. Today most of these complications are considered to be the result of arteriosclerosis and involve the heart or the head: myocardial infarction or thrombotic brain infarction. These so-called arteriosclerotic complications of mild and moderate hypertension have become relatively more frequent as the overall severity of hypertension has decreased during the last few decades. In the past, when severe hypertension was more common, complications, related more directly to elevated blood pressure, were also more common. These complications were renal failure, cerebral hemorrhage and congestive heart failure in the presence of an elevated pressure.

The three major topics considered in this chapter are as follows:

1. Major complications of hypertension: the conditions under which they occur, their frequency and their course. The treatment designed to prevent them is discussed under pharmacologic therapy in Chapters 4–6.

2. Antihypertensive therapy after the occurrence of complications: how useful is it, when is it indicated and finally how does it differ from the standard therapy described in Chapters 4–6.

3. Complications of therapy itself: When dealing with pharmacologically active agents, complications of treatment are bound to occur, and these complications merit discussion since their frequency and severity bear on who should be treated and how enthusiastically.

II. Complications, hypertensive and arteriosclerotic

The major complications associated with hypertension are renal failure, intracerebral hemorrhage, heart failure, myocardial infarction and atherothrombotic brain infarction. The first three are considered true hypertensive complications and occur in patients with severe hypertension, while the other two are really arteriosclerotic complications that develop as a result of long-established and usually mild hypertension. In addition to the major complications, there are less severe and less persistent manifestations of hypertension such as angina pectoris and transient ischemic attacks, which could be considered warnings of major complications to come. There are also asymptomatic indications of potential problems, such as progression to more severe hypertension and development of electrocardiographic evidence of left ventricular hypertrophy.

A. Hypertensive complications of severe high blood pressure

Renal failure can either precede and cause hypertension, a course of events which is not considered here, or it can be an end result of severe hypertension; the latter type of renal failure is a true complication and does warrant discussion here. When malignant hypertension was more frequent, renal failure was the cause of death for more than half of untreated patients with that diagnosis. Once a diagnosis of malignant hypertension was made, the process was rapidly progressive, with a median survival time of less than six months. The pathologic hallmark of malignant or accelerated hypertension is fibrinoid necrosis of the arterioles throughout the body, but particularly in the kidney. Lesser hypertension is associated with a different, more slowly progressive renal lesion, arteriolar nephrosclerosis, which is characterized by gradual diminution in the size and function of the kidneys. Although some degree of arteriolar nephrosclerosis occurs with any long-standing hypertension, it seldom progresses to renal failure and demise unless the hypertension is severe.

Most strokes result from (intra)cerebral hemorrhage or (athero)thrombotic brain infarction. The former tends to be associated with severe hypertension, the latter with moderate or mild hypertension. According to data from the Framingham Study [1], thrombotic strokes are four times as common as hemorrhagic strokes; however, this predominance may partly be due to the fact that with the milder, less rapidly progressive thrombotic strokes, more patients survive to reach the hospital and are thus included in the statistics. Hemorrhagic strokes can rupture either into the subarachnoid space or into the substance of the brain. Subarachnoid hemorrhages are apparently the more common, but the typical hemorrhagic stroke of severe hypertension is intracerebral and is manifested by sudden appearance of a neurologic deficit, usually of severe degree. It often progresses rapidly to coma and death. Characteristically there is bloody spinal fluid, which has been used as a criterion to distinguish hemorrhagic from thrombotic strokes. Thrombotic strokes manifest similar symptoms, but they tend to be milder and less rapidly progressive.

Before effective antihypertensive treatment became available in the early 1950s, congestive heart failure was apparently the most common cause of death among hypertensive patients. Yet the human heart is a very effective pump which does not fail unless the hypertension is very prolonged and severe or the heart is seriously compromised by a separate pathologic process. Severe hypertension can now be treated and controlled, and thus fatal heart failure in hypertension should occur only when mild hypertension is accompanied by significant underlying disease, usually arteriosclerotic coronary disease.

B. Arteriosclerotic complications of moderate and mild hypertension

Although myocardial infarctions, like thrombotic brain infarctions, are really arteriosclerotic events, more than half of them occur in mild hypertensives who have had their disease long enough for significant arteriosclerosis to have developed. In addition to typical myocardial infarction, coronary artery disease can be manifested by angina pectoris from symptomatic but reversible myocardial ischemia or by asymptomatic electrocardiographic changes. In the United States an estimated 1.5 million myocardial infarctions occur annually. Half of recognized infarctions are recurrent attacks. Death within three weeks occurs in 30% of subjects with their first infarction but in 50% of subjects with recurrent infarctions. Since 1900 there has been a marked change in the pattern of myocardial infarction. Figure 1 indicates the United States mortality, from heart disease corrected for age, during the last 80 years. Although there have been

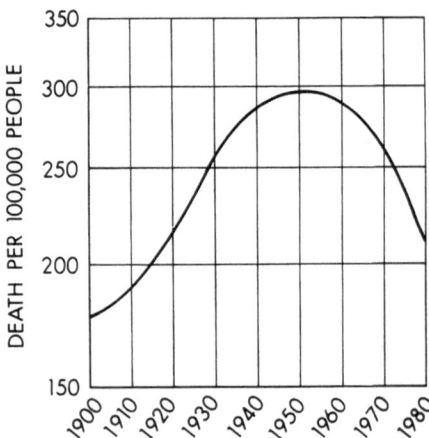

Figure 1. Annual mortality from 'heart disease' in the United States from 1900 to 1980 (visually smoothed curve corrected for the change in age of the population). The recent changes in mortality are largely due to what is here termed 'myocardial infarction.' The heart disease rubric was used to avoid problems associated with changes in the official terminology. Thus, 'angina pectoris' was replaced by 'diseases of the coronary arteries' in 1930, by 'arteriosclerotic heart disease' in 1949, and by 'ischemic heart disease' in 1968 [2].

some changes in terminology during this period, the primary cause of death has been myocardial infarction. After reaching a maximum in the 1950s and 60s, the mortality fell 30% during the 1960s [2]. The decline did not happen everywhere at once; it began in California in the late 1950s, long before it appeared in most of the rest of the country, and gradually spread, with the southeast being the last area to be involved. The explanation for this decrease is unknown, but we must be doing something right.

Although thrombotic brain infarction and myocardial infarction are both generally considered arteriosclerotic complications, they sometimes behave differently. For instance, antihypertensive treatment prevents most strokes but seems to have little effect on the incidence of myocardial infarction. There may be additional, poorly understood differences in the apparently similar arteriosclerotic complications of mild and moderate hypertension, with those of mild hypertension being less responsive to treatment than those of moderate hypertension.

III. Course of hypertension and its complications

A. Natural history of untreated hypertension

The natural history of untreated hypertension is known from studies conducted before effective drug treatment was available. One of the last such studies was reported in 1950 by Smith, Odel and Kernohan, who selected 376 cases of varyingly severe untreated hypertension from the Mayo Clinic autopsy records [3]. Using Keith, Wagener and Barker's severity criteria based on findings in the ocular fundi, the 376 patients were divided into four groups (Table 1). The cause

Table 1. Cause of death for varyingly severe hypertension

Keith Wagener and Barker Fundal groups	Causes of death					Mean age at death (years)
	Congestive heart failure	Coronary heart disease	Cerebro-vascular accident	Uremia	Other non cardio-vascular causes	
Group I	21	7	9	3	60	62
Group II	26	20	17	2	35	60
Group III	39	12	18	16	15	54
Group IV	21	1	16	59	3	45

Legend: The table lists the percentages of patients dying of various cardiovascular causes as a function of the severity of their hypertension (based on Keith Wagener and Barker fundal changes). Cerebrovascular accidents include both hemorrhagic and thrombotic strokes. Data are from a study by Smith, Odel and Kernohan of a Mayo Clinic series of untreated hypertensives [3].

of death was strongly dependent on the severity of hypertension. Most patients with mild hypertension died of causes unrelated to cardiovascular disease, such as pneumonia or automobile accidents; whereas most patients with malignant hypertension died of renal failure.

As the severity of hypertension increased, the percentage of cardiovascular deaths increased and of other deaths decreased. Arteriosclerotic complications appeared first in the form of myocardial infarctions and thrombotic strokes; however, with severe hypertension, the complications were primarily hypertensive, renal failure and hemorrhagic stroke. Congestive heart failure was common with hypertension of all degrees of severity. Presumably, however, for mild hypertension, the basis of the failure was underlying coronary artery disease, whereas, for more severe and rapidly progressive hypertension, arteriosclerosis had had less time to develop and the cardiac failure was primarily due to the very high pressure.

In addition to differences in cause of death, severity of hypertension is strongly related to both length of survival and age at death. Severe hypertension is a disease of youth and its survival time is short, for malignant hypertension an average of less than six months from time of diagnosis. This combination of young patients and rapid demise gave an average age at death of 45 years for malignant hypertension. Mild hypertension, in contrast, is often found in somewhat older individuals, usually appearing in the forties or fifties and its average survival time is measured in decades. Finally, to complete the contrast between the mildest and most severe types of hypertension, at least 30 million people in the United States are currently estimated to have mild hypertension but fewer than 3000 have malignant hypertension.

Perera, in a study that began long before antihypertensive drugs became available, followed 500 untreated hypertensives of all degrees of severity (ranging down to casual diastolic pressures less than 90 mmHg and no prior complications) until their deaths [4]. Thirty percent were first seen before the onset of hypertension, which appeared at a mean age of 32 years. These subjects spent an average of threequarters of their hypertensive lives free of complications, but most eventually succumbed to them. Mean survival for this group was 20 years, and the average age at death was 52 years – this was 15–20 years less than normal life expectancy. Usually survival was directly related to the appearance of hypertensive complications (Table 2).

B. Complications of hypertension as treatment evolved

The Framingham Study examined what happened without specific intervention to a primarily white community-based population of more than 5000 subjects [1]. The importance of blood pressure level in the development of arteriosclerotic

Table 2. Complications of untreated hypertension

Complication	Percent affected	Mean survival after complications (years)
Cardiac		
Hypertrophy by x-ray	74	8
Hypertrophy by ECG	59	6
Congestive failure	50	4
Angina pectoris	16	5
Encephalic		
Encephalopathy	2	1
Stroke	12	4
Renal		
Proteinuria	42	5
Azotemia	18	1
Accelerated hypertension	7	1

Legend: Data from a study by Perera of 500 cases of untreated hypertension of all degrees of severity (including 30% who were first seen before hypertension developed). The cases, all without prior complications, were followed until death [44].

complications is evident. Men between the ages of 30 and 39 with the lowest level of mild hypertension (diastolic pressure 90–94 mmHg) have about twice the normal risk of developing a myocardial infarction. The risk is a smooth function of diastolic pressure over the range from 60 to 120 mmHg, although the curve becomes somewhat flattened below 85 mmHg (Table 3). Systolic pressure is also a very strong predictor for coronary heart disease, but other risk factors are also important, including smoking, cholesterol level, family history and ECG evidence of cardiac compromise. As age increases blood pressure becomes a less marked risk factor. Although their absolute risk is much lower than the risk in men, hypertensive women demonstrate a greater *relative* risk in comparison to normotensive women (Table 3) [1].

For stroke, the Framingham data demonstrated that increased blood pressure was indeed a major risk factor; this was true when cerebral vascular accidents were considered as a whole or when they were divided into cerebral hemorrhage and thrombotic brain infarction. For both men and women, the annual stroke incidence was approximately 0.1% if the diastolic pressure was normal, 2 or 3 times that if it was borderline (80–89 mmHg), and $7\frac{1}{2}$ times that if it was elevated.

C. Treatment-induced changes in severe and moderate hypertension (Veterans Administration VA Trial)

Effective control of hypertension has now been available for over 30 years. The critical question is how has control altered the course of hypertension: Which

Table 3. Incidence of coronary heart disease

	30–39 Men	Women	40–49 Men	Women	50–59 Men	Women
Normotension <80	128	56	287	102	386	188
Borderline 80–89	241	91	279	182	635	300
Hypertension >90	312	165	506	274	729	509

Legend: Twenty-four year incidence per 1000 people at risk of coronary heart disease, from the Framingham Study [1].

complications are affected and to what extent? Definitive answers can only be found in randomized, double-blind, placebo-controlled trials that compare the courses of treated patients with those of their untreated 'matches'. The untreated matches would be expected to behave similarly to the untreated pre-1950 population, and in general they do, although the very severe hypertensives, who make up the upper part of the pre-1950 distribution, are lacking in recent studies. As indicated in Table 4, for the VA Study the total event rate was twice as great in severe as in moderate hypertension and three times as great in severe as in mild hypertension [5–7]. The ratio of hypertensive to arteriosclerotic events (complications) was also a function of the severity of the hypertension: For severe hypertensives, there were twice as many hypertensive as arteriosclerotic complications; whereas, for mild and moderate hypertensives, there were about equal numbers of the two types of complications.

The primary importance of the VA Study, however, was in demonstrating that treatment decreased both morbid and mortal events, both hypertensive and arteriosclerotic, in those with moderate and severe hypertension. On the other hand, the arteriosclerotic complications of mild hypertension are less amenable to treatment. Perhaps it is the small numbers in the VA trial, but treated mild hypertensives actually had a higher complication rate (almost five events per 100 patient-years of exposure) than treated moderate or severe hypertensives (between one and two events per 100 patient-years) (Table 4). There are several possible explanations for this unexpected observation: First, the complications associated with moderate and severe hypertension, even those listed as arteriosclerotic, are more closely related to the hypertension and less to long-standing arteriosclerosis as indicated in Table 4, while the complications of mild hypertension are primarily related to long-standing arteriosclerosis. Alternatively the 'mild' hypertensives in the VA population, which is generally considered to have been sicker than other studied populations, had enough additional 'other' disease to explain the anomaly. The vitally important lesson from this table is that patients with diastolic pressures greater than 105 mmHg must be treated, whereas the situation is much less clear for those with mild hypertension [5, 6].

Table 4. Type and frequency of complications in varyingly severe hypertension

Untreated patients				Treated patients	Treated and untreated patients
Number of patients	Severity of hypertension	Hypertensive to atherosclerotic events (ratio)	Events per 100 pt-yrs	Events per 100 pt-yrs	Therapeutic efficacy ratio
73	Severe (115)	2.1	23	1.6	14
110	Moderate (105–114)	1.2	11	1.3	8.5
84	Mild (90–104)	1.1	9.3	4.7	2.0

Legend: The relative frequencies of hypertensive and arteriosclerotic complications and the yearly event (i.e., complication) rate for untreated (placebo) patients in the VA Study [7]. For purposes of comparison, the yearly event rates of the treated patients in the same study are tabulated to the right as a therapeutic efficacy ratio, defined as the ratio of the event rate for the active patients divided by the event rate for the placebo patients. The randomization process rendered the treated and untreated populations very similar in age, race and other characteristics.

Table 5. Comparison of antihypertensive treatment in the presence or absence of complications

	Patients with prior event		Patients without prior event	
	Number of patients	New event	Number of patients	New event
Placebo	36	17 (47%)	158	39 (25%)
Treated	39	9 (23%)	145	13 (9%)
Protection	47/23 = 2.0		25/9 = 2.8	

Legend: The numbers of new events that occurred in treated and untreated (placebo) patients with and without pretreatment myocardial infarction or cerebrovascular accident [5].

D. Benefit of treatment in mild hypertension (VA and later trials)

The problem of when mild hypertension should be treated is still unresolved. In brief, of the published double-blind, placebo-controlled studies, only the Australian Study is large enough and long enough to use differences in morbid and mortal events – rather than surrogates for them – to demonstrate that treatment is beneficial. Moreover that study only demonstrated a need to lower the diastolic pressure to 95 mmHg; there is no evidence that lowering it further provides additional benefit [8]. The Hypertension Detection and Follow-up Program (HDFP) has been interpreted as indicating benefit from lowering the diastolic pressure into the low '80s,' but that interpretation is open to serious question because both groups of participants in the trials were treated, but by different therapists and different regimens [9]. Unpublished HDFP data have been presented suggesting that two-thirds of the lowered mortality rate in the mild 'special care' group results from antihypertensive therapy, but the assumptions are considerable and the explanation for the remaining one-third of the effect is still uncertain. In contrast to HDFP, the similarly designed 'Multiple Risk Factor Intervention Trial' (MRFIT) has so far failed to even suggest any benefit from lowering the diastolic pressure below 95 mmHg (the same 'cutoff' level as was observed in the Australian Study) [10]. Thus, until further data become available, it would seem better to individualize the recommendation for treatment of mild hypertension, basing the decision on the degree and immediacy of risk and, especially in young patients, on the desire for treatment since compliance is all important. When considering whether to treat mild hypertensives, other risk factors, such as age and target organ damage, should be considered because they increase morbidity and mortality. There is no question that mild hypertension increases the risk of stroke and heart attack, the question is whether treatment lowers this risk and whether it has inherent risks of its own [11].

IV. Antihypertensive treatment after the occurrence of complications

A. Benefits in VA Study of mild and moderate hypertension

It is critical to know whether treating persistent hypertension is more useful or less so after a complication has occurred. In other words, in the presence of one complication, how effective is treatment in preventing additional complications. Because it dealt with a seriously ill population, many of whom had hypertensive complications, the VA Study provides some information on this point. Of its 380 subjects with mild and moderate hypertension, 75 had had prior myocardial infarction or stroke (Table 5). Of the untreated patients with prior events, 47% had new events; whereas, of the treated patients with prior events, only 23% had new events. Thus treatment of those with prior events appeared to lower the subsequent event rate by half, but the numbers are very small so there is considerable uncertainty (Table 5).

The table also indicates the relative benefits of treating those with and without prior complications. In patients without prior events, treatment lowered the event rate by almost two-thirds, so the percentage benefit appeared to be even greater than the 50% lowering in the group with prior events. Finally, a somewhat different answer is obtained if the data are considered in terms of the absolute numbers of patients who might expect to benefit by treatment. Thus, if one had 100 patients with a prior event and 100 without a prior event, treatment of the first group would lower the event rate from 47% to 23% and so prevent (or delay) complications in 24 patients. Treating 100 patients without a prior event would lower the subsequent event rate even more percentage wise, i.e., from 25% to 9%, but would only benefit 16 patients (Table 5) [11].

B. Benefits of treating subjects with completed strokes

A randomized, double-blind, placebo-controlled study of stroke recurrence, in patients with mild and moderate hypertension reported that treatment did not lower the incidence of a second stroke, nor did it raise it – and there had been some worry that lowering the pressure might lower blood flow and lead to additional infarction. The only morbid event that was changed significantly was congestive heart failure which was reduced in the actively treated group [12].

A more recent, but less rigorous trial involving 124 severely hypertensive (average blood pressure before treatment 195/120 mmHg), relatively young (<65 years of age), white 'stroke survivors' reported 11 recurrent strokes within two years in the 70 males all of whom were treated. The pretreatment blood pressures were similar for the 11 patients with recurrences and the 59 without them, but the blood pressures achieved during treatment were significantly higher for the former than the latter (184/109 versus 167/101 mmHg), suggesting that lowering the blood pressure was preventive. Even in the nonrecurrent group, however, the pressure was not well controlled [13].

C. Benefits of treating subjects with myocardial infarction

Two randomized, double-blind, placebo-controlled trials have demonstrated that beta-blocking agents can reduce the incidence of both sudden death and a second myocardial infarct in subjects with a recent myocardial infarction (5–28 days before treatment began) [14, 15]; most of these subjects were normotensive, but hypertensive subjects were included and fared no differently from others. In the initial trial involving nearly 2000 subjects, there was a 'placebo mortality' rate of 15% in 24 months; beta-blockade reduced this mortality by almost 40%. The comparable reduction in the reinfarction rate was almost 30%. The patients in this trial were men and women with an average age of 61 years. About 20% were taking antihypertensive agents [14]. Very similar results were reported from a similar study involving somewhat younger subjects, some of whom were black, and using propranolol instead of timolol as the beta-blocking drug [15]. An apparent difference between the two trials was the number of months of protection afforded by the beta-blockade; in the first, protection lasted for more than two years after the original infarct, while in the second it seemed to persist for only one year.

An earlier similarly designed trial, using the now unobtainable beta-blocking agent practolol, suggested that beta-blockade induced a significant reduction in both total deaths and sudden deaths but only in normotensive subjects. The benefit was apparently limited to approximately half of the population with diastolic pressures less than 79 mmHg; there was no protection for the half with higher pressures [16].

Despite the practolol trial, if there are no contraindications to beta-blockade, it seems reasonable to choose a beta-blocking agent as an antihypertensive agent whenever one is concerned about the possibility of myocardial infarction, i.e., in the presence of angina pectoris, electrocardiographic changes suggestive of ischemia, a family history of myocardial infarction or other risk factors such as smoking, elevated cholesterol or diabetes mellitus. Under these circumstances beta-blockade could be added to a diuretic, or used as initial therapy if the circumstances warrant. (*Note:* the benefit of anturane treatment to prevent myocardial infarction is set forth separately in Chapter 12.)

D. Treatment recommendations for patients with complications

Individuals with myocardial infarction or stroke who have diastolic pressures which persistently average more than 110 mmHg deserve to have their blood pressures lowered. It must be emphasized, however, that such a patient is a high risk patient and liable to develop trouble as a result of therapy, but he is probably even more likely to have problems if no attempt is made to control his blood pressure. Treatment should be carried out according to the same general plan that is advocated for other patients; current 'Joint National Committee' recommendations still favor diuretics first, with an adrenergic blocker and then a vasodilator added as needed [17]. It should be remembered, however, that such patients are often in delicate cardiovascular balance and may be unusually sensitive to antihypertensive drugs. If possible, no more than half of the maximum dose recommended for the patient without complications should be used. If this is not effective, however, and if the physician thinks the patient is liable to get into difficulty otherwise, the cautious use of larger doses is not only appropriate but mandatory. Obviously any symptoms associated with therapy which is suggestive of an incipient event, such as a neurologic deficit or anginal pain, require that therapy be deminished. Although parenteral medication may be indicated for the individual with markedly elevated pressures or when there is a problem taking things by mouth, peroral therapy is usually sufficient and should ordinarily begin with a diuretic. However, for the individual who has had a myocardial infarction and has no contraindication to beta-blockade, a beta-blocker seems the most reasonable second-step agent. For such a patient, a third-step agent should be avoided if possible, since any peripheral vasodilator can cause an increase in pulse rate and cardiac work. For individuals who have had a stroke without myocardial compromise, a third step agent should cause no problems.

Acute congestive heart failure in the presence of marked hypertension will respond dramatically to parenteral antihypertensive drugs. For patients with chronic congestive failure, oral antihypertensive treatment is sufficient. In my experience, chronic failure associated with a diastolic pressure over 110 mmHg is very likely to respond to antihypertensive therapy. In contrast, failure in association with a diastolic pressure below 100 mmHg is unlikely to respond. In the intermediate range of 100–110 mmHg, antihypertensive therapy may or may not help. Finally, it should be noted that in the Veterans Administration Trial, subjects less than 60 years of age did not develop heart failure; after 60 it was not uncommon in the untreated (placebo) group, but it was completely prevented by treatment [7].

In summary, it should be reemphasized that even after a major complication, lowering an elevated pressure is usually indicated, and there are no data which indicate that it is harmful. Whenever possible, however, a markedly elevated pressure should be lowered carefully and cautiously if a significant complication is present. There is a real risk in treating such a patient, but the risk of not treating is generally greater.

V. Complications of therapy

Untreated hypertension has very serious sequellae resulting in disability and death; it is the most important risk factor for myocardial infarction and stroke which between them account for more than one-fourth of all deaths in the United States. Chronic treatment of hypertension can prevent or significantly delay many of these sequellae; in fact, antihypertensive agents are among the few drugs which, when used chronically, have actually been demonstrated to decrease morbidity and mortality. To achieve this beneficial effect, however, requires very prolonged usage and therefore entails an unusual risk of toxic and/or undesirable effects (Table 6). The first antihypertensive drugs dramatically demonstrated this unusual risk. Not only did they induce side effects which were often intolerable, but they also induced very serious toxic reactions. Of the two original agents, methonium compounds are well known for their universal and indiscriminate autonomic blockade; but it is often forgotten that in addition they rarely produced an almost always fatal fibrinous pneumonitis in mildly azotemic malignant hypertensives [18]. Hydralazine, the second of the original agents, has significant but less serious side effects and is still widely used; however, it too was associated with a major complication, the first frequent and predictable 'drug-induced lupus' [19, 20]. Other early agents also were associated

Table 6. Unwanted actions of antihypertensive drugs

Drug	Undesirable effect	Demonstrated toxicity	Comment
1. Hexamethonium		Fatal fibrinous pneumonitis	Malignant hypertensives with azotemia but not uremia
2. Mecamylamene		Reversible tremor & mental changes from depression to coma	Most of same population as above who were challenged
3. Thiazides & thiazide-like diuretics	Lowers potassium Raises cholesterol Raises glucose		'Wrong way' chemical changes without evidence of increased morbidity
4. K-sparing diuretics		Hyperkalemia	
5. Beta-blockers	Decreases cardiac contractility Broncho-constrictor Vasoconstrictor Masks hypoglycemia		
6. Practolol		Peritoneal fibrosis	Not induced by other beta-blockers
7. Reserpine		Depression	But only with 10–100 × present dose
8. Methyldopa	Coombs positivity	Hemolytic anemia Hepatitis	Positive Coombs in 30%, but anemia in only 1 of 30,000
9. Clonidine	Rebound hypertension		
10. Guanethidine	Postural hypotension and impotence		With therapeutic doses side effects approach 100%
11. Prasozin	Syncope		
12. Hydralazine		Rheumatoid arthritis	Nondeforming arthritis No lupus changes in kidney or brain
		Lupus erythematosus	Reversal on withdrawal of drug
13. Minoxidil	Fluid retention		
14. Captopril		Agranulocytosis Marked proteinuria	

Legend: Some undersirable and toxic effects, but no side effects, of commonly used oral antihypertensive agents.

with toxicity. Of particular interest, since it seems to be staging a 'comeback,' is reserpine which, in daily doses of 10–100 times the current recommended maximum dose (2.5–25 mg/day), produced severe depression [21, 22]. With the current recommended maximum dose of 0.25 mg/day, there have been no further documented depressions, and now an even smaller dose (0.05 mg/day) seems to have almost the same antihypertensive efficacy [23].

The next generation of antihypertensive drugs was associated with less frequent and less severe side and toxic effects. For instance, methyldopa can cause an auto-immune hemolytic anemia but is estimated to do so only once in about 30,000 exposures. It can also induce hepatic dysfunction, but this is usually limited to asymptomatic increases in blood levels of liver enzymes, although significant hepatitis can rarely occur, usually in association with preexisting liver disease [24]. 'Rebound hypertension' has been reported when clonidine is discontinued [25], however, such rebound apparently causes few difficulties, since many noncompliant patients must surely discontinue the drug daily, yet few problems are reported (Table 5).

A. Thiazides and related diuretics

The antihypertensive agent which is currently causing the greatest concern as a *possible* cause of significant toxicity is the thiazide diuretic. Except for a rare suggestion of difference, the thiazide-like diuretic, chlorthalidone, has been considered to behave as a thiazide; this assumption has been made here. These agents have long been the preferred first step in antihypertensive treatment [17]. Even if a thiazide is not effective by itself, it potentiates other antihypertensive agents and so decreases their side effects while causing relatively few of its own. Many physicians, particularly in the United States, still prefer thiazides as initial therapy because of their low cost and flat dose–response curve (meaning that little dose-titration is needed), but some concerns have begun to be heard.

Although originally thought to be almost free of undesirable effects, there has been a gradually increasing awareness of thiazide-induced, 'wrong-way' chemical changes which are asymptomatic for the patient but disturbing to the physician. The most worrisome of these is hypokalemia. The minimum acceptable potassium level is 3.0 mEq/l, and it occurs in about 20% of thiazide-treated patients [26]. Many consider a level between 3.0 and 3.5 mEq/l as the minimum acceptable level. It must be remembered, however, that plasma contains only 2% of the body's potassium, and thus it is an unreliable index of cardiac potassium, the parameter we would really like to measure. Hypokalemia has been reported to induce disturbing cardiac arrhythmias that wax and wane as a function of plasma potassium concentration [27]. It should be emphasized that to date no increased morbidity or mortality has been demonstrated with hypokalemia;

however, with life-long therapy, the possibility of late toxicity cannot be excluded.

Recently, the unexpected failure of MRFIT to confirm the HDFP findings has raised the spectre of detrimental effects from the thiazides. Although MRFIT was limited to high risk patients and was seeking the effects of reducing other risk factors as well as blood pressure, the two trials were otherwise similar in design. HDFP was interpreted as showing benefit from lowering the diastolic pressure into the 'low 80s'. In contrast, MRFIT showed no such trend; in fact patients with baseline diastolic pressures below 95 mmHg seemed to do less well with 'special intervention' than those with 'usual care'. The excess deaths in MRFIT seemed to have been sudden deaths and so suggested arrhythmias associated with hypokalemia. It has been suggested that 'special intervention patients' in MRFIT had larger doses of hydrochlorothiazide than 'usual care patients'; it has also been suggested that MRFIT relied heavily on hydrochlorothiazide and HDFP on chlorothalidone [9, 10].

Unfortunately in view of the question raised about thiazides, neither HDFP nor MRFIT can provide information on possible thiazide toxicity; all patients in both trials were subject to treatment, and there were no control (placebo) groups. Although there are many other interpretations besides a detrimental effect of hydrochlorothiazide, the 'Australian Study' could be interpreted as suggesting, in addition to the beneficial antihypertensive effects, a deleterious effect from thiazides that increased morbidity and mortality and was observable when treatment failed to lower blood pressure [8]. Among treated subjects, those whose postrandomization diastolic pressures were poorly controlled (in the 95–99 or the over 100 mmHg ranges) while on active drugs had a much higher morbid event rate than those with the same pressures on placebo (Figure 2). One aspect of the VA Study could be similarly interpreted [7]. The fact that actively treated patients after diastolic pressures in the '90s' had the same event rate as actively treated patients with diastolic pressures in the '70s' could also be due to a competing deleterious effect when treatment was pushed too enthusiastically. Again it must be emphasized, however, that although this interpretation is possible, there is no real evidence that thiazides have a harmful as well as their very well authenticated helpful effect.

The second 'wrong way' change associated with thiazide therapy is a small increase in total cholesterol, averaging only 10 mg/100 ml, which is probably of little clinical significance. The primary effect is on low-density lipoprotein cholesterol. There is no increase in high-density lipoprotein cholesterol, and there is an associated but more variable increase in triglycerides. This 'lipid effect' has been carefully examined in a randomized, placebo-controlled, double-blind study of over 1000 patients with mild hypertension [28]. It appears relatively early and persists with little change for at least two years. It is a function of baseline cholesterol, being greatest for those with the lowest baseline levels; the

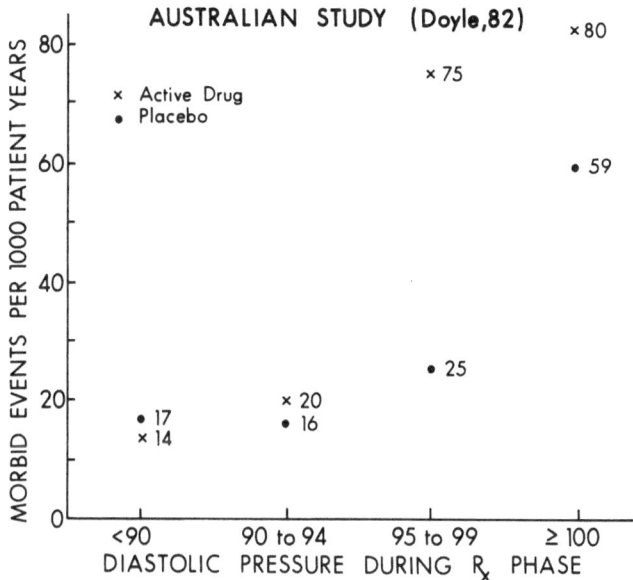

Figure 2. Relationship between morbid event rate and level of treated blood pressure in the Australian Study. Here the placebo and active drug patients are divided into the four diastolic pressure categories on the basis of their pressures at the end of the trial, and the morbid event rates have been calculated for that category.

effect is also larger for young patients, but the relationship with age is almost entirely explained by the tendency of the young to have low baseline levels. Although an average increase of 5% of total cholesterol is small, logistic regression equations from the Framingham Study estimate that a difference of 10 mg/100 ml in cholesterol levels implies a 12% difference in the risk of coronary heart disease in a 37.5-year-old man [1]. However, a series of large scale trials has indicated that lowering circulating cholesterol has no demonstrable effect in lowering the incidence of myocardial infarction [29–31]; it therefore seems reasonable to question whether an induced increase in cholesterol will increase the incidence of myocardial infarction. In any case so far there is no evidence that the thiazide-induced increase in cholesterol has been associated with any change in morbidity or mortality.

A third 'wrong-way' chemical effect of thiazide is on carbohydrate metabolism. After a year of thiazide (chlorthalidone) exposure, it was manifested by an average increase of less than 5 mg% in fasting blood glucose [26]. A recent small study from Dollery's group, however, suggests that glucose tolerance worsened markedly after long-term treatment with thiazides and partially reversed after discontinuation of the drug [32]. After 14 years of uninterrupted thiazide therapy, the average two-hour postprandial blood glucose was 45% higher than it had originally been; the ten patients who discontinued thiazides after 14 years, fell half way back to the pretreatment level after seven months. The thiazide-treated patients with carbohydrate changes had a moderately lowered average plasma potassium level, but it is difficult to tell how much of the intolerance may have been related to hypokalemia – or how much was due to 14 years of aging. To get a better picture of the magnitude of the problem, much larger numbers are needed.

Thiazides frequently induce hyperuricemia, with about 15% of patients having uric acid levels above 9 mg/100 ml. This change is probably of little general significance; secondary gout is an infrequent occurrence since the induction of arthritis requires protracted disruption of uric acid metabolism, with the accumulation of large uric acid stores. Finally, thiazides induce an increase in circulating renin, the clinical significance of which is unknown.

B. Beta-blocking agents

Because of the demonstrations that beta-blockade prevents recurrent myocardial infarctions and sudden death in patients who have had an infarct, and because of the concern about thiazides, there has been increasing use of beta-blocking agents as the first antihypertensive drug. For patients who are considered at high risk for myocardial infarction, it seems reasonable to use these agents; however, there are strong contraindications in large groups of the mildly hypertensive population: chronic obstructive pulmonary disease, history of congestive heart failure and significant peripheral vascular diseases. In addition, beta-blocking agents are relatively contraindicated in diabetic patients primarily because they can mask the symptoms of hypoglycemia, and in patients with bradycardia because of their tendency to further slow the heart. Finally there are rare instances when sudden withdrawal has seemed to precipitate cardiac problems.

In addition to patients considered to be at high risk for myocardial infarction, beta-blocking agents have been recommended for patients with 'high renin' hypertension, but the advantage seems insufficient to warrant very expensive 'renin profiling' (Table 6).

VI. Treatment of hypertensive emergencies

Two genuine hypertensive emergencies demand immediate attention: hypertensive encephalopathy and left heart failure in the presence of a markedly elevated diastolic pressure. 'Hypertensive encephalopathy' is a poorly defined term that has been used to describe three quite different pathological conditions: (1) edema of the brain, (2) small infarctions of the brain occurring over a period of time, and (3) localized arteriolar spasm. The term should really be limited to the last of these three. The spasm is apparently a response to greatly increased intraluminal pressure; the result is localized edema that may progress to necrosis if the spasm is sufficiently severe and persistent. Hypertensive encephalopathy is rare, perhaps because effective treatment prevents it, and even ineffective treatment may prevent the full-blown recognizable symptom complex. Excluding the encephalopathy of eclampsia and preeclampsia which are considered in Chapter 13, hypertensive encephalopathy is ordinarily seen only in those who have severe and relatively acute hypertension. The symptoms include severe headache, confusion, varying degrees of loss of consciousness and finally epileptiform convulsions, all in association with a markedly increased diastolic pressure, usually in the 130–140 mmHg or higher range. Headache, as the sole symptom, in combination with a marked elevation in pressure, should trigger a search for etiologies other than hypertensive encephalopathy. When the headache is excruciating or there is diminished consciousness or convulsions, the markedly elevated diastolic pressure must be rapidly lowered.

If intensive care facilities are available with minute-to-minute monitoring, nitroprusside by an intravenous drip provides the most effective antihypertensive medication and permits minute-to-minute control of the blood pressure since the response is extremely rapid and the effect extremely short. The average adult dose is 3 μg/kg/min and the maximum recommended dose is 800 μg/min; however, in a closely monitored situation, it is safe and appropriate to try higher doses if you are the physician of last resort. When a very high pressure is to be lowered, normotension should not be the immediate goal; the pressure should be lowered to the range that corrects the dramatic cerebral symptoms, and ordinarily any diastolic pressure below 120 mmHg will do this. Thus, an immediate goal of 110 mmHg for parenteral agents is reasonable; if it is not quite achieved, the result will still be below the range that causes rapid damage and, more importantly, if there is an overshoot of 20 mmHg or even more, serious hypotension should not occur. Moreover a goal of 110 mmHg permits a relatively simply substitution of oral agents for the initial parenteral one. This is done by using a lower goal diastolic pressure for oral agents and adding them until the average diastolic pressure has been lowered another 10–20 mmHg, at which point the parenteral agent can be discontinued. It is important to remember two facts. First, in general, the more urgent it is to lower blood pressure, the more sensitive the patient is to antihypertensive medications; it is wise therefore to start with a small test dose and then rapidly increase the dose as necessary. Second, disastrous hypotension can result if two antihypertensive drugs are started simultaneously. Therefore, almost without exception when treating severe hypertension, the effect of the first drug should be tested before the second antihypertensive drug is added. Finally, it is worth remembering that even before effective antihypertensive agents were available, hypertensive encephalopathy, although a frightening syndrome, was rarely fatal.

When it comes to treating congestive heart failure in a severly hypertensive patient, few things in medicine are more dramatic than abruptly lowering the diastolic pressure preferably with nitroprusside. Symptoms melt away within minutes, and digitalis is rarely needed if the hypertension remains under control.

Mild azotemia in a patient with a very high pressure is not a real hypertensive emergency, in the same sense, but it is the next thing to it. It indicates markedly compromised renal function and requires that the pressure be lowered promptly, not within minutes, but certainly within a few days if not a few hours. The physician should remember that a high pressure can destroy renal parenchyma very rapidly. Even a week of a very high pressure in an individual with borderline renal function can be the difference between needing or not needing dialysis or transplantation. If intensive care facilities are not available, even a very high diastolic pressure can be lowered within hours by successively doubled doses of intramuscular hydralazine, beginning with 5 mg, every half hour. Other anti-hypertensive drugs can also be used effectively, but every effort should be made to avoid compromising renal blood flow; even so, any mild azotemia that is present will probably worsen for a week before it returns to its pretreatment level.

VII. Summary

The major complications of hypertension itself are renal failure, (intra)cerebral hemorrhage, and congestive heart failure in the uncontrolled hypertensive. These complications occur in severe hypertension and are less common now than in the past because severe hypertension is usually treated and at least partially controlled. The major complications of mild and moderate hyper-tension are myocardial infarction and (athero)thrombotic brain infarction. They are considered arteriosclerotic; in general they occur after a much longer period of hypertension than hypertensive complications. The evidence is conclusive that treatment of severe and moderate hypertension can prevent (or delay) compli-cations, but evidence for preventive benefit from treating mild hypertension is much less clear.

The VA Trial suggests that treating patients with complications prevents additional complications. Moreover, it seems very likely that hypertensive pa-tients presenting with prior myocardial infarctions benefit by beta-blockade. For patients with prior strokes, the available data are less convincing. Nonetheless, the usual recommendations for patients with complications is to treat, but to treat cautiously.

All effective drugs have the potential for unwanted effects. Of greatest con-cern today, among antihypertensive drugs; is the thiazide diuretic, which has been shown to cause several 'wrong-way' chemical changes, particularly hypokalemia. The significance, if any, of these changes is not yet clear; to date there is no evidence of a harmful effect.

Markedly elevated diastolic pressure may lead to two hypertensive emergencies: hypertensive encephalopathy and congestive heart failure. For both, emergency treatment with careful but effective use of parenteral antihypertensive drugs yields good results.

References

1. Dawber TR: The Framingham Study. Cambridge, Mass, Harvard University Press, 1980.
2. Stallones RA: The rise and fall of ischemic heart disease. Sci Am 243(5):1980.
3. Smith DE, Odel HM, Kernohan JW: Causes of death in hypertension. Am J Med 9:516–527, 1950.
4. Perera GA: Hypertensive vascular disease: description and natural history. J Chronic Dis 1:33–42, 1955.
5. Veterans Administration Cooperative Study Group on Antihypertensive Agents: Effects of treatment on morbidity in hypertension. 1. Results in patients with diastolic blood pressures averaging 115 through 129 mmHg. JAMA 202:116–122, 1967.
6. Veterans Administration Cooperative Study Group on Antihypertensive Agents: Effects of treatment on morbidity in hypertension. II. Results in patients with diastolic blood pressure averaging 90 through 114 mmHg. JAMA 213:1143–1152, 1970.
7. Veterans Administration Cooperative Study Group in Antihypertensive Agents: Effects of treatment on morbidity in hypertension. III. Influence of age, diastolic pressure, and prior cardiovascular disease: further analysis of side effects. Circulation 45:991–1004, 1972.
8. Reader R (Study-Director): A report by the Management Committee in the Australian Therapeutic Trial in Mild Hypertension untreated mild hypertension. Lancet 1:158, 1982.
9. Five-year findings of the Hypertension Detection and Follow-up Program. I. Reduction in mortality of persons with high blood pressure, including mild hypertension. JAMA 242:2562, 1979.
10. The Multiple Risk Factor Intervention Trial. JAMA 248:1465, 1982.
11. Perry HM Jr: Mild Hypertension – when and how to treat it. Praxis 71:265, 1982.
12. Hypertension – Stroke Cooperative Study Group: Effect of antihypertensive treatment on stroke recurrence. JAMA 299:409–418, 1974.
13. Johnston JH et al: The importance of good blood pressure control in the prevention of stroke recurrence in hypertensive patients. Postgrad Med J 57:690–693, 1981.
14. The Norwegian Multicenter Study Group: Timolol-induced reduction in mortality and re-infarction in patients surviving acute myocardial infarction. N Engl J Med 304(14):801–807, 1981.
15. B-Blocker Heart Attack Study Group: The B-blocker Heart Attack Trial. JAMA 246(18): 2073–2074, 1981.
16. Multicenter International Study: Supplementary report: reduction in mortality after myocardial infarction long-term beta-adrenoceptor blockade. Br Med J [Clin Res] 2:419–421, 1977.
17. The 1980 report of the Joint National Committee on Detection, Evaluation and Treatment of High Blood Pressure. Arch Int Med 40:1280, 1980.
18. Perry HM Jr, O'Neal R, Thomas WA: Pulmonary disease following chronic chemical ganglionic blockade: a clinical and pathological study. Am J Med 22:37, 1957.

19. Perry HM Jr, Schroeder HA: Syndrome simulating collagen disease caused by l-hydrazin-ophthalazine (Apresoline). JAMA 154:670, 1954.
20. Perry HM Jr: Possible mechanisms of the hydralazine-related lupus-like syndrome, arthritis and rheumatism 24; 8:1093–1105.
21. Schroeder HA, Perry HM Jr: Psychosis apparently produced by reserpine. JAMA 159:839, 1955.
22. Freis ED: Mental depression in hypertensive patients treated for a long period with large doses of reserpine. N Engl J Med 251:1006, 1954.
23. Veterans Administration Medical Centers: Low doses vs standard dose of reserpine. 248: 2471–2477, 1982.
24. Goldstein GB, Lam KC, Mistilis SP: Drug-induced active chronic hepatitis. Am J Dig Dis 18:177–184, 1973.
25. Geyskes GG, Boer P, Dorhout Mees EJ: Clonidine withdrawal. Mechanism and frequency of rebound hypertension. Br J Clin Pharmacol 7:55–62, 1979.
26. Goldman AI, Steele BW, Schnaper HW, Fitz AE, Frohlich ED, Perry HM Jr: JAMA 244:1691, 1980.
27. Holland AB, Nicon JA, Kuhnert L: Diuretic-induced ventricular ectopia activity. Am J Med 70:762, 1981.
28. Perry HM: VA-NHLBI Study Group for Cooperative Studies on Antihypertensive Therapy: Mild hypertension. Circ Res 40:I–180, 1977.
29. Leren P: The Oslo Diet-Heart Study. Circulation 42:935, 1970.
30. The Coronary Drug Project Research Group: Clofibrate and niacin in coronary heart disease. JAMA 231:306, 1975.
31. Oliver MF, Heady JA, Morris NN, Cooper J: A cooperative trial in the primary prevention of ischemic heart disease using clofibrate. Br Heart J 40:1069, 1978.
32. Murphy MD, Kohner E, Lewis PJ, Schuber B, Dollery CJ: Glucose intolerance in hypertensive patients treated with diuretics: a fourteen-year follow-up. Lancet 2:1293–1295, 1982.

11. Heart failure and hypertension

JAMES FOERSTER

Before the advent of effective antihypertensive drugs, physicians interested in hypertension respected the heart because the majority of their patients died of heart failure. As effective drugs were developed, flagrant heart disease became less common, and lesions developed in other organs besides the heart; in particular, renal failure and stroke increased.

At this point, some conventional cardiologists became interested in vasodilators. They were late entrants into the field because hypertension specialisits had been using vasodilators in a thoughtful manner to manage blood pressure in a variety of circumstances. The cardiologists, however, felt that they had discovered vasodilators. In fact, what they had done was to discover a very important application of vasodilators to ordinary garden-variety heart disease. This application has excited the people in the cardiological community to a considerable extent and changed, in a fundamental way, their thinking about heart failure.

It is, therefore, now quite appropriate – whereas ten years ago it would have been much more forced – for a cardiologist to consider certain conceptual links between the failing heart and the management of blood pressure in general and the reduction of peripheral vascular resistance in particular. Just as the cardiologist has had to discover some of what physicians managing patients with hypertension have learned, the hypertension specialist should become aware of how antihypertensive management may impinge on the underlying heart disease that he is trying to prevent or at least minimize.

I would like to begin this discussion with a consideration of the pathophysiological aspects of congestive heart failure and then progress to the clinical pharmacology of managing congestive heart failure.

The sarcomere is the architectural building block of the myocardial cell. When the heart is functioning normally, contraction occurs because the actomoycin filaments in the muscle are pulled past each other, with ATP providing the energy for this contractile shortening. If the muscle is fixed at either end, the attempt to shorten results in an increase in force. If the muscle is allowed to change its geometry, the contractile energy is translated into actual shortening of the muscle or contraction of the heart.

There are other elements of the myocardial cell that are worth thinking about briefly: the cell membrane which allows calcium to enter the cell, the sarcoplasmic reticulum which takes the calcium up in a bound form and terminates the contraction and the mitochondria which are the energy source for these activities. The heart is exquisitely dependent on aerobic metabolism. Under physiologic conditions, ATP for all cardiac contraction is confined to the mitochrondria, where it is manufactured by oxydative metabolism of fatty acids and carbohydrates; in addition, however, some limited glycolytic metabolism is possible. When myocardial muscle is contracting, bridges between the thick and the thin filaments in the sarcomeres are being rapidly made and broken and ATP is split into ADP and phosphate. Thus, when the heart contracts repetitively, it consumes ATP and in so doing converts chemical energy into mechanical energy.

It is well recognized that the mitochrondria are the energy source for contraction, and preservation of their function is vital. Many years ago there was a strong flurry of interest regarding the basis of heart failure; it was claimed that there was something wrong with the mitochrondria that caused the failure in the usual types of congestive heart failure. This idea did not stand the test of time, and we do not yet know what combination of specific chemical, biochemical and organ defects are responsible for congestive heart failure. We do know if we poison the mitochrondria, impair the cross bridging of the myofibrils or block the calcium transport mechanism, we can stimulate failure in animal models. That does not mean that these derangements occur during failure in human beings. Statistically, in the Western world, human congestive heart failure is largely the result of coronary artery disease which has expressed itself as repetitive myocardial infarction, as microinfarcts with fibrosis, or as pathologically recognizable, but poorly understood, phenomena in which fibrotic replacement occurs differently throughout the heart without localized frank infarction in any single region. Although cardiomyopathy and valvular heart disease are important, coronary artery disease is the most common cause of heart failure in our population. From a statistical point of view, if a patient enters the hospital with heart failure, with or without associated hypertension, the probabilities are high that he has underlying coronary artery disease.

Let us consider some mechanical aspects of heart muscle. If heart muscle is suspended in a muscle bath and its rate of shortening observed, this rate can be extrapolated to the situation in which the muscle is lifting no weight and therefore is shortening as fast as possible. This maximum rate of shortening is designated 'V max'. If a load is put on the muscle, it will shorten less rapidly and its contractile elements will be doing work. If the contractility is changed by adding norepinephrine in the bath, the 'force versus velocity' curve shifts, and both the actual velocity of contraction and the extrapolated V max are increased. This approach has proved useful in providing an experimental method for looking at contractility as influenced by mechanical factors and drugs.

In the intact heart, the function of the left ventricle is determined by several factors that impinge on these underlying physiological relationships. The contractility of the heart muscle is a major determinant of how well it will perform as a pump. In the intact state, the heart that is exposed to catecholamines, digitalis glycosides, glucagon, or a number of other agents with positive inotrophic effects, will become a more effective pump. It will do more work.

When the muscle is stretched, as happens when the ventricle is distended, a larger opportunity is provided for cross bridges to be made between actomyosin binding sites. So, when the muscle is stretched the ventricle is distended. Thus, distension in the intact heart, increases the movement of blood which is the hearts primary function. This is the Frank Starling mechanism. The energy cost of this is modest, neither trivial nor excessive.

Obviously, if the heart is trying to pump blood against an infinitely high impedence or resistance, no blood will be ejected because the pressure gradient cannot be overcome even though the heart muscle is perfectly healthy. Thus, performance is influenced to a very large extent by afterload. For a given physiological state of the myocardium, stroke volume is determined very largely by the impedance. Of course, heart rate is also a major determinant of how much cardiac output can be achieved, or in other words, of how much perfusion of the peripheral organs, including the heart itself via the coronary circulation, can be achieved.

In a patient with failure, these factors must be manipulated in order to improve the effective performance of the heart, such that perfusion of organs throughout the body, including the heart itself, is maximized. Preload can be adjusted, contractility can be stimulated, afterload can be modified and heart rate can be manipulated, but there is a price.

Since most patients with congestive heart failure have underlying coronary disease, the availability of oxygen to their heart muscle is not infinite. In fact, it is not infinite even in a normal individual because there is a maximum attainable value of coronary flow associated with a peak delivery of oxygen by the blood.

Several well-known factors are major determinants of myocardial oxygen consumption (Table 1). Heart rate is one. When the heart performs external work, most oxygen consumption is associated with systole. Obviously, if the

Table 1. Determinants of myocardial oxygen consumption

Heart rate
Contractility
Preload (ventricular wall tension during diastole, determined by diastolic volume)
Afterload (ventricular wall tension during systole)

heart beats once a minute, it consumes little oxygen compared to its needs if it beats 100 times per minute.

The contractile state of the heart is probably the most important determinant of oxygen consumption since in biochemical terms increased contractility means increased conversion of chemical energy via oxydative metabolism to physical work. Therefore, when contractility is stimulated, the oxygen costs to the tissue increase.

It costs the heart a great deal of energy just to prevent itself from 'blowing up.' The Laplace Relationship, where wall tension equals pressure multiplied by radius, is easily visualized if one considers a balloon. When you start to blow up a ballon, you must blow hard to begin to inflate it. As inflation proceeds and the radius increases, the pressure required to maintain any given wall tension decreases in inverse proportion to the radius. Conversely, as the balloon enlarges, more wall tension is needed to balance any fixed pressure. Since the heart is subject to the same forces as a balloon, when it becomes distended, resulting in a large volume at the beginning of systole, the oxygen cost to make ATP must rise in order to generate the additional wall tension needed to prevent even greater distension. Thus, increased preload increases oxygen consumption of the heart.

When the pressure within the ventricle increases at any given volume, as it must to meet an increased blood pressure, the Laplace Relationship requires that the wall tension must again be increased. Thus, increasing 'preload' will increase ventricular radius, and increasing 'afterload' results in higher intraventricular pressure; both changes increase oxygen cost. Wall tension, as determined by both preload and afterload, is a major determinant of oxygen consumption by the heart.

Therefore if cardiac output is to be improved in the patient with a failing heart by taking advantage of the Frank-Starling mechanism and increasing preload, we are increasing wall tension as well and hence the oxygen requirement. If cardiac output is increased by stimulating contractility or speeding up heart rate, we are again increasing the oxygen requirement. If the patient does not have sufficient reserve coronary blood flow to meet the oxygen cost of the increased burden, our efforts are doomed to failure: even though they are physiologically useful, they are biochemically unattainable.

Consider now one last physiological aspect of the balance between oxygen supply and demand, the determinants of coronary flow. If asked what factors control coronary flow, there is a tendency to say the diastolic pressure because 90% of left ventricular coronary flow occurs during diastole when the coronary arterioles are open. The perfusion pressure for coronary flow, however, is not determined by diastolic blood pressure alone; it is reduced by the left ventricular diastolic pressure. A patient, with congestive heart failure and a diastolic blood pressure of 70 mmHg and a left ventricular end diastolic pressure (LVEDP) of 20 mmHg, has a coronary perfusion gradient of 50 mmHg. If the same patient has a diastolic blood pressure of 70 mmHg and an LVEDP of 5 mmHg, his perfusion gradient is 65 mmHg, 30% higher. So, it must be remembered that perfusion pressure is not simply the diastolic pressure. It is the diastolic pressure minus the LVEDP and may be improved by vasodilators which reduce LVEDP more than diastolic blood pressure.

Coronary blood flow is also influenced by active coronary vascular tone, and many drugs used by the cardiologist have an effect on the coronary vascular bed. For example, cardiac glycosides have recently been shown to affect the coronary arteries just as they have been known for many years to affect the peripheral vasculature. In the days when intravenous acetyl strophanthadine was used as a diagnostic tool, its use was accompanied by modest increases in blood pressure due to increases in peripheral vascular resistance. Cardiac glycosides have vasoconstrictor effects on the coronary bed as well as on the peripheral arterial bed; these vasoconstrictor effects can be blocked by phentolamine, suggesting that there is a reflex basis for them involving alpha-adrenergic efferent activity. All glycosides produce some coronary vasoconstriction when they are administered intravenously. When they are taken orally, the effect is much less marked and may not occur at all.

Although antihypertensive drugs may do wondrous things for the periphery, if such a drug blocks the ability of the heart to support its own nutrition and oxygenation requirements, it will not be very useful. Propranolol, for instance, by blocking the beta-adrenergic receptor and leaving the alpha receptor unopposed, may also induce a net increase in vascular resistance, including coronary vascular resistance, with a resultant decrease in coronary blood flow. There is some recent evidence, however that the tone of the coronary vasculature is regulated in a very different way when the myocardium is ischemic.

Manipulation of afterload is a particularly attractive way of approaching heart failure because lowering afterload, i.e., decreasing peripheral resistance, will do all of the right things. It will allow the heart, at a given contractile state and rate, to eject blood against a lower pressure and, therefore, lower the oxygen requirement associated with wall tension; at the same time it will allow maintenance of adequate perfusion to the periphery without increasing myocardial oxygen requirements. In modern centers, today's primary treatment of congestive heart failure involves vasodilation and reduction of afterload. Moreover, it is now recognized that even modest hypertension, in the presence of borderline cardiac functional status, can be very deleterious and can precipitate or exacerbate congestive heart failure.

In patients hospitalized with an acute myocardial infarction, efforts are being made to reduce infarct size by vasodilator therapy. Presently, the only patients clearly known to benefit from such pharmacologic intervention are those with significant hypertension. Their oxygen requirements are excessively high and reducing afterload should be beneficial; judging from several criteria, it is.

Reducing the afterload in a patient with mitral regurgitation who is *in extremis* can produce dramatic improvement; such a patient can sit up and say that he feels fine. Of course, it is naive to think that we have really solved an underlying problem; we have adjusted conditions so that the patient is comfortable even though the underlying cardiac dysfunction remains [1].

Thus, cardiologists treating congestive heart failure from all causes have become progressively more interested in vasodilators. There is a selection of them, with some being effective in one setting and some in another.

Nitrates constitute an interesting class of direct acting vasodilators, which relax the smooth muscle of veins and arteries by an unknown mechanism. Even though it can be demonstrated that they also dilate resistance arterial vessels, these agents are more effective venodilators and they should be thought of as venodilators. As such they induce a marked fall in right atrial pressure, as well as fall in the pulmonary artery end diastolic pressure which is a reflection of left ventricular filling pressure (LVED). The class consists of nitroglycerin, isosorbid dinitrate and other cogeners that are closely related chemically to these compounds.

What does venodilatation do in the case of the patient with heart failure? It pools blood on the right side of the circulation. reducing the influx into the lungs and the left heart. Pulmonary edema should therefore lessen as a result of the lower pressure in the pulmonary bed. The left ventricular filling pressure decreases as the venous return is reduced. The heart size gets smaller thereby reducing the myocardial oxygen requirement.

What happens to systemic arterial blood pressure and heart rate under these circumstances? Ideally blood pressure should drop slightly as right-sides venous pooling reduces the left ventricular filling pressure. If cardiac output drops sharply, however, the blood pressure may fall significantly, leading to a striking reflex tachycardia which is a serious complication of therapy and must be avoided [2].

Adrenergic blocking agents are vasodilators that affect the pre- and post-synaptic adrenergic receptors and possess arterial effects. The mechanisms of action are not the same for all of them. Let us consider for a moment the relative function of pre- and post-synaptic adrenergic receptors. We are accustomed to thinking about postsynaptic receptors that can be blocked by either beta-receptor antagonists, such as propranolol, or alpha-receptor antagonists such as phentolomine. We are much less accustomed to thinking about presynaptic receptors, but such receptors are important because they regulate the intraneuronal synthesis of neurotransmitter. When this presynaptic receptor 'sees' norepinephrine in the cleft, it blocks the liberation of more norepinephrine; when it does not, it causes new norepinephrine to be produced. This phenomenon explains the tachycardia that occurs with phentolomine. Phentolomine blocks both pre- and post-synaptic receptors. The norepinephrine that is synthesized and released cannot combine with the target organ, so there is no peripheral vasoconstriction. In the heart, the norepinephrine cannot combine with the presynaptic receptor. It therefore intensifies the neuronal synthesis of norepinephrine. The result is an excess of norepinephrine which causes tachycardia by a beta effect which is not blocked by phentolomine. Thus, in addition, to the reflex tachycardia induced by the vasodilatory effect as it decreases left ventricular filling pressure, phentolomine causes tachycardia by leading to stimulation of beta receptors.

Vasodilators include a number of different drugs with quite different pharmacological properties. The very old fashioned *veratrum alkaloids* are interesting in that they produce reflex vasodilatation. *Thiazides* may well have their effect by a sodium mechanism involving the vascular wall, although it has proved difficult to demonstrate. They almost certainly do not work exclusively by producing total body sodium depletion, because they still reduce blood pressure after sodium balance has been restored.

Whereas *phentolomine* is an indirect acting vasodilator because of its alpha-antagonistic effect, *nitroprusside* is a direct acting arterial vasodilator. Maroko et al. used these vasodilators to study the effect of increasing heart rate during experimental myocardial infarction [3]. When dogs were studied in the pre-occlusion state by multiple site EKG tracings, ST-segment elevations were trivial. After coronary occlusion, there was a marked increase in ST-segment elevation. The animals were then given phentolamine and the ST-segment elevation increased even more, but the heart rate increased from 117 to 130 beats/min. Under these circumstances, the beneficial effects of phentolomine in reducing afterload and cardiac work were more than offset by the increase in myocardial oxygen consumption caused by the increased heart rate. The same deleterious effects were found with nitroprusside, but to a lesser degree because the increase in heart rate was somewhat less. When the rate was accelerated by ventricular pacing to what it had been with phentolomine, the ST-segment elevation was the same. The difference, then, in apparent benefit between phentolomine and nitroprusside, modest as it was, became obliterated by equalizing the heart rates. We should learn from this that when vasodilators are used in patients with congestive failure, hypertension and probable underlying coronary disease, care must be taken to avoid inducing reflex tachycardia. Even if the agents themselves do not cause problems directly, reflex tachycardia is a serious problem with almost all the vasodilators if the left ventricular filling pressure falls too low and decreases the cardiac output too much.

Hydralazine is another vasodilator that has been well studied and found to be useful. It accelerates the heart rate by releasing catecholamines from the atrial myocardium in the vicinity of the SA node, and its cardio-accelerating effect can be blocked by propranolol. Even in a denervated heart, it produces a mild cardioaccelerator effect which is sympathetically mediated through this local release. In patients with congestive heart failure, however, Chatterjee et al. [4] found that a single dose of hydralazine did not increase heart rate, presumably because his patients started off with very high left ventricular filling pressures which did not fall below the optimal level for maximum cardiac output and thus did not initiate reflex cardioacceleration. Hydralazine acts on the arterial side of the circulation; its primary effect is to decrease peripheral vascular resistance. This is associated either with an increase or no change in left ventricular filling pressure because blood flow is augmented in the systemic circuit; hence, there is no harmful compensatory increase in heart rate. Hydralazine is therefore a good drug to use; it increases cardiac index and stroke volume, perfusion is favored and oxygen requirement is not increased.

Prazosin is an interesting drug in that it blocks the postsynaptic receptor, but it does not block presynaptic receptors. The cell can therefore respond appropriately to the amount of neurotransmitter which is synthesized. Patients with congestive failure who are given prazosin reduce their systemic vascular resistance and blood pressure; at the same time they increase stroke work and cardiac index [5]; thus, the heart performs better. There is a controversy about how long the effect persists; some investigators feel that tachyphylaxis develops very rapidly, while others disagree. It seems likely that circulating levels of catecholomines and overall sympathoadrenal stimulation determine whether or not tachyphylaxis occurs. In any event, this drug does not induce reflex tachycardia at the local level because the presynaptic receptor can respond to local norepinephrine concentration.

Phosphodiesterase inhibitors are relatively new drugs which have quickly become widely used throughout Europe. They allow the accumulation of cyclic AMP in vascular tissue. This is the presumed mechanism underlying their vasodilatory properties, although some phosphodiesterase inhibitors are not vasodilator and some drugs with phosphodiesterase inhibitory properties, such as prazosin, do not work by that particular mechanism. *Verapamil* is the usual drug of choice for supraventricular tachyarrhythmias. It is also the drug of choice for many other kinds of ventricular dysrhythmias and in many patients with angina. It is an effective vasodilator because it blocks calcium influx into the vascular smooth muscle cell and thereby deprives the contractile apparatus of the calcium that is needed to permit actomyosin bridge formation to occur. The same thing happens in the heart. Thus, one of the side effects of verapamil is negative inotropy, but the effect in the vessels is much more dominant, such that the drug is primarily a vasodilator and an antiarrhythmic. *Nifedipine* and *diltiazem* are alternative calcium channel blockers with a different spectrum of clinical properties.

Dopamine and *dobutamine* are the last agents to be considered. Most authorities would classify them as cardiac stimulants, but they are indeed also vasodilators. Tuttle and Mills, as well as others, observed that substitutions in the catecholamine structure produced differential biological actions, and they created some very specific and interesting compounds [6]. The beta-hydroxyl group is responsible for the cardioaccelerating action of the catecholamine structure. Thus, dopamine and dobutamine, which do not have a beta-hydroxyl group, are less likely to cause increases in heart rate even though they have adrenergic effects throughout the body. There are dopaminergic receptors in vessels which lead to specific vasodilitation of the splenic bed and the renal artery. If a patient with profound heart failure is given dopamine, there will be abrupt and dramatic increases in urine output because of a very specific renal vasodilation even if the hemodynamic status of the patient as a whole does not improve substantially. Dobutamine, which is an even newer drug, does not have this dopaminergic action on the renal vessels. Both of these drugs stimulate the beta receptors in the heart, increasing contractility. They both cause vasodilitation in the periphery by a beta-adrenergic mechanism and therefore decrease peripheral vascular resistance. It has been shown that this vasodilitation can be blocked with phenoxybenzamine, an alpha antagonist, just as the vasodilitation of epinephrine is blocked. This indicates, simply, that dopaminergic effects on vessels and the heart are mediated by the same receptors as when those effects are due to conventional catecholamines.

Coronary blood flow can be remarkably well preserved in experimental myocardial infarction. It has been demonstrated that animals subjected to left anterior coronary occlusion after dobutamine possessed much more homogeneous perfusion between the ischemic and nonischemic beds than without dobutamine. In other words, during the coronary ligation, there was an improvement in coronary perfusion of the ischemic region because of more favorable pressure relationships in the left ventricle. In the clinical setting, Sobel and colleagues demonstrated that dobutamine increased cardiac index, lowered the pulmonary wedge pressure and caused virtually no change in heart rate and only a slight increase in systolic blood pressure, apparently because of the dominance of the cardiostimulatory effect and despite the vasodilatation. Moreover dobutamine did this without extending the apparent infarction, as judged from enzymatic indices [7].

In summary, congestive heart failure, in an acutely ill patient in a coronary care unit, is now reason for the judicious use of selected vasodilators. In ambulatory care medicine, the management of patients with congestive heart failure is shifting in the same direction because of the biological advantages noted above. The intimate relationship between the level of blood pressure, the level of peripheral vascular resistance and the function of the heart was recognised long ago. It was evident when hypertension was a frequent presenting sign of profound congestive failure. Once hypertension was avoided in this setting, the heart was neglected. It is now time to again consider the whole patient when one is dealing with heart failure in a hypertensive and to use agents that influence hemodynamics, coronary perfusion, left ventricular oxygen requirement and cardiac function as well as blood pressure.

References

1. Mason DT (ed): Symposium on vasodilator and inotropic therapy of heart failure. Am J Med 65:101, 1978.
2. Williams DO, Amsterdam EA, Mason DT: Hemodynamic effects of nitroglycerin in acute myocardial infarction: decrease in ventricular preload at the expense of cardiac output. Circulation 51:421, 1975.
3. Maroko PR, Kjekshus JK, Sobel BE: Factors influencing infarct size following experimental coronary artery occlusions. Circulation 43:67, 1971.
4. Chatterjee K, Parnley WW, Massie B, Greenberg B, Werner J, Klausner S, Norman A: Oral hydralazine therapy for chronic refractory heart failure. Circulation 54:879, 1976.
5. Miller RR, Awan NA, Maxwell KS, Mason DT: Sustained reduction of cardiac impedance and preload in congestive heart failure with the antihypertensive vasodilator prazosin. N Engl J Med 279:303, 1977.
6. Tuttle RR, Mills J: Development of a new catecholamine to selectively increase cardiac contractility. Circ Res 36:185, 1975.
7. Gillespie TA, Ambos HD, Sobel BE, Roberts R: Effects of dobutamine in patients with acute myocardial infarction. Am J Cardiol 39:588, 1977.

12. Antiplatelet drugs

SOL SHERRY

Introduction

Hypertension is one of the most important risk factors in the development of vascular disease, which predisposes the patient to a variety of acute vascular events; prominent among these is the appearance of an acute thrombosis.

There are two major classifications of thrombi: those that form in areas of slow flow and low pressure and those that form in the presence of rapid flow and high pressure. Although there may be some overlap in the biochemical and physiological mechanisms producing these entitites, it is recognized that a thrombus, which forms in the veins (slow flow, low pressure) and to which the hypertensive patient is not predisposed, is primarily a coagulation thrombus and consists mostly of red blood cells and fibrin. By contrast, those which occur in the systemic arteries (rapid flow, high pressure) and to which the hypertensive patient is predisposed, consist of a prominent 'white' head composed of platelets, which have adhered to and aggregated at a site of injured or destroyed endothelium, and a variable amount of superimposed fibrin-red cell coagulum. Since the systemic arterial type of thrombus is the one most likely to be affected by antiplatelet drugs, the focus of this chapter will be on a review of the results of studies with these drugs on two major acute cardiovascular complications in hypertensive patients, i.e., acute coronary events and stroke.

Sulfinpyrazone, aspirin and dipyridamole will be the only drugs under consideration. All three have undergone investigation and continue to be extensively investigated for their antithrombotic effects in arterial vascular disease. Each of them, despite differences in their pharmacological actions, influences platelet activity through prostaglandin-mediated pathways. Other drugs, e.g., clofibrate and beta-blockers, have also demonstrated platelet-inhibitory activity, but they will be excluded from this review because their mechanism of action is unclear, or they have not undergone extensive testing, or the rationale for their use in various trials was unrelated to their platelet effects.

Cardiac studies on prevention of acute coronary events

In recent years there has been considerable interest in testing whether agents that affect prostaglandin metabolism, and thereby inhibit the ability of platelets to aggregate at sites of vascular injury, might decrease the risk of a coronary death. The rationale is that the two major immediate causes of 'coronary death', i.e., sudden cardiac death (presumably due to an acute fatal arrhythmia) and the more classical myocardial infarction, may, in large part, be due to platelet phenomena. In sudden cardiac death – platelet thrombi readily form on the injured coronary vessels which frequently occur in coronary artery disease – and these thrombi are also likely to shed platelet emboli. Such thrombi and emboli can readily produce areas of transient ischemia both by physical obstruction and by the vasconstrictive properties of the released serotonin and thromboxane A_2; the resulting ischemia can precipitate an arrhythmia sufficient to cause sudden death. Myocardial infarction can be caused when, in areas of *more extensive* injury to a coronary artery (such as a sudden crack, fissure, or ulcer in an atheromatous plaque), a plug of platelets rapidly fills the lesion and serves to initiate a larger arterial thrombus, often sufficient in size to occlude the entire vessel and cause an extensive transmural infarction. Thus there is reason to suspect that agents that inhibit platelet function could significantly influence the incidence of major coronary events.

Secondary prevention of death in ischemic heart disease

To test the hypothesis that treatment with antiplatelet drugs could prevent death from acute coronary events or their sequelae, several large-scale secondary intervention trials have been undertaken in patients with chronic ischemic heart disease. The population chosen for study were patients who had experienced one or more acute myocardial infarctions – an almost certain indicator of ischemic heart disease. In addition, this population has the advantage for study of being at higher risk of mortality from subsequent acute coronary events, thus providing a better opportunity for assessing the efficacy of these drugs.

In North America, aspirin, alone or in combination with dipyridamole, and sulfinpyrazone have each recently been the subject of intensive investigation in large multicenter studies of patients with previous myocardial infarction, with the results of all three studies being published in 1980. Other controlled, clinical trials have also been conducted, especially with aspirin. Still other clinical studies are being planned or are in progress.

1. Clinical trials with aspirin alone
More studies, dating back to earlier times, have been conducted with aspirin than with the other drugs.

a. Retrospective studies. Interest in the possible role of aspirin for coronary events was first expressed by Craven in the early 1950s when he reported that in 1465 sedentary, overweight men, aged 45–65 years, placed on a daily regimen of 300 mg of aspirin over a seven-year period, no coronary occlusion or insufficiency occurred [14]. Cobb et al [11] did not speculate on the association of aspirin therapy and the unexpectedly low incidence of myocardial infarction as the cause of death in the autopsy findings of a large series of patients dying with rheumatoid arthritis at the Massachusetts General Hospital. However, their observations, in retrospect, could be interpreted as providing evidence for Craven's view. However, it is only in the last decade that Craven's remarkable claims, albeit in an uncontrolled study, have found any support in subsequent studies.

In an epidemiological survey reported in 1974 [6], the *Boston Collaborative Drug Surveillance Group* found that the percentage of patients who had regularly (usually daily, but of undetermined dosage) taken aspirin during the month before hospitalization was significantly lower in 325 patients hospitalized with acute myocardial infarction than in 3807 patients hospitalized for other causes (0.09% versus 4.9%). In an update of their retrospective data published two years later in 1976 [7], the group reported that this negative association between aspirin use and risk of myocardial infarction was maintained with the accumulation of approximately twice the original data. Because of the nature of this study, the findings could not be taken as conclusive, but they provided important impetus for several subsequent controlled prospective studies.

Another study was an *American Cancer Study* survey of records of over 1,000,000 men and women maintained during a five-year period [24]. A review of these records showed that the rate of death from coronary heart disease was no lower for those who took aspirin 'often' than for those who took the drug 'seldom' or 'never'. Unfortunately, the use of aspirin and the cause of deaths were loosely defined in the records surveyed.

b. Prospective studies. In an early attempt to study the issue prospectively, no benefit was found for aspirin. In a Finnish double-blind, prospective study conducted for a year in 430 aged people (all more than 70 years of age; mean, 79), no difference was found in morbidity (hospitalization) or mortality between the aspirin-treated (1 gm daily) and control (placebo) groups [27]. However, later studies have shown somewhat more interesting results.

(1) *Medical Research Council Studies.* More direct support for aspirin's role in the secondary prevention of mortality from myocardial infarction came with the publication in 1974 of the results of a prospective, randomized, controlled Medical Research Council study conducted in England by Elwood et al. [17]. In a double-blind trial, the investigators compared the effects on mortality of daily treatment with 300 mg of aspirin for two years with those of placebo in 1239 men

who had a confirmed diagnosis of myocardial infarction. The low dosage of aspirin was chosen on the basis that it was well above the level needed to inhibit collagen- or ADP-induced platelet aggregation. In the aspirin-treated group, reductions in total mortality of 12% and 25% over that in the placebo group were found at six and 12 months, respectively. These reductions were not statistically significant. However, when the results were analyzed in respect to the interval between myocardial infarction and admission to the study, a stronger difference was found. Approximately half the patients entered the study less than six weeks after myocardial infarction. The mortality rate for the aspirin-treated group which entered the study within six weeks after myocardial infarction was 7.8% as compared to a 13.5% rate in the placebo group.

The same investigators recently completed another *Medical Research Council Study* of a similar multicenter, randomized, double-blind design [18]. For this study, however, a higher daily dosage of aspirin, 900 mg (300 mg three times daily), was used for a period of just one year. Moreover, women were included in the study and comprised 15% of the total 1682 patients in the study.

In addition to total mortality, mortality from ischemic heart disease and rehospitalization resulting from myocardial infarction, ischemic heart disease without myocardial infarction or other causes were measured. The investigators attempted to measure compliance, on the basis of tests for salicylate made at unannounced home visits, and they estimated it to be at least 72% and probably much higher.

Although the withdrawal rate, primarily due to side effects, was high, it was evenly distributed (228 patients, or 27%, from each group), and the withdrawals were included in the analysis.

The total mortality rate in patients given aspirin was 12.3%, as compared to a rate of 14.8% in those receiving placebo. The 17.3% reduction in mortality attributable to aspirin was not statistically significant. However, these data may have been influenced by the fact that two factors strongly prognostic of death, pulmonary congestion and cardiac enlargement, were more common in the aspirin-treated group. The analysis of specific mortality resulting from ischemic heart disease suggested a greater, statistically significant reduction in the aspirin-treated group, but, when this rate was adjusted for slight age differences between the groups, it was no longer significant.

There were only slight differences between the treatment groups in numbers of rehospitalizations for ischemic heart disease without myocardial infarction or for other causes. However, 7.1% of the aspirin-treated group was readmitted for infarction as compared with 10.9% for the placebo group – a 34% reduction that was statistically significant. The total mortality, when combined with the nonfatal ischemic heart disease morbidity, increased with age in men but not consistently so in women; the combined rate was significantly reduced in the aspirin-treated group by 28% (p < 0.05) in all patients. However, in their report of their findings, the investigators note that the data on nonfatal reinfarctions were limited and uncertain.

The investigators found that, although inconclusive, the results consistently suggested a smaller benefit from aspirin for women than for men. Moreover, they noted that their data 'suggested that the difference between the treatments emerges very early and about three months after infarction little further difference developed.' Again, their findings in this respect could not be considered conclusive.

(2) *Coronary Drug Project Aspirin Study*. The Coronary Drug Project Aspirin Study, completed in 1975, evaluated total mortality, cause-specific mortality, nonfatal events, and combinations of fatal and nonfatal events in aspirin-treated and control (placebo) groups [12].

The study population was selected from groups who had been receiving dextrothyroxine or estrogen therapy in another Coronary Drug Project Study, but had terminated treatment. The 1529 patients, all male, had had at least one documented myocardial infarction; one-third had had serious complications or more than one infarction. Five or more years had elapsed since the last infarction for approximately 75% of the patients, and more than 60% of them were over 35 years of age.

The patients were randomly assigned, on a double-blind basis, to daily treatment with 972 mg of aspirin (324 mg three times per day) or placebo, for a period ranging from ten to 28 months. Patients were evaluated at four-month intervals and compliance was monitored.

Overall mortality was 5.8% in the aspirin group and 8.3% in the placebo group (an observed difference of 30%). In regard to cause-specific mortality, the aspirin group had a reduction relative to the placebo group of 27% for coronary death and 19% for sudden cardiovascular deaths (i.e., deaths occurring within 60 min after onset of symptoms).

The incidence of definite nonfatal myocardial infarction was only slightly lower in the aspirin group (3.7%) than in the placebo group (4.2%). The largest clinical difference in definite or suspect nonfatal cardiovascular events was for the development of hypertension since entry, which occurred in 12.2% and 9.6% of the aspirin and placebo groups, respectively – an incidence that was 27% higher in the aspirin group.

All observed side effects were reported more frequently by the aspirin group than by the placebo group. The largest difference was for stomach pain; twice as many aspirin patients complained of such pains as did placebo patients (12.5% for aspirin, 6.3% for placebo).

(3) *German-Austrian Multicenter Study*. In a German-Austrian, multicenter, prospective study, completed in 1977, aspirin was compared with phenprocoumon or placebo for the secondary prevention of myocardial infarction or sudden death [8, 9]. Of the 946 patients admitted to the study four to six weeks after their

qualifying infarction, 78.5% were male. Patients were randomly allocated to one of three treatment groups: aspirin, 1.5 gm daily; placebo; or phenprocoumon.

Phenprocoumon, an anticoagulant widely used in Germany and Austria for the prevention of reinfarction, was given at a dosage adjusted individually to maintain prothrombin time values between 15% and 25% or thrombotest values around 10%. The trial was double-blind regarding treatment with placebo or aspirin but open regarding treatment with phenprocoumon. Randomization was within strata, including hospital, age, sex, secondary infarction, cardiac failure and hyperlipidemia or cholesterolemia.

Over a two-year observation period, patients received clinical and laboratory evaluations at two- to four-week intervals. Compliance was checked in subgroups through urine salicylate. Nonfatal myocardial infarction and sudden death, as well as total and cardiac mortality, were selected as endpoints for the trial, and patients experiencing a nonfatal event were not enrolled as participants in the trial thereafter.

A final analysis of the data has not yet been published. However, some results have been reported [8]. A total of 61 patients died of verified myocardial infarction or sudden death during the trial. Most of these died during the first half year. The highest numbers of coronary deaths occurred in the phenprocoumon group with 26 and placebo group with 22, whereas only 13 such deaths occurred in the aspirin group. This reduction reaches a level of statistical significance close to a p value of 0.05. When compared to the placebo, the benefit from aspirin was restricted to the first six months, although, because of the relatively small numbers of deaths during this period, a statistically significant benefit could not be established.

The investigators analyzed risk factors in relation to their results and found that for death the most relevant risk factors were reinfarction as the qualitying event for entry into the study and heart failure within four weeks after the initial infarction.

Side effects occured most frequently in the aspirin group, especially gastrointestinal complaints.

(4) *Aspirin Myocardial Infarction Study* (AMIS). By far the largest prospective trial of aspirin for the secondary prevention of death from myocardial infarction has been the recently completed Aspirin Myocardial Infarction Study [4]. This double-blind, controlled study, sponsored by the National Heart, Lung, and Blood Institute and conducted at 30 clinical centers in the United States, was designed to test whether the regular administration of aspirin to patients who had experienced at least one documented myocardial infarction would result in a significant reduction of total mortality over a three-year period. Secondary objectives, such as cause-specific mortality and nonfatal cardiovascular events, were also evaluated.

Over a 13-month period, 4524 patients with a previous, documented myocardial infarction were entered into the study. Of these, 4021 (89%) were men. The patients were between the ages of 30 and 69 years, with a mean age of 54.8 years. In a double-blind fashion, patients were randomly assigned to treatment with aspirin or placebo. Based on the experience of the Coronary Drug Project Aspirin Study [12], a total daily dosage of 1.0 gm (0.5 gm twice daily) of aspirin was selected.

The time of entrance into the study after the qualifying myocardial infarction ranged anywhere from eight weeks to as long as five years, with a mean of 25 months. Results were further compromised by the fact that, as a happenstance of the randomization process, seven baseline characteristics were distributed unevenly enough between the two groups to make the discrepancies statistically significant. These risk factors included previous heart failure, angina pectoris, cardiomegaly and histories of using digitalis, nitroglycerin, propranolol or 'other drugs'. For all seven, the inferred risk fell more heavily on the aspirin group.

During the minimum three-year follow-up period, the initial baseline characteristics were reviewed at four-month intervals. Various biochemical measurements were also recorded during the course of the study. Compliance was checked and estimated to be very good.

Fatal events were analyzed with the Cox statistical procedure (based on a proportional hazard model). For nonfatal events, such as recurrent myocardial infarction, angina pectoris, stroke, intermittent cerebral ischemic attacks, and cardiovascular surgery, a 2×2 table analysis was employed. All randomized patients were included in the analysis.

In terms of the study's primary endpoint, total mortality, no significant benefit from aspirin was found. The total mortality rate after 38 months of follow-up was 10.8% in the aspirin group and 9.7% in the placebo group. On the other hand, the cardiovascular-morbidity tallies favored the aspirin-treated group. The percentage of nonfatal myocardial infarction was 6.3% in the aspirin group versus 8.1% in the placebo group.

(5) *Single-Dose Study*. Another study, sponsored by the Medical Research Council in England, investigated the effects upon mortality of a *single* dose of aspirin, 300 mg, given to patients who have experienced acute symptoms suggestive of myocardial infarction upon mortality within three days. In an analysis of 1705 such patients [19], no benefit upon mortality within 28 days was found.

c. Other studies in progress or unpublished. An open, randomized study of the effects of aspirin (1.5 gm daily) versus those of oral anticoagulants on reinfarction and cardiac death in patients with myocardial infarction has been conducted in 15 hospitals in France under the Institut National de la Santé et de la Recherche Médicale (INSERM), but details of the study have not yet been published. An enrollment of 1500 patients is called for, which will be followed for two years [44].

No other studies known to us are presently in progress for the investigation of treatment with aspirin alone for the *secondary* prevention of death in patients with ischemic heart disease, as indicated by prior myocardial infarction. However, two studies have been started in order to study the effects of aspirin on myocardial infarction and death in patients with unstable angina pectoris.

One double-blind, randomized study, being conducted in ten Veterans Administration hospitals in the United States, compared the effects of low doses of aspirin (324 mg) and of placebo given daily for 12 weeks [45]. The patients are men who have been admitted to a coronary care unit for new or worsening angina and have evidence of coronary artery disease but not acute myocardial infarction.

The other double-blind, randomized study, sponsored by the medical Research Council of Canada and designed to cover a two-year follow-up period will measure the effects of aspirin (1.3 gm daily) and sulfinpyrazone (800 mg daily), singly and in combination, versus placebo in 700 patients admitted to a coronary care unit with unstable angina pectoris. The study, scheduled for completion in 1984, will have acute myocardial infarction and death as its endpoints (M. Gent, personal communication).

A large study of aspirin in the primary prevention of death and cardiovascular events (stroke, heart attack) is being conducted in 4200 healthy subjects (all physicians) in England [45]. Patients have been randomly allocated to a control (untreated) group or treatment with aspirin, 500 mg daily.

Comment. The results of the various prospective studies with aspirin alone in reducing cardiac mortality following an acute myocardial infarction remain inconclusive. In those trials where aspirin was tested early after an infarction, there appears to be a beneficial effect in reducing the high mortality observed during the early postrecovery period. In general, the findings are reminiscent of those more clearly established with sulfinpyrazone in the Anturane Reinfarction Trial (see below).

When beneficial results have been claimed, they have been observed with doses of aspirin varying from 0.3–1.5 gm daily; this suggests that the dosage of aspirin may not be as critical in vivo as postulated on the basis of in vitro studies.

2. Clinical trials with dipyridamole and aspirin

The rationale for combined treatment with dipyridamole and aspirin is based on a possible synergistic effect, since aspirin inhibits production of the platelet-aggregating substance, thromboxane A_2, while dipyridamole enhances the action of prostacyclin, an inhibitor of platelet aggregation [32], which is inhibited by aspirin. The recent Persantine-Aspirin Reinfarction Study (PARIS) compared the effects of combined treatment with dipyridamole (Persantin) and aspirin with those of aspirin alone or placebo on mortality and morbidity in patients with previous myocardial infarction [36].

In the double-blind trial conducted at 20 clinical centers in the United States and England, 2026 patients, aged 3074 years, of whom 1759 (87%) were men, were randomly allocated to one of the following treatments given three time daily: dipyridamole, 75 mg, and aspirin 324 mg; aspirin, 324 mg, and one placebo tablet; and two placebo tablets. There were 810 patients allocated to each of the two active treatment groups and 406 to the placebo group.

Patients were entered into the trial anytime from eight weeks to as long as five years after a myocardial infarction documented by ECG changes and enzyme elevations. The primary endpoints evaluated were total mortality, coronary mortality and coronary incidence (coronary death or definite but nonfatal myocardial infarction).

Of the total 2026 patients, 1666 completed the trial. Another 224 patients were reported deceased. The remaining 136 patients withdrew from the study; of these one was known to have died, 128 were known to be alive and the fate of seven was unknown at the time the results were reported.

Follow-up visits were scheduled at one month after entry into the study and at four-month intervals thereafter, for an average follow-up period of 44 months. Compliance was monitored at these visits by tablet count and urine treating for drugs and was found to be similar in the three groups.

Total mortality was 16% and 18% lower in the dipyridamole/aspirin and aspirin groups, respectively, than in the placebo group. Three-quarters of the deaths were coronary in nature. There were 24% and 21% fewer coronary deaths in the dipyridamole/aspirin and aspirin groups, respectively, than in the placebo group. Coronary *incidence* was reduced by 25% and 24% in these groups. The aspirin group had the highest incidence of sudden coronary death, with 5.6% of the group's patients dying within one hour after the onset of symptoms. On the other hand, the aspirin group showed the lowest incidence of nonsudden coronary death – 2.5%, compared to 5.7% and 4.0% in the placebo and dipyridamole/aspirin groups, respectively.

None of the above differences were statistically signifficant at a Z value greater than 2.6, the critical value chosen for the study. However, significant differences in coronary *incidence* between the dipyridamole/aspirin and placebo groups were found after 4, 8, 12, 16, 20 and 24 months of treatment.

Patients enrolled in the study within six months after myocardial infarction had fewer deaths in the active treatment groups, a reduction of 44% in the combination group and 51% in the aspirin group. However, the number of patients enlisted so soon after myocardial infarction was limited (179 in the dipyridamole/aspirin group, 173 in-the aspirin group and 95 in the placebo group).

Both active treatment groups showed a reduction in incidence of definite nonfatal MI, angina pectoris requiring hospitalization, and stroke; however, both showed a higher incidence of acute coronary insufficiency than the placebo group. The largest difference occurred for congestive heart failure; both active treatments showed a lower incidence than the placebo group, but neither difference was statistically significant.

Several additional analyses were conducted to assess the occurrence of angina during the trial. Between-group differences were small, with no detectable effect (adverse or beneficial) of either active treatment.

The expected aspirin-related side effects appeared in both active treatment groups. These reactions included stomach pain, heartburn, nausea, gastrointestinal irritation and gastrointestinal bleeding. The combination group also showed a significant increase in incidence of headaches.

Because of the marked reductions in total and coronary deaths in patients entering the PARIS trial within six months after infarction and treated with aspirin and dipyridamole, another large-scale study is being undertaken by the same investigators in patients within four months after myocardial infarction. This study will compare the combination treatment with placebo only.

Comment. While this study did not show a statistically significant benefit from treatment with aspirin alone or in combination with dipyridamole, nevertheless, in contrast with the results of the Aspirin Myocardial Infarction Study (AMIS), it does suggest an appreciable reduction in fatal coronary events and in combined fatal and nonfatal coronary episodes (coronary incidence). Furthermore, this beneficial effect could more readily be demonstrated among those patients who entered the trial within six months of their qualifying myocardial infarction, i.e., during a period of increased mortality risk (early postrecovery period). In this respect, the findings in the aspirin group of PARIS are reminiscent of the observations previously reported in the Elwood studies [17, 18] and the German-Austrian multicenter trial [8, 9].

Whether the addition of dipyridamole to aspirin in the dosages employed provided any additional benefit over that claimed for aspirin alone is not answered by this trial. While some of the clinical endpoints appeared to favor the combination therapy, others favored aspirin alone.

3. Clinical trials with sulfinpyrazone

Sulfinpyrazone, a uricosuric agent used since the 1950s for the treatment of gout, was first reported to have platelet-regulating action in 1965 [40]. In the ensuing decade, its effects were studied in the prevention of arteriovenous shunt thrombosis [28], recurrent venous thrombosis [41] and thromboembolism in patients with prosthetic cardiac valves [42]. In 1975, in a double-blind, placebo-controlled study of 291 elderly male patients, sulfinpyrazone was reported to significantly reduce mortality from vascular causes in a subgroup of 166 atherosclerotic patients [5].

a. Anturane Reinfarction Trial. In 1975 a large-scale, double-blind study was undertaken of the effects of sulfinpyrazone on cardiac mortality in patients with a recent myocardial infarction [2, 3]. The study, conducted over a three-year period at 26 clinical centers in the United States and Canada and designated the Anturane Reinfarction Trial, compared sulfinpyrazone, 800 mg daily (200 mg four times per day), with placebo for an average period of 16 months. Patients were enrolled in the study 25–35 days after the occurrence of a documented myocardial infarction.

In contrast with previous 'intent-to-treat' trials, the Anturane Reinfarction Trial was designated as a 'clinical efficacy' study. This was considered possible without influencing bias for the following reasons: (a) sulfinpyrazone could not be differentiated from the placebo by either patient or physician on the basis of taste, color or appearance; (b) sulfinpyrazone would produce no unique symptoms or signs that would allow it to be identified either by patient or physician; (c) all laboratory determinations were carried out in a central laboratory and, in addition, uric acid determinations were blanked out from any laboratory assays conducted on trial patients at the respective participating institutions; (d) all criteria for analyzability were set forth clearly in the protocol and operations manual before the trial was initiated; (e) the accuracy of the data collected was reviewed both during the trial and retrospectively during several audits carried out at different levels by independent groups with expertise in the conduct of such audits; and (f) all decisions were made on a blind basis without knowledge of drug assignment, and all such decisions were reviewed at three independent levels.

Therefore, it was deemed feasible to establish beforehand that the primary analysis would be only of cardiac deaths among eligible patients with analyzable events, according to clearly defined criteria for eligibility and analyzability established before the inception of the trial. Thus, prior to the start of the trial, specific criteria were established for the classifications of death as 'sudden death', 'myocardial infarction', or 'other cardiac' deaths. 'Sudden death' was an unobserved death or one that occurred within 60 min of the onset of symptoms. 'Myocardial infarction' had to be documented at autopsy, or by clinical evidence of pain, electrocardiographic findings and by elevation of a serum enzyme (serum glutamic oxaloacetic transaminase, lactic dehydrogenase or creatinine phosphokinase) to twice the normal level. The 'other cardiac' category included congestive heart failure, arrhythmia or cardiogenic shock.

All deaths in eligible patients were further classified as analyzable or nonanalyzable. A death was considered nonanalyzable if it occurred within seven days after the initiation or termination of therapy or in a patient who did not comply with instructions, or if it could be attributed directly to surgery without association with a nonfatal event occurring during treatment. Analyzable deaths formed a basis for the primary analysis of the efficacy of sulfinpyrazone.

Of the original 1629 patients entered into the study, 1143 (73%) completed the protocol as planned and were included in the primary analysis. Of the remainder,

415 withdrew prematurely for various medical and nonmedical reasons, and 71 were excluded from analysis by the study's Policy Committee because they were judged, on a blind basis, not to meet the protocol criteria.

Follow-up visits were scheduled at 4, 8, 10, 14, 16, 20 and 22 months after entry into the study. Eighty-seven percent of the patients consistently took at least 80% of their medication, as measured by tablet counts at these visits. Serum uric acid levels were also measured as an indication of compliance with sulfinpyrazone therapy.

Side effects were recorded at each visit according to frequency, severity and duration. Thromboembolic events were reported in 36 patients (5%) receiving placebo and only 19 patients (2%) of those receiving sulfinpyrazone. Gastro-intestinal problems were reported by 214 patients taking sulfinpyrazone and 185 placebo-treated patients. Side effects were reported by 84% of the placebo-treated patients and 81% of those receiving sulfinpyrazone. Fifty-eight patients withdrew from the trial because of these events, but these were equally distributed between the groups.

All 106 analyzable deaths reported in the study were cardiovascular in nature, 105 were cardiac (the primary endpoint), and one was cerebrovascular. At 24 months the observed reduction in cardiac mortality from sulfinpyrazone treatment was approximately 32% (p = 0.058).

Over half of the deaths were sudden cardiac deaths and the reduction in this category was mainly responsible for the overall reduction. There were 37 sudden deaths in the placebo group versus 22 in the sulfinpyrazone-treated group, a reduction of 43% (p = 0.041). This advantage occurred during the first six months of treatment when the rate of analyzable sudden deaths was 7% in the placebo group versus 1.8% in the sulfinpyrazone-treated group, a highly significant reduction of 74% (p = 0.003). Thereafter, however, the rates of sudden death were comparable for the two groups (2.0% with placebo versus 2.3% with sulfinpyrazone treatment).

The reduction in sudden deaths, when nonanalyzable sudden deaths were included, was 68% at six months for the sulfinpyrazone-treated group. By this time, the majority of sudden deaths had already occurred. For the entire 24-month observation period, the reduction rate was 41%.

Sulfinpyrazone had no effect upon analyzable deaths from myocardial infarction, there being 18 such deaths in the placebo group and 17 in the sulfinpyrazone group after 24 months.

In reporting these findings, the investigators noted that the first six months after myocardial infarction are a period of high risk (particularly from sudden death) directly related to the previous myocardial infarction, and it is during this period (early postrecovery period) that sulfinpyrazone exerts its effect. They also noted that while the study was undertaken because of sulfinpyrazone's known effects upon platelet function, the fact that it was effective in reducing sudden

cardiac deaths, but not deaths from myocardial infarction, suggested that another, yet to be elucidated, mechanism of action exists.

b. Anturane Reinfarction Italian Study. A trial, similar in design to the Anturane Reinfarction Trial and designated 'The Anturane Reinfarction Italian
Study' (ARIS), is just reaching completion.

This study differed from the larger American counterpart in several respects
[37]. The daily dosage of sulfinpyrazone, 800 mg, was given in two doses of 400
mg/day instead of four 200-mg doses. Moreover, patients were enrolled into the
study a week or two earlier after their qualifying infarction – 10–20 days. In
addition to fatal reinfarction and sudden cardiac death, nonfatal myocardial
infarction serves as an endpoint for the study. Finally, platelet function tests
were performed during the course of the study to see if a correlation exists
between therapeutic effects and effects on platelet function.

The study was designed for a population of 650 patients of both sexes, which
will be followed for a period of at least one year. A preliminary report described
details of 400 patients enrolled at the time and preliminary findings of the platelet
function studies [13]. Final results have yet to be published.

c. Other sulfinpyrazone studies. It is our understanding that a very modest-sized
trial involving three compartments (placebo, aspirin and sulfinpyrazone) has
been completed in South Africa. No details of the trial design are available, and
no report has been issued as yet.

As mentioned in a previous section, a large Canadian study comparing the
effects of sulfinpyrazone and aspirin, singly and in combination, in patients with
unstable angina is currently in progress.

Comment. A great deal of publicity has been given to sulfinpyrazone, since the
Anturane Reinfarction Trial is the only study which has claimed a major benefit
for an agent in reducing cardiac mortality following an acute myocardial infarction, by virtue of a striking reduction in sudden death during the first six months
or high-risk early postrecovery period following discharge of the patient from
the hospital. This claim was made possible because of the unique features of trial
design, i.e., as a clinical efficacy study. By avoiding the various dilution factors
inherent in 'intent-to-treat' trials, this study allowed for a quantitative assessment of the drug's actual effect in compliant patients. In addition, because of the
early and narrow entry window (25–35 days post qualifying infarction), the trial
studied the effect of this drug on the natural history of mortality among recent
survivors of an infarct by both period and cause.

Considering the negative results of the Aspirin Myocardial Infarction Study
(AMIS) and the inconclusive results of the Persantine-Aspirin Reinfarction
Study (PARIS), it is not surprising that the trial has come under considerable
criticism. More recently, the US Food and Drug Administration has raised

serious questions as to the classification of certain of the deaths (sudden, myocardial infarction, other cardiac) within each treatment group. A review of the deaths by an outside independent panel of cardiologists recently convened for this purpose may clarify this issue.

While the emphasis on the reduction of sudden death alone may or may not require modification, the overall reduction in cardiac mortality during the early postrecovery period is not dissimilar to the beneficial trends ascribed to aspirin during this period in both the Elwood studies [18, 19], the German-Austrian multicenter trial [8, 9] and for those patients receiving the combination of aspirin and dipyridamole in the Persantine-Aspirin Reinfarction Study who were entered within the first six months of their qualifying infarction.

The claim that sulfinpyrazone reduces the incidence of sudden death and not fatal myocardial infarction has stimulated research on other actions of this drug which could account for this finding. Since most sudden deaths are due to the appearance of a lethal ventricular arrhythmia, the effect of this drug on experimentally induced ventricular arrhythmias arising from an inschemic myocardium in animals has been under study and already a number of interesting observations have been made [29, 34, 38]. Since an observation of a similar action by aspirin was reported previously [33], an effect of these agents on prostaglandin pathways other than platelets may be involved in any possible beneficial therapeutic effect.

The striking effects of the Anturane Reinfarction Trial require confirmation. Consequently, great interest can be attached to the results of the Italian study. Unfortunately, the size of this trial (approximately 650 patients) is probably too small to yield statistically significant differences even if the differences observed are similar to those described in the Anturane Reinfarction Trial. Therefore, the importance of this study probably will relate more to whether the various period and cause mortality rates are or are not influenced in a similar fashion to that described in the North American study.

Cerebrovascular disease studies

Secondary prevention of transient ischemic attacks (TIAs), stroke, and death in patients with TIAs

Cerebral transient ischemic attaks (TIAs) are known to be frequent precursors of stroke and death [15] and thromboembolism is thought to play a major role in their pathogenesis [23]. An early, double-blind study [1] of the effect of dipyridamole in 169 patients with cerebral ischemia, however, showed no benefit from treatment with the drug. The first evidence for an effect by platelet-active drugs came in 1972 in the form of case reports [26, 35] of two patients and one patient, respectively, with amaurosis fugax. Aspirin was found to reduce, or, in the latter case, abolish attacks of transient blindness in these patients. When dipyridamole was given to one of these patients, it had no effect.

In 1973 Dyken et al. [16] reported on their retrospective study of patients with TIAs, in which they found that 15 patients treated with aspirin had a marked reduction in subsequent TIAs compared to nine patients who did not receive aspirin.

In 1972, Evans [20] published findings of a 12-week, double-blind crossover comparison of sulfinpyrazone (200 mg four times daily) and placebo in 20 patients with amaurosis fugax. He found that treatment with sulfinpyrazone significantly reduced the number of subsequent TIAs.

Another double-blind study comparing sulfinpyrazone and placebo, conducted by Blakely and Gent [5], included 99 elderly institutionalized men who had a stroke. In these men a significant reduction in death from vascular causes was found in the sulfinpyrazone-treated group. Steele et al. [43] reported a marked reduction in subsequent TIAs in 19 TIA patients treated with sulfinpyrazone when compared with six untreated patients over an average 27-month period. Similarly, in a prospective, double-blind trial conducted in Heidelberg [39], aspirin (1500 mg/day) caused a significant reduction in TIAs and cerebral infarcts in 31 patients with carotid TIAs, when compared to placebo over a 24-month period.

1. The Canadian Cooperative Study: aspirin and sulfinpyrazone

The Canadian Cooperative Study Group [10] assessed the relative efficacy of aspirin and sulfinpyrazone, singly and in combination, in the reduction of recurrent transient ischemic attacks, stroke or death. In their trial, conducted at 24 clinical centers in Canada, 585 patients with threatened stroke (defined as at least one cerebral or retinal ischemic attack within the preceding three months) were studied for an average period of 26 months. Patients were stratified for each clinical center on the basis of the presumed site of ischemia and the presence or absence of a residual deficit, prior to random assigment on a double-blind basis, to one of four treatment groups. In approximately 65% of the patients, the symptoms of the ischemic attack were referable to the carotid circulation, in 25% to the vertebrobasilar, and in 10% to both. More than half of the patients for each site were free of residua.

The four regimens, each to be taken four times daily, were: sulfinpyrazone, 200 mg, plus a placebo; aspirin, 325 mg, plus a placebo; sulfinpyrazone, 200 mg, plus aspirin, 325 mg; and two placebos. Because sulfinpyrazone was believed to require one week to produce a biologically significant effect, any events occurring in the first week of therapy with any of the four regimens were excluded from the analysis of the results. Since the reason for withdrawal of any patient from the trial might be a deterioration in their neurological status, patients who withdrew were followed for six months and any events occuring were charged against the corresponding study regimen. Any bias caused by their inclusion would, of course, be against showing a benefit of treatment.

The endpoints were TIA and stroke or death. The latter were grouped together on the basis that those who died could not proceed to stroke.

Follow-up visits were scheduled at one and three months after entry into the study and every three months thereafter. Pill counts were made, and the final follow-up visit compliance was estimated to be 92%. The average follow-up period was 26 months.

Aspirin produced a risk reduction of 19% for all events – continuing TIAs, stroke or death. For the clinically more important events of stroke or death, aspirin produced an observed risk reduction of 31%, with a 48% reduction occurring in men. The greatest response (a reduction of 62%) was found in the 331 aspirin-treated men who entered the study without a previous myocardial infarction. There was no significant reduction in women.

Of the total population included in the study, 114 patients suffered stroke or death, or both. There were 23 additional events of stroke or death which were ruled ineligible because they occurred within the first seven days of treatment or more than six months after withdrawal from the study. If these 23 events were included in the main analysis, the statistical significance of the observed aspirin effect would increase.

No statistically significant reductions in TIAs or stroke or death occurred in the sulfinpyrazone-treated group as compared to the placebo group, nor in the group treated with a combination of aspirin and sulfinpyrazone as compared to aspirin alone. However, among the men in the study, the fewest events (strokes or deaths) occurred in the group receiving combined treatment. No statistically significant differences were found to be associated with the different sites of ischemia, the presence or absence of residua, single and multiple attacks, amaurosis fugax, age, smoking, obesity, hypercholesterolemia and hypertension.

Among the various side effects reported at the three-month follow-up visits, pain in the upper abdomen and heartburn were more common among patients allocated to aspirin-containing regimens. A total of 41% of the patients entered in the study withdrew from treatment. Of these 24% were due to side effects, and 72% of those withdrawing because of side effects were receiving aspirin.

2. AITIA study: aspirin

The Aspirin in Transient Ischemic Attacks (AITIA) study compared the effects of aspirin with those of placebo upon reduction or prevention of TIAs, cerebral infarction, and stroke-related mortality in patients with carotid TIAs [21, 22].

The study, conducted at ten clinical centers in the United States, included only patients who had experienced TIAs of the hemispheric type or attacks of monocular blindness (Amaurosis fugax). Upon entry into the study, a clinical decision regarding surgical intervention was made for each patient. The patient was then assigned to either a medical or surgical group. Within each group, patients were randomly allocated in a double-blind fashion to treatment with aspirin, 1300 mg daily (650 mg twice a day), or placebo. The medical group consisted of 178 eligible patients and the surgical group 125.

The absolute endpoints were total mortality and cause-specific mortality (from stroke and cardiovascular causes) and both cerebral and retinal infarction.

In additon, the number of carotid TIAs occurring within the three months prior to randomization was compared with the number reported in the first six months of follow-up. Based on this comparison, and in combination with the absolute endpoints, the patient's response was classified as either 'favorable' or 'unfavorable'. Those patients who did not complete the full six months of observation were labeled as 'less than six months follow-up'.

Follow-up visits were scheduled monthly for the first six months and at three-month intervals thereafter. Compliance was checked by pill counts and urine salicylate testing.

The results of the 178 medically treated patients were reported as follows [21]: an analysis for the first six months of follow-up showed that within the placebo group, 34 of 77 cases (44.2%) were classified as unfavorable because of continuing TIAs, whereas only 15 of 78 cases (19.2%) were classified as unfavorable in the aspirin group. This difference was considered statistically significantly. When analysis was extended from six to 12 months, 48 out of the 178 patients (24 in each of the treatment groups) could not be classified as 'favorable' or 'unfavorable' because of a lack of follow-up. Because of the large number of such cases (27%), further analysis of the TIA results was confined to six months.

The analysis of absolute endpoints showed no significant difference for the aspirin and placebo treatments. It was when patients having as many TIAs in the first six months of follow-up as they had had in the three months prior to randomization were included with those having an absolute endpoint in the first six months that aspirin emerged as the superior treatment.

Within the subgroup of patients diagnosed as having stenotic lesions of the carotid artery, significantly fewer (29.3%) absolute endpoints were reached in the aspirin treated group. When the occurrence of carotid TIAs in six months of follow-up was also considered in this subgroup, the difference was even more pronounced in favor of aspirin.

Various side effects reported by the medically treated patients included upset stomach, weakness, dizziness and urticaria, but none was of sufficient magnitude to cause withdrawal from the study.

Results for the 125 patients who had carotid TIAs and one or more accessible carotid lesions and underwent reconstructive surgery of the carotid artery were reported separately [22]. Most of these patients (60–70%) were randomized to either aspirin or placebo treatments within one week of surgery.

Results and analyses for the surgical patients were generally consistent with findings reported for the medical group. Life-table analysis of absolute end-points for 24 months follow-up did not reveal a statistically significant difference between the aspirin and placebo treatments. When deaths which were not stroke-related were eliminated from the life-table analysis, a significant difference was observed in favor of aspirin. Because of the small number of patients and the short period of follow-up, however, it was not possible to conclude that aspirin has an effect in preventing cerebral infarction.

Eight patients from the placebo group suffered brain infarcts as absolute endpoints within 24 months. Among aspirin-treated patients, there was one cerebral infarct and six cardiovascular deaths. This occurrence of cardiovascular mortality was claimed to be related to the much higher percentage of patients with cardiovascular risk factors remaining in the aspirin group 12 months after randomization.

The absolute level of cases having an unfavorable outcome in the surgical treatment group was about half of those reported for the medically treated patients.

Comment. There is little question that TIAs represent an excellent model for testing platelet-active drugs. Thromboembolic phenomena have long been implicated as playing a prominent role in most cases of TIA and stroke; anti-coagulation has been shown to be a useful secondary intervention in selected situations [30, 31]; and the importance of platelets in the pathogenesis of these morbid events is as important as (if not more important than) fibrin formation. This is in contrast to acute coronary events where the significance of thrombo-embolic phenomena precipitating sudden death or myocardial infarction is much less clear, where the effects of anticoagulation are still controversial and where the role of platelets in these episodes remains to be clarified.

From early observations and the more recent large double-blind controlled trials, reasonable evidence has not been provided that aspirin at a dosage of 1300 mg daily has a therapeutic effect in males suffering from transient ischemic episodes; clearly it reduces the incidence of subsequent ischemic episodes and also appears to lessen the occurrence of strokes and stroke-related mortality. Quite surprising is the lack of benefit from this medication in females [10]. A biological, pharmacological or clinical basis for the difference is unclear at present.

As for the other platelet-active drugs, dipyridamole given alone appears to have no effect. Whether it will act synergistically with aspirin, as it does in improving platelet survival [38], remains to be clarified.

The sulfinpyrazone data are conflicting. The observations of Evans [20], Steele [43], and Blakely and Gent [5], that a significant reduction in thromboembolic phenomena primarily due to decreased incidence of TIAs and strokes was found in the sulfinpyrazone group, all suggest a positive effect for this agent. On the other hand, sulfinpyrazone had no demonstrable effect when used alone in the Canadian Cooperative Study, although there is a suggestion of some benefit, in terms of hard endpoints, when sulfinpyrazone was combined with aspirin. Although no further studies with sulfinpyrazone are contemplated at present, the issue of its effectiveness (or lack thereof) remains unresolved.

Concluding comments and future prospects

The investigation of drugs affecting prostaglandins as antithrombotic agents, particularly for preventing acute arterial vascular catastrophies, has opened a new and exciting chapter in medical therapeutics. While a clear picture of their usefulness in various selected clinical situations still remains to be defined, it is evident that benefits can be ascribed to their use. In some situations, as described in this chapter, their value appears to be established, while in others much further work is required to determine whether there is an effect and, if so, to what extent.

The agents so far investigated not only vary in their effect on various prostaglandins but also have additional pharmacological actions that may influence the final clinical result. Consequently, we need to know much more about the differing effects of these drugs and what may be expected from each of these agents either singly or in combination with others.

Particularly relevant to the investigation of these agents is the need to establish optimal dosages, to improve on trial design and to clarify whether there are sex differences in responsiveness.

Furthermore, we still do not know whether dipyridamole by itself has any antithrombotic effect in vivo or whether, when used in combination with aspirin, the clinical effect is greater than that with aspirin alone. One could also speculate that the combination of dipyridamole with sulfinpyrazone, from a theoretical standpoint, may well be superior to that of dipyridamole with aspirin. Considering that, in the last analysis, arterial thrombosis involves both the interaction of platelets with the vessel wall and the coagulation of blood with fibrin formation, it is likely that maximal benefits will not be achieved until platelet-active drugs are tested in combination with anticoagulants.

The explosion of knowledge concerning both platelet and endothelial cell function and the mediators of their regulation will undoubtedly lead to the development and testing of many new drugs in the future. One can only hope that the scientific basis for their evaluation will be more firmly established than the empiricism that appears to dominate our current approach.

If the platelet-vessel wall interaction proves to be the key or initiating step in the pathogenesis of arteriosclerosis, then the research which has begun in this field may ultimately lead to primary preventive measures rather than the secondary interventions that appear to be the goal of most of our current endeavors for the major catastrophic vascular accidents.

References

1. Acheson J, Danta G, Hutchinson EC: Controlled trial of dipyridamole in cerebral vascular disease. Br Med J 1:614–615, 1969.
2. The Anturane Reinfarction Trial Research Group: Sulfinpyrazone in the prevention of cardiac death after myocardial infarction. N Engl J Med 298:289–295, 1978.
3. The Anturance Reinfarction Trial Research Group: Sulfinpyrazone in the prevention of sudden death after myocardial infarction. N Engl J Med 302:250–256, 1980.
4. Aspirin Myocardial Infarction Study Research Group: A randomized controlled trials of aspirin in persons recovered from myocardial infarction. JAMA 243:661–669, 1980.
5. Blakely JA, Gent M: Platelets, drugs, and longevity in a geriatric population. In: Hirsh J, Cade JF, Gallus AS, Schonbaum E (eds) Platelets, drugs, and thrombosis. Basel, S. Karger, pp 284–291, 1975.
6. Boston Collaborative Drug Surveillance Group: Regular aspirin intake and acute myocardial infarction. Br Med J 1:440–443, 1974.
7. Boston Collaborative Drug Surveillance Program: Regular asprin use and myocardial infarction. Br Med J 2:1057, 1976.
8. Breddin K, Uberla K, Walter E: German-Austria multicenter two years prospective study on the prevention of secondary myocardial infarction by ASA in comparison to phenprocoumon and placebo. Sixth International Congress on Thrombosis and Haemostasis. Thromb Haemost 38:168, 1979 (abstract).
9. Breddin K, Loew D, Lechner K, Uberla K, Walter E: Secondary prevention of myocardial infarction: comparison of acetylsalicylic acid, phenprocoumon and placebo. Thromb Haemost 40:225–236, 1979.
10. The Canadian Cooperative Study Group: A randomized trial of aspirin and sulfinpyrazone in threatened stroke. N Engl J Med 299:53–59, 1978.
11. Cobb S, Anderson F, Bauer W: Length of life and cause of death in rheumatoid arthritis. N Engl J Med 249:553–556, 1953.
12. The Coronary Drug Project Research Group: Aspirin in coronary heart disease. J Chronic Dis 29:625–642, 1976.
13. Cortellaro M, Fassio G, Boschetti C, Basagni M, Polli EE: Controlled ex-vivo effect of sulfin-pyrazone on platelet function of myocardial infarction patients. Haematologia 64:173–189, 1979.
14. Craven LL: Experiences with aspirin (acetylsalicyclic acid) in the nonspecific prophylaxis of coronary thrombosis. Miss Valley Med J 75:38–44, 1953.
15. Didisheim P, Fuster V: Actions and clinical status of platelet-suppressive agents. Sem Haematol 15:55–72, 1978.
16. Dyken ML, Kolar OJ, Jones FH: Differences in the occurrence of carotid transient ischemic attacks associated with antiplatelet aggregation therapy. Stroke 4:732–736, 1973.
17. Elwood PC, Cochrane AL, Burr ML, Sweetnam PM, Williams G, Welsby E, Hughes SJ, Renton R: A randomized controlled trial of acetylsalicylic acid in the secondary prevention of mortality from myocardial infarction. Br Med J 1:436–440, 1974.

18. Elwood PC, Sweetnam PM: Aspirin and secondary mortality after myocardial infarction. Lancet 2:1313–1315, 1979.
19. Elwood PC, Williams WO: A randomized controlled trial of aspirin in the prevention of early mortality in myocardial infarction. J R Coll Gen Pract 29:413–416, 1979.
20. Evans G: Effect of drugs that suppress platelet surface interaction on incidence of amaurosis fugax and transient cerebral ischemia. Surg Forum 23:239–241, 1972.
21. Fields WS, Lemak NA, Frankowski RF, Hardy RJ: Controlled trial of aspirin in cerebral ischemia. Stroke 8:301–316, 1977.
22. Fields WS, Lemak NA, Frankowski RF, Hardy RJ: Controlled trial of aspirin in cerebral ischaemia. Part II: Surgical group. Stroke 9:309–319, 1978.
23. Genton E, Barnett HJM, Fields WS, Gent M, Hoak JC: XIV. Cerebral ischemia: the role of thrombosis and of antithrombotic therapy. Stroke 8:150–175, 1977.
24. Hammond EC, Garfinkel L: Aspirin and coronary heart disease: findings of a prospective study. Br Med J 2:269–271, 1975.
25. Harker LA, Slichter SJ: Studies of platelet and fibrinogen kinetics in patients with prosthetic heart valves. N Engl J Med 283:1302–1305, 1970.
26. Harrison MJG, Marshall J, Meadows JC, Ross Russell RW: Effect of aspirin in amaurosis fugax. Lancet 2:743–744, 1971.
27. Heikinheimo R, Järvinen K: Acetylsalicylic acid and arteriosclerotic-thromboembolic diseases in the aged. J Am Geriat Soc 19:403–405, 1971.
28. Kaegi A, Pineo GF, Shimizu A, Trivedi H, Hirsh J, Gent M: Arteriovenous shunt thrombosis. N Engl J Med 290:304–306, 1974.
29. Kelliher GJ, Dix RK, Jurkiewicz N, Lawrence TL: Effects of sulfinpyrazone on arrhythmia and death following coronary occlusion in cats. In: McGregor M, Mustard JF, Oliver M, Sherry S (eds) Cardiovascular actions of sulfinpyrazone: basic and clinical research. Miami, Symposia Specialists, 1980, pp 193–209.
30. Link H, Lebram G, Johansson I, Rodberg C: Prognosis in patients with infarction and TIA in carotid territory during and after anticoagulant therapy. Stroke 10:529–532, 1979.
31. Millikan CH, McDowell FH: Treatment of transient ischemic attacks. Stroke 9:299–308, 1978.
32. Moncada S, Korbut R: Dipyridamole and other phosphodiesterase inhibitors act as antithrombotic agents by potentiating endogenous prostacyclin. Lancet 1:1286–1289, 1978.
33. Moschos C, Haider B, DeLaCruz C Jr, Lyons MM, Regan TJ: Antiarrhythmic effects of aspirin during nonthrombotic coronary occlusion. Circulation 57:681–684, 1978.
34. Moschos CB, Escobinas AJ, Jorgensen DB: Effects of sulfinpyrazone on ischemic myocardium. In: McGregor M, Mustard JF, Oliver M, Sherry S (eds) Cardiovascular actions of sulfinpyrazone: basic and clinical research. Miami, Symposia Specialists, 1980, pp 175–191.
35. Mundall J, Quintero P, von Kaulla KN, Harmon R, Austin J: Transient monocular blindness and increased platelet aggregability treated with aspirin: a case report. Neurology 22:280–285, 1972.
36. The Persantine-Aspirin Reinfarction Study Research Group: Persantine and aspirin in coronary heart disease. Circulation 52:449–461, 1980.
37. Polli EE, Cortellaro M: Anturane Reinfarction Italian Study Research Group (letter). N Engl J Med 298:1258–1259, 1978.
38. Povalski HJ, Olson R, Kopia S, Furness P: Comparative effects of sulfinpyrazone and aspirin in the coronary occlusion-reperfusion dog model. In: McGregor M, Mustard JF, Oliver M, Sherry S (eds) Cardiovascular actions of sulfinpyrazone: basic and clinical research. Miami, Symposia Specialists, 1980, pp 153–171.
39. Reuther R, Dorndorf W: Aspirin in patients with cerebral ischemia and normal angiograms or non-surgical lesions. Results of a double-blind trial. In: Breddin K, Dorndorf W, Loew D, Marx R (eds) Acetylsalicylic acid in cerebral ischemia and coronary heart disease. Stuttgart, FK Schautlauer, Verlag, 1978, pp 97–106.

40. Smythe HA, Ogryzlo MA, Murphy EA, Mustrad JF: The effects of sulfinpyrazone (Anturane) on platelet economy and blood coagulation in man. Can Med Assoc J 92:818–821, 1965.
41. Steele PP, Weily HS, Genton E: Platelet survival and adhesiveness in recurrent venous thrombosis. N Engl J Med 288:1148–1152, 1973.
42. Steele P, Weily H, Davies H, Pappas G, Genton E: Platelet survival time following aortic valve replacement. Circulation 51:358–362, 1975.
43. Steele P, Carroll J, Overfield D, Genton E: Effect of sulfinpyrazone on platelet survival time in patients with transient cerebral ischemic attacks. Stroke 8:396–398, 1977.
44. Verstraete M: Registry of prospective clinical trials. Third report. Thromb Haemost 39:759–767, 1978.
45. Verstraete M: Registry of prospective clinical trials. Fourth report. Thromb Haemost 43:176–181, 1980.

13. Pregnancy, oral contraceptives and hypertension

GRETA H. CAMEL, MICHAEL J. GAST and H. MARVIN CAMEL

Hypertension and pregnancy

Hypertensive disorders in pregnancy are a serious threat to the mother and to the fetus, who is often delivered prematurely, either following a spontaneous delivery or by therapeutic termination of pregnancy. In the past 40 years, the maternal death rate in the United States has been reduced by 95% because of specific advances made in combatting hemorrhage and infection. Unexpectedly, maternal mortality due to hypertensive disorders has also decreased proportionately even though its management remains empiric [1]. The plaque on the colonnade of Chicago Lying-In Hospital that has been reserved for the discoverer of the basic etiology of eclampsia is still blank as of this date [2].

Incidence and definitions

At present, hypertension is the most common medical disorder seen in pregnancy. The prevalence of all hypertensive disorders in pregnancy is probably 6% [1]. In the Obstetrical Statistical Cooperative study involving 11 hospitals, the incidence of hypertension varied from 1.6% to 12.6%. Varying clinical diagnostic criteria and the type of population selected as to geographical location, race and socioeconomic factors have added to the problem of arriving at an accurate figure.

The Committee on Terminology of the American College of Obstreticians and Gynecologists [3] has specified four criteria for the diagnosis of gestational hypertension:

1. A sustained rise of 30 mmHg or more in the systolic pressure.
2. A sustained rise of 15 mmHg or more in the diastolic pressure.
3. A sustained systolic pressure of 140 or more.
4. A sustained diastolic pressure of 90 or more.

'Sustained' means blood pressure readings on at least two occasions six or more hours apart.

Page [56] proposed the use of mean arterial pressure (MAP) as a means of following the hypertensive pregnant patient. MAP is equal to the diastolic pressure plus one-third of the pulse pressure (systolic pressure minus diastolic pressure). Page proposed 107 as the maximum acceptable figure. Chesley feels this is too high [1]. The Toxemia Task Force of the National Institutes of Health in 1978 felt that 95 was the maximum acceptable number during the first and second trimester of pregnancy [4] (Figure 1).

We concur with Welt and Crenshaw [2] that the classification of hypertensive disorders in pregnancy as proposed by the Committee on Terminology of the American College of Obstetricians and Gynecologists and by DeAlvarez shows little correlation to the classifications used by internists such as Kaplan [5].

We propose the following simplified Classification of Hypertensive Diseases of Pregnancy:
1. Gestational hypertension.
2. Chronic hypertension.
3. Pregnancy-induced hypertension: (a) primary (b) superimposed on chronic hypertension.

Definitions
1. Gestational hypertension. This term refers to elevated blood pressure levels or changes in blood pressure as described above that occur *without* proteinuria or abnormal edema. It also implies a return to normal blood pressure levels within ten days after delivery [6].

2. Chronic hypertension. This is a descriptive term that applies to any hypertensive disease antedating pregnancy. The most common is primary essential hypertension, labile or sustained, etiology unknown. It actually may appear for the first time during pregnancy. Less common is secondary hypertension due to underlying renal disease, endocrine disorders, such as thyrotoxicosis, Cushing's syndrome, hyperaldosteronism, pheochromocytoma or vascular abnormalities involving increased cardiac output [2, 7].

According to Barnes [8], the 'chronic hypertensive diseases' make up one-third to one-half of all cases of hypertension in pregnancy. Zuspan and O'Shaughnessy found an incidence of 51.0% of chronic hypertensive disease and 1.1% of chronic renal disease when they reviewed the discharge diagnoses of 7.893 cases with documented clinical hypertension at Chicago Lying-in Hospital at the University of Chicago. Hypertension is generally defined as a blood pressure greater than or equal to 140/90 mmHg.

3. Pregnancy-induced hypertension (PIH). This term is synonymous with preeclampsia, eclampsia or toxemia of pregnancy [8]. Although it can complicate any pregnancy, the syndrome of PIH occurs more commonly in a small sector of the population: the young, poor, malnourished primigravida, and is more likely to occur in an urban population.

The Obstetrical Statistical Cooperative study, involving 11 hospitals, as reported by Chesley [1], used uniform clinical noninvasive guidelines as to diagnosis and yet the reported incidence of preeclampsia ranged from 48% to 92%.

PIH occurs in about 15% of obstetric patients who present themselves for outpatient clinic care at teaching institutions and is much lower (1%–1.5%) in obstetric patients seen by physicians in private practice. The incidence is about 5% for the entire U.S.A. Sixty-five percent of cases of preeclampsia-eclampsia occur during the first pregnancy. This incidence is increased even more if the primigravida is under 17 or over 35 [11].

PIH can be superimposed on an underlying chronic hypertension. The diagnosis based on purely clinical symptoms must be made carefully and is fraught with error. By light microscopy, the most reliable morphological change related to preeclampsia is intracapillary swelling and vacuolization. The glomerular tufts are swollen and apt to protrude into the neck of the proximal convoluted tubule. The characteristic renal lesion is swelling of the endothelial cell in the glomerular capillary. Within the cytoplasm of the endothelial cell, there may be amorphous fibrinous degradation product laid against the basement membrane. There may be similar deposit in the subendothelial space. These changes markedly narrow, and at times completely obliterate, the capillary lumen. The clinical picture of preeclampsia correlates poorly with the finding of typical renal lesions. Even in young primigravidas Smythe et al. [10] found that ten of 56 had arteriolar nephrosclerosis, rather than the pathological findings characteristic of preeclampsia. McCartney [5] carefully selected 62 primigravidas known to be clinically normal in early and midpregnancy and who developed classical signs of preeclampsia in the third trimester. Only 71% had the renal lesion of preeclampsia, 21% had chronic glomerulonephritis.

Prognosis

The Toxemia Task Force of the National Institutes of Health examined the course of some 50,000 pregnant women and found a sharp rise in perinatal mortality when the blood pressure rose above 125/70 mmHg. They therefore concluded from their data that instead of 140/90 mmHg, a more reasonable upper limit of blood pressure would be 130/80 mmHg [4].

Dunlop [12] found perinatal mortality rates to be normal in mild uncomplicated hypertension (2.6%). The rates worsened with progressively severe disease to 23%, primarily due to premature delivery but also due to growth retardation and abruptio placenta. With superimposed preeclampsia the perinatal mortality rose to 29.7%. On the other hand, Chesley [1], reporting on a series of 2366 cases of mild preeclamptics over a period of 15 years, reports a perinatal mortality of 4.27%. Over the same period of time, there were only 215 cases of severe eclampsia with a perinatal mortality of 6.5%.

The maternal mortality from chronic hypertension is less than 1% [13] and is usually due to cerebral hemorrhage or congestive heart failure caused by superimposed PIH. According to Wingate [14], maternal morbidity and mortality, particularly in patients with underlying chronic hypertension and superimposed preeclampsia, is 3–10%.

Hemodynamic changes of pregnancy

The normal woman retains approximately 900 mEq of sodium throughout pregnancy, with water retention of about six liters. This normal saline solution is distributed throughout the mother, the products of conception and the hypertrophied organs of pregnancy. It includes a 1.5-liter increase in plasma volume, about 40% above the prepregnancy level. Despite the increases in plasma volume and cardiac output, studies of normal women indicate that the diastolic pressure is lowered by an average of 5–10 mmHg during most of pregnancy and rises to exceed the level existing prior to pregnancy during the third trimester (Figure 1) [15]. The reduction in blood pressure in the face of increased cardiac output is due to a marked reduction in peripheral vascular resistance. Such a decrease in peripheral resistance has been measured. The expansion in plasma volume is thought to compensate for the shunting of effective blood volume through the placenta.

The mechanism of sodium retention during pregnancy is more complicated. It is the end result of many forces, some of which increase sodium loss:

1. Increased glomerular filtration.
2. Reduced renal vascular resistance.
3. The natriuretic action of progesterone.

Others tend to cause sodium retention:

1. Increased estrogen acting alone or via an increase in plasma renin activity.
2. Increased aldosterone, almost certainly secondary to the increased renin levels.
3. Decreased effective circulating blood volume because of the increased venous distensibility.
4. The decrease in oncotic pressure of the plasma.
5. Fetal and amniotic fluid sequestration in the growing uteroplacental bed.

In addition the enlarged uterus interferes with the venous return to the heart and increases the formation of dependent pedal edema in women in the third trimester. As a result, peripheral edema nearly always appears in pregnant women who are otherwise normal. Significant edema was found in 40–60% of women who remained normotensive troughout their pregnancies [1, 5].

Renal function

The glomerular filtration rate (GFR) is increased approximately 50% from a normal nonpregnant range of 80–120 cm^3/min to 120–200 cm^3/min, returning to normal postpartum. Renal plasma flow, as estimated by paraaminohippurate clearance, is raised by 200–250 ml/min above that of nonpregnant subjects throughout early and mid-pregnancy and returns to the normal range near term [16].

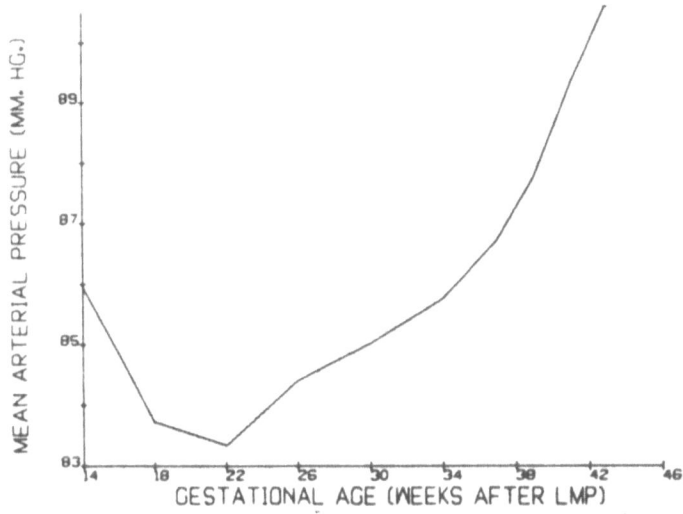

Figure 1. Mean arterial blood pressure by gestational age for term white single live births. (From E.W. Page and R. Christianson: Am J Obstet Gynecol 125:742, 1976.)

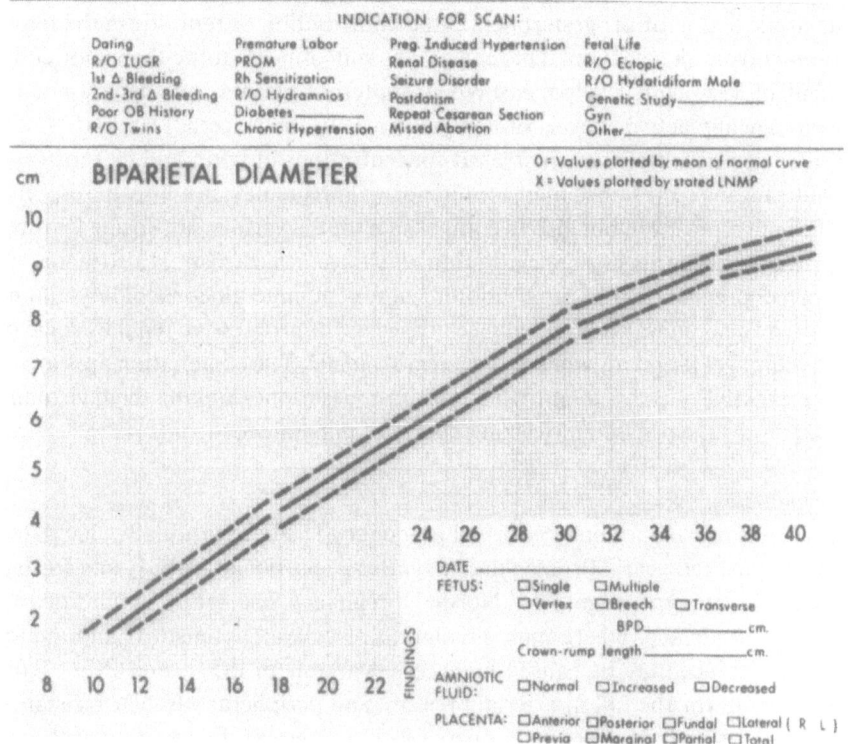

Figure 2. Standard curve for growth of fetal biparietal diameter during pregnancy (Ultrasound report, Washington University Perinatal Laboratory).

Hemodilution secondary to the increase in GFR and increases in tubular secretion result in a decrease in serum creatinine and blood urea nitrogen. In a normal pregnancy the creatinine values range from 0.5 to 0.7 mg/100 ml and BUN 7–10 mg/100 ml.

Uric acid levels are similarly decreased, the level in normal pregnancy being 3–5 mg/100 ml. For that reason, hyperuricemia is often utilized as an early sign of maternal vasoconstriction. However, it must be remembered in hypertensive patients that diuretics can also cause hyperuricemia.

The total 24-hr urine protein excretion in the pregnant woman rises from a normal of 40–120 mg daily to 250–300 mg daily [1, 16].

Renin angiotensin aldosterone system

Plasma renin activity, renin concentration and renin substrate are all increased in normal pregnancy. Levels of renin activity and concentration are elevated in part as a consequence of the estrogen-induced stimulation of renin substrate. Two other facts almost certainly contribute: (1) the various hemodynamic and renal changes described above, which tend to activate the release of renin, including the fall in blood pressure, the dilatation of the vascular bed, and the natriuretic action of progesterone; (2) the contribution of renin from the fetus, probably from the chorion. This chorionic renin appears to be the major component of very high levels measured in maternal plasma, but it may not be physiologically active. Levels of angiotensin II in the maternal circulation are elevated as a result of these increased concentrations of renin and its substrate.

Aldosterone secretion is increased in normal pregnancy, not only in response to the high renin level, but also to compensate for the various salt-losing features of pregnancy. The plasma concentration of deoxycorticosterone is also increased in normal pregnancy. The large amounts of potent mineralocorticoids would be expected to maintain sodium balance at the cost of progressive renal wastage of potassium, yet pregnant women are normokalemic. The explanation appears to be a protective effect of their high levels of progesterone, making them virtually refractory to the potassium-wasting action of mineralocorticoids [1, 5].

Prostaglandins

The role of prostaglandins in normal pregnancy has been gradually elucidated over the past ten years. Prostaglandin synthesis, particularly PGI_2 and PGE_2, increase in human pregnancy. Normal pregnancy has many similarities to Bartter's Syndrome, where high circulating plasma angiotensin II and angiotensin resistance may be caused by excess synthesis of PGE_2 and PGI_2. This may account for the fall in arterial pressure and peripheral vascular resistance which occurs early in pregnancy. Increases in urinary PGE_2 and 6-keto-$PGF_{1\alpha}$ have been documented in the urine of pregnant women. An increased synthesis of PGI_2 has been demonstrated from endothelial cell cultures of umbilical arteries from human pregnancy. The rise in renin secretion, which is unrelated to changes in sodium balance, may reflect resistance to angiotensin II caused by vascular synthesis of PGI_2 or it may be a direct effect of renal prostaglandin synthesis on renin secretion [1, 5].

Pathophysiology

1. Chronic hypertension

Arterial hypertension represents an interaction of many components mediated finally through alterations of blood flow and peripheral resistance. Increases in volume or resistance or vasoconstriction will cause the same end result: an elevated blood pressure. Different forms of arterial hypertension may have increases of either blood volume, peripheral resistance, or high cardiac output as the predominant abnormality. In chronic hypertension, gestational decreases in blood pressure may not always occur. Chesley and Annito [17] analyzed 301 pregnancies of women with documented chronic hypertension and found that in only 40% was the blood pressure significantly reduced until the third trimester.

The theories of low renin (volume dependent) versus high renin (vasoconstrictive) causes of essential hypertension cannot be applied to pregnancy in view of the estrogen-induced increases in plasma renin-angiotensin concentration in normal pregnancy. Although there is a wide individual variation as to what constitutes normal plasma volume in pregnancy, there are several reports that show a relatively reduced blood volume in chronically hypertensive patients. Moreover, the reduction in blood volume seems to be correlated not only to the severity of hypertension, but also related to the degree of intrauterine growth retardation if present. Arias [18] feels that a failure to expand plasma volumes from a prepregnancy level of approximately 45 cm^3/kg body weight to a level beyond 60 cm^3/kg body weight will clearly identify those pregnancies leading to growth retardation or fetal death. The etiology of this failure to expand blood volume has not been worked out. It may possibly involve the renal handling of sodium.

The uteroplacental blood flow has been shown to be decreased in all hypertensive disease, the decrease being in proportion to the severity of the hypertension. Histologically, the uteroplacental arteries have been found to be remarkably sensitive to the development of hyperplastic arteriosclerotic lesions, over a relatively short time. The severest and most extensive uteroplacental arterial lesions are found in patients with essential hypertension complicated by PIH [1].

II. Pregnancy-induced hypertension

Pathophysiology of PIH is characterized by intense vasospasm of peripheral arterioles. The initiating event in the development of this vasospastic hypertension is unknown. It may be related to alterations in vascular sensitivity to endogenous hormones, that is, angiotensin II, catecholamines, or a drop in PGI2 levels, possibly mediated through changes in arteriolar wall sodium concentrations. Whatever the cause, the end result is acute vasospastic hypertension with contraction of the circulating plasma volume in proportion to the severity of vasospasm in peripheral arterioles and capacitance vessels. Decreases of plasma volume of up to 40% have been reported in the most severe cases.

The vascular reactivity of patients with PIH is increased in response to angiotensin and catecholamine infusions. Apparently the process begins long before it becomes apparent clinically. Primary hypovolemia, hypotension, and hypoperfusion may be the cause of the increased vascular reactivity, subsequently producing hypertension. The reverse may also be true, that is, primary vasospasm produces first a contracted plasma volume and then elevation of blood pressure. Sensitivity to angiotensin II can be seen as early as 20 weeks gestation, long before the development of overt hypertension. One report showed significantly diminished plasma volumes at 26 weeks gestation in a small number of patients who later developed PIH [1, 5, 11].

Other theories have been proposed

1) Uteroplacental inadequacy. The uteroplacental unit is inadequate and elaborates a substance which produces vasospasm and vascular injury. This is a restating of the uterine ischemia theory proposed by numerous investigators during the 1930s and 1940s. Two new pieces of evidence support this theory; by inducing chronic uterine ischemia Hodari [19] produced a syndrome in the pregnant dog resembling preeclampsia; Gant et al. [20] found that the metabolic clearance of dehydroisoandrosterone sulfate is partly dependent on placenta function and is diminished in those women who are destined to develop preeclampsia. As with their increased sensitivity to angiotensin, this decrease in placental function can be detected weeks before the syndrome appears. In addition to this evidence for derangement in placental function, the morphology of the placenta changes in preeclampsia, that is, increased numbers of syncytial sprouts on the villi appears to reflect an attempt to respond to hypoxia [1].

2) Intravascular coagulation can be found in many preeclamptics. Certain characteristic pathologic features, such as endothelial swelling and fibrin deposition can be reproduced experimentally by infusion of thromboplastin. The placenta is rich in thromboplastin. The presumably pathognomonic renal glomerular lesion has been ascribed to the deposition of fibrin. The lesion consists of deposits underneath the basement membrane and within the swollen cytoplasm of endothelial cells and an increase of intercapillary cells. The decrease in glomerular filtration rate and other renal functions would largely reflect this mechanical blockade. The characteristic liver lesion is thrombosis in the small vessels of the periportal system, resulting in hemorrhagic necrosis and fibrin deposits. In the myocardium are found fibrin thrombi, focal necrosis and subendothelial hemorrhages. Cerebral edema is present and in 20% of patients there are cerebral hemorrhages involving the pons, basal ganglia and subcortical areas [1, 5, 11].

3) Loss of immunologic barrier. The trophoblast must normally perform a major role in preventing immunological rejection of the fetus. This role appears to depend at least in part on the presence of a layer of acid mucopolysaccharide containing sialic acid, which gives the cell surface a strong negative charge. Since the maternal lymphocytes also possess a strong negative charge, the cell-to-cell contact required for detection of the trophoblastic antigen would not normally occur. Petrucco [21] found that immunoglobulins IgM and IgG are deposited in the glomeruli of preeclamptic women in proportion to the severity of the disease. Feeney et al. [5] suggest that the disease is related to initial exposure of the patient to foreign antigen and consequently there is a decreased incidence of preeclampsia in women who have had a previous pregnancy or blood transfusions.

4) Prostaglandin. The decrease in urine, blood flow and fibrin deposits may also be due to an aberration in the balance of PGI2 synthesis in the blood vessels and thromboxane in the platelets. Decreases in production of PGI2 lead to an increase in angiotensin sensitivity. Increased angiotensin sensitivity may be the cause of the hypertension seen in toxemia [1, 5, 11].

Work-up of the chronic hypertensive pregnant patient
The initial work-up of the patient must include a detailed history of previous blood pressure readings, urinary tract infections or 'childhood' history of kidney problems or repeated streptococcal infections and the incidence of a family history of essential hypertension. Further clues to underlying chronic hypertension in pregnancy (CHP) would be an obstetrical history of abruptio placenta, premature labor, growth retardation, previous stillbirths and late abortions.

Physical examination must include a funduscopic examination, evaluation of heart size, the presence or absence of an abdominal bruit and simultaneous palpation of the femoral and radial pulses to rule out coarctation. In establishing an accurate baseline blood pressure, the following points must be kept in mind:

1. The patient should sit quietly with the arm unconstricted for 5 min or more prior to measurement.
2. The size of the cuff must be appropriate for the dimensions of the arm.
3. The manometer must be accurate.

4. The arm must be at heart level.
5. Keep in mind situations that may artificially raise or lower blood pressure, such as noisy surroundings, exertion, anxiety, pain, cold, bladder distension or drugs.
6. For ease of clinical evaluation the American Heart Association recommends as standards the first and fifth sounds, i.e., the initial sound of systole and the last sound of diastole.

In cases where labile hypertension is suspected, serial measurements of the blood pressure at home may better reflect the true status. The home readings of greatest interest are a basal value one-half hour after arising, a late afternoon reading, and a determination before retiring in the evening.

Laboratory evaluation

Hemoglobin or hematocrit is routinely assessed. A decrease in the hematocrit determination in early pregnancy and a slow return by mid-third trimester are normally expected. A rapid increase in the hematocrit determination may signal a restricted intravascular volume.

The chest x-ray during pregnancy generally shows a normal variation, i.e., the heart is displaced with straightening of the upper left border and prominence of the pulmonary conus. In a patient with CHP, increased pulmonary markings and left ventricular hypertrophy are indicative of hypertensive cardiovascular disease of considerable duration and severity. The left ventricular hypertrophy may be confirmed by an ECG. However, a 15 degree left axis deviation on the ECG is normal in pregnancy.

A routine urinalysis, including a microscopic examination, must be done. Blood chemistries should include serum electrolytes, uric acid, blood sugar, BUN, serum creatinine and a liver profile. In patients suspected of having underlying renal disease, it is important to obtain a mid-stream urine culture and a 24-hr creatinine clearance, including potassium, sodium and protein levels [1, 5, 11].

Therapeutic management

The known hypertensive patient should start prenatal care as early as possible. The patient should be followed every two weeks until the thirtieth week of gestation, after which time she should be seen weekly until delivery [2, 7].

A diet containing at least 90 gm of protein per day is fundamental for adequate growth of the fetus. Some investigators believe the question of salt content a useless cause for worry, whereas others recommend a 4–6 gm sodium chloride diet [1, 7].

Daily periods of bed rest, at least one hour every midday, should be encouraged beginning early in pregnancy and increased late in gestation. Presumably bed rest improves uteroplacental perfusion and nutrient supply to the fetus and is felt to increase renal blood flow and glomerular filtration rate in the mother. Therapeutic abortion is rarely necessary, unless uncontrollable hypertension or progressive renal failure is present [1, 2, 7].

Drug therapy
No studies are available in the group of patients with CHP whose blood pressure falls to normal levels in the first and second trimester as to whether drug therapy should be initiated during this period of time. In the 50–60% of patients with CHP whose blood pressure does not increase, constant monitoring of the drug regimen and flexibility in altering drugs and dosages will yield the best results. Drug therapy is recommended when the diastolic pressure is greater than 100 mmHg or the systolic pressure is greater than 150 mmHg. Control in the range of 90 mmHg, plus or minus 5 mmHg, diastolic, or a mean arterial blood pressure (MAP) reading of less than 105, is the goal of therapy (22).

Diuretics
The volume-depleting effects of the benzothiadiazides have made them extremely valuable as adjunctive therapy in patients receiving both adrenergic blockade and arteriolar dilators. This very effect makes them potentially dangerous for use in pregnant hypertensive patients.

Gant et al. [23] have shown that volume depletion induced by the thiazides or furosemide leads to a decrease in dehydroandrosterone (DHAS) clearance by the placenta. These studies and the findings of Arias [24] and of Soffronoff et al. [25] suggest that the outcome of pregnancy may be poorer in the volume-depleted patient. Thiazides should be used only after significant hypervolemia has been documented or is encountered secondary to the antihypertensive agent used.

The sympatholytic agents reserpine, guanethidine, and methyldopa maintain prolonged periods of dilatation of capacitance vessels, thereby allowing an increase in intravascular volume without jeopardizing systemic blood pressure. Reserpine is so long-acting that it can cause respiratory depression and nasal stuffiness in the newborn. Nasal stuffiness, peptic ulcer, and increased sensitivity to seizures may occur in the mother. The main objection to guanethidine is postural hypotension in the mother and paralytic ileus in the newborn. Methyldopa produces simulation of alpha-adrenergic receptor sites in the hypothalamus and other portions of the central nervous system. It competitively inhibits the actions of dopadecarboxylase (which results in decreased production of norepinephrine) and is converted to alpha-methylnorepinephrine, a false neurotransmitter. The side effects of methyldopa therapy include drowsiness, fluid retention and postural hypotension. In addition, a significant number of patients on methyldopa therapy will develop a positive Coomb's test in the nonpregnant state. This does not seem to be as great a problem in the pregnant patient, but if it occurs it can be confusing in patients in whom isoimmunization might be expected. Methyldopa is thought to have no effect on cardiac output and uterine blood flow seems to be unchanged during its usage. Because of extensive experience with its use during pregnancy, methyldopa remains the drug of choice for the treatment of the pregnant hypertensive patient. Methyldopa, 500–2000 mg in divided dosages, is given orally to keep diastolic blood pressures below 100 mmHg [7].

Of the alpha blockers, phenoxybenzamine is used only in the rarely occurring cases of pheochromocytoma because of its short duration of action and intolerable side effects. Clonidine is an effective alpha blocker, but its side effects of drowsiness, postural hypertension and its tendency to cause marked rebound hypertension if abruptly discontinued do not make it a drug of choice [2, 26].

Vasodilators [25]
By direct arterial dilation these drugs decrease vascular resistance and increase blood flow. The resultant intravascular volume increase and reflex tachycardia may necessitate the use of an adrenergic agent and a diuretic. The three most widely used are hydralazine, the drug of choice; diazoxide; and nitroprusside. Hydralazine acts to decrease blood pressure by direct relaxation of arteriolar smooth muscle. This action occurs primarily on precapillary resistance vessels and resistance on the coronary, splanchnic, and renal circulations and is reduced more than that in skin and muscle. There is no direct action on the autonomic nervous system. Orthostatic hypotension seldom occurs. The effect of hydralazine on uteroplacental circulation is uncertain at this time.

Oral hydralazine, 40–200 mg in divided doses, does not provide effective blood pressure control unless it is used in conjunction with methyldopa or beta-blocking agents in the pregnant patient. However, hydralazine is particularly effective when utilized by the intravenous or intramuscular routes for the acute control of pregnancy-induced hypertension at or near term [1, 2].

Diazoxide may cause a precipitous drop in blood pressure, endangering uterine perfusion. Nitroprusside must be given intravenously and carries with it the danger of cyanide poisoning when used over more than 36 hr.

Certainly, one of the most significant controversies in perinatal medicine today is the use of beta-adrenergic antagonists as antihypertensive agents in pregnancy [27, 28]. Among the most common of these agents is propranolol, although other beta agents with more specific beta-1 activity, such as metoprolol, have been gaining in popularity recently. These agents are thought to act in three ways in the pregnant patient. They decrease renin secretion, decrease cardiac beta stimulation resulting in decreased cardiac rate and output, and act directly on the central nervous system where unopposed alpha stimulation can produce a decrease in the arterial pressures. These agents are thought to be most useful in those patients with increased cardiac outputs and what is termed 'hyperdynamic circulation' of pregnancy. Beta-blockers are contraindicated in pregnant diabetic patients because they mask the neural mediated signs and symptoms of hypoglycemia. Glyconeogenesis and insulin production are believed to be under beta-2 control. Therefore, in stable diabetics and asthmatics, beta-1 selective blockers, such as metaprolol, can be used cautiously if needed. Chronic administration of beta-adrenergic antagonists has been associated in some studies with intrauterine growth retardation (IUGR) and neonatal hypoglycemia and bradycardia [28]. Other authors have suggested that there is a decrease in fetal reserve function secondary to a loss of sympathetic tone following maternal administration of beta antagonists, which appear to cross the placenta extremely well. In our experience, the beta-adrenergic antagonists have provided us with an excellent first-line drug for the treatment of hypertension in pregnancy without significantly affecting maternal and fetal mortality and morbidity.

It must be remembered that blood pressure measurement may be misleading. Regardless of the control achieved, intensive fetoplacental monitoring must be instituted.

Pregnancy management

Making the diagnosis of chronic hypertension in pregnancy requires either a well documented history of blood pressure elevation, greater than 140 mmHg systolic or 90 mmHg diastolic, outside of pregnancy or documentation of the same degree of hypertension prior to the 20th week of gestation. The first half of pregnancy is a period in which the patient is unlikely to develop pregnancy-induced hypertension in the absence of multiple gestation or molar pregnancy. Page and Christianson [15] showed that the average mean arterial pressure in early pregnancy is approximately 85 or 86 mmHg. This decreases to about 83 mmHg at 20 weeks' gestation and rises to a level of approximately 90 mmHg by term (Figure 1).

Administration of antihypertensive medications to women with mild to moderate chronic hypertension in pregnancy is a highly debated issue. The European literature contains a variety of examples showing that, in patients with mean arterial pressures in the 100 mmHg range, efforts at reduction of blood pressure produced no significant decrease in maternal or fetal mortality or morbidity [29]. Other authors believe that treatment of blood pressures even at relatively low values of mean arterial pressure in the first trimester and continuing through pregnancy can decrease the incidence of intrauterine growth retardation, placental abruptions and stillbirths. It is not known whether treatment of chronic hypertension in pregnancy can reduce the incidence of superimposed, pregnancy-induced hypertension or change its severity.

Fetal well-being can be monitored by a variety of techniques. One of the most popular and valuable techniques to be developed in the last 10 years is diagnostic obstetrical ultrasound. Utilizing both the static and real-time methods one may evaluate fetal growth based upon serial measurements of the biparietal diameter (BPD) [30] (Figure 2).

The biparietal diameter displays a predictable pattern of growth during normal pregnancy. In the absence of adequate uteroplacental function, intrauterine growth retardation (IUGR) can develop. This is perhaps the most common fetal abnormality affecting the pregnancies of hypertensive gravida.

It is impossible to make a diagnosis of IUGR without a comparison of the head to abdominal circumference ratio, which should be markedly elevated in the growth-retarded fetus. Other sonographic abnormalities which are characteristic of hypertensive pregnancy include premature senescence of the placenta and premature decrease in the volume of amniotic fluid.

Another measure of fetal well-being is provided by nonstressed antepartum fetal heart rate monitoring (NST). This procedure is initiated at 32 weeks (or earlier if there are signs of marked intrauterine growth retardation). The patients arrive at the perinatal laboratory at scheduled intervals. The fetal heart rate is monitored by external Doppler techniques for 20–120 min. Signs of fetal well-being include a normal amount of variability in the baseline fetal heart rate and rises in the fetal heart rate of 15 beats/min or more lasting 15 or more seconds in response to gross fetal movements. Two or more of these elevations in fetal heart rate (which we call the fetal heart reactivity) allow us to predict with 98% accuracy that the fetus under study will survive in utero for one more week in the absence of any extreme change in the maternal condition.

A second technique which evaluates fetal placental reserve is called the contraction stress test (CST). Mild uterine contractions can produce significant stress for the inadequate fetal placental unit. During CST, uterine contractions are induced with intravenous infusion of the posterior pituitary hormone, oxytocin. A compromised fetus will display characteristic heart rate decelerations following contractions and requires immediate delivery. At this time, most centers utilize nonstress testing as their primary antepartum fetal monitoring technique with contraction stress tests as a backup if the fetus does not show appropriate reactivity in the nonstress test.

Biochemical monitoring of the fetal placental unit, that is, urinary estriol levels and serum human placental lactogen levels, has fallen into disfavor in many centers in recent years, having been largely replaced by weekly or twice-weekly antepartum fetal heart rate monitoring.

Delivery

Delivery of the hypertensive gravida should be no different from any other pregnant patient. Delivery by the vaginal route is preferred in the absence of maternal or fetal indications for Cesarean section. Induction of labor is a useful technique in those patients who show evidence of instability of their blood pressures following attainment of fetal-lung maturity. In those gravidas who show stable blood pressures and normal fetal growth with adequate antepartum fetal heart rate monitoring, delivery can await the onset of normal labor in the absence of other obstetrical complications.

Diagnosis and treatment of PIH

The syndrome of pregnancy-induced hypertension can occur either in the presence or the absence of chronic hypertension or underlying renal disease. It is characterized by any or all of the following signs and symptoms: accelerated hypertension (a rise of 15 or more mmHg in diastolic blood pressure), rapid weight gain, edema, proteinuria or signs of rapidly occurring severe volume constriction.

Laboratory findings in PIH

Among the changes that are most prominent in pregnancy-induced hypertension are an increase in the hematocrit, serum uric acid and blood urea nitrogen values. These changes are all secondary to extreme hemoconcentration and are among the most sensitive and earliest changes found in PIH. Serum creatinine and hepatic enzymes also increase. These are both secondary to concentration and end organ phenomena and will often be slightly delayed when compared to changes in uric acid and urea nitrogen levels. Another laboratory index that can be of value in PIH is the decrease that is found in platelets and clotting factors. Of these, the platelet count is the easiest and most rapid test which may be obtained. Platelet counts that are significantly below 100,000 indicate an increased severity of preeclampsia, even in the absence of other clinical and laboratory signs. Disseminated intravascular coagulation is an uncommon but ominous manifestation of the preeclamptic disease.

Management of PIH

It is helpful to break pregnancy-induced hypertensive patients into two classes. This is not based on the etiology of the disease, but rather on the severity of the hypertension and other pathophysiologic events that are occurring in the patient.

1. Mild disease is characterized by slight increases in blood pressure, five or more pound weight gain in a single week, and/or evidence of minimal to moderate (less than 1 gm/24 hr) degree of proteinuria. These patients will often display a moderate degree of hyperreflexia and should show some of the biochemical signs of vasospasm. They often respond extremely well to bed rest (in the lateral recumbent position) alone and in instances where fetal-lung immaturity is suspected, conservative management is preferable to delivery. In those patients who are at or near term, particularly in those patients whose cervices are compatible with the induction of labor, immediate delivery in the treatment of choice.

2. Moderate to severe preeclampsia is characterized by blood pressure with diastolics in the 110 mmHg range or proteinuria greater than 1 gm/hr, or symptoms of end organ failure such as right upper quadrant pain or tenderness, severe headaches, visual disturbances, or oliguria. Although brief trials of bed rest and sedation may be attempted in these patients, the large majority will not respond to such conservative therapy and should be delivered as soon as possible for maternal indications. Recently some authors have suggested utilizing bed rest, magnesium sulfate and antihypertensives in those patients remote from term, attempting to mature the fetal lungs through administration of corticosteroids through the mother. This technique, although promising, needs to be evaluated on a larger scale to assess accurately any difference in maternal and fetal morbidity during the three- to four-day intervals required to realize an effect from maternal steroid administration. Attempts to deliver a severely preeclamptic patient should initially be undertaken via the vaginal route with Cesarean section being reserved only for those patients with maternal or fetal indications for abdominal delivery or failed inductions. Some signs of fetal distress in these patients are common (e.g., decreased beat-to-beat variability, late decelerations) secondary to decreased uteroplacental blood flow resulting from marked vasospasm. The fetal scalp pH is an effective technique for helping to adequately evaluate these fetuses, but should be used somewhat judiciously since the infant of the severely preeclamptic mother will often display a mild to moderate degree of thrombocytopenia. It is also not uncommon for maternal preeclampsia to worsen as the labor process goes along, many times reaching its peak severity in the period of time just prior to delivery and in the intrapartum period.

Drug therapy of the moderate to severe preeclamptic should always include utilization of magnesium sulfate as delineated in another section of this chapter. When blood pressures rise above 110 mmHg diastolic, we customarily administer either IV or IM hydralazine, 5–20 mg/dose, for temporary and moderate decreases of maternal pressures. It is important to remember that too severe a reduction in infusion of the uterus can result in an equally severe reduction in the ability of the fetus to transfer waste products back to the mother via the uteroplacental route. This can lead to severe distress in a fetus that is tolerating labor well prior to maternal blood pressure reduction.

Several drugs have been useful in the treatment of maternal seizure activity should it occur. Perhaps the most popular drug in recent years in treating maternal seizure activity is diazepam. Diazepam has the advantage of acting quickly to break existing seizure activity and is a familiar drug for many of the physicians managing the seizing patients. The drug, however, has several disadvantages. First, it can readily cross the placental barrier where it can cause profound and persistent fetal depression because it is not well metabolized by the fetal liver. Second, it can cause profound maternal respiratory depression in doses very close to those required to break the seizure activity. When utilizing diazepam to control maternal seizure activity, it is always advisable to have personnel and equipment immediately available for the intubation and respiratory support for those patients who will undergo respiratory arrest secondary to the drug. We generally utilize magnesium sulfate (4 gm IV bolus) as our first drug to prevent and stop maternal seizures.

Magnesium sulfate is the agent of choice in patients with adequate urinary function for prevention of seizures in pregnancy-induced hypertension. Its use for that purpose and the documentation of its efficacy in doing so goes back over 50 years. Magnesium sulfate probably acts in two locations: the neuromuscular junction in opposition to calcium, and centrally to depress nervous system irritability. The drug is rapidly excreted through the maternal kidney and as the magnesium concentration in the plasma increases so does the renal clearance of the drug. Magnesium sulfate therapy is capable of significant depressions of maternal serum calcium levels. Although magnesium in high concentrations can depress myometrial contractility both in vivo and in vitro, this does not interfere significantly with the induced labor of severely preeclamptic patients. Similarly, although the drug has been implicated in the depression of neonatal respiratory and neuromuscular function, it is rapidly cleared in the newborn. Clinically, therapy with magnesium sulfate may be followed by watching patellar reflexes, hourly urine outputs and the degree of ankle clonus, if present. Patellar reflexes provide a good clinical indication of when magnesium sulfate dosage is reaching adequate therapeutic serum levels. Absent patellar reflexes, however, are not a good indication of the imminent onset of respiratory depression. The higher the urine output the more aggressive the administration of magnesium sulfate must be to maintain the magnesium levels at the therapeutic range.

Magnesium blood levels of 1–2 mEq/l are considered in the normal range; 3–4 mEq/l can provide adequate coverage for many women with mild to moderate preeclampsia but do not guard against eclamptic seizures in patients with moderate to severe disease; 5–6 mEq/l of magnesium is considered within the therapeutic range although some authors believe that 8–10 mEq/l is a more appropriate level; 8–10 mEq/l is the approximate range where patellar reflexes begin to become completely absent. When serum magnesium levels reach 12–15 mEq/l respiratory paralysis can and does occur. These levels, however, are unlikely in the face of conventional therapy when urine output remains adequate.

If the initial administration of a 4 gm bolus of magnesium sulfate does not produce adequate decrease in patellar reflex and ankle clonus function, another 2–4 gm may be administered as a second bolus. This is often accompanied by flushing, a sensation of extreme warmth (second to peripheral vasodilation) and by nausea and vomiting. These effects can be minimized by prolonging the duration of the administration of the initial bolus, but must be weighed against the need to control impending seizure activity. Bolus administration is followed by the administration of magnesium sulfate in a continuous drip to obtain adequate depression of reflex function. Serum magnesium levels must be checked to ensure that patients remain in therapeutic range. The dose of magnesium sulfate required to maintain adequate serum levels may be as high as 3–4 gm/hr, depending on urinary output.

Delivery

Our preference for anesthetic management of the preeclamptic patient is local or small regional blocks such as paracervical and pudendal anesthesia. Narcotics can further depress the fetus and unless extremely experienced anethesiologists are present, the use of spinal or epidural anesthesia carries with it the great danger of volume compromise (secondary to broad sympathetic block) of an already compromised vascular space. For that reason a paracervical block is the anesthesia of choice in those patients with preeclampsia who need anesthesia. Similarly, for delivery of the preeclamptic patient by Cesarean section general anesthesia has proved to be satisfactory.

Postpartum

The postpartum care of the preeclamptic patient is generally unremarkable. It should be recalled that although the majority of seizure activity and other complications of severe preeclampsia occur in the antepartum and intrapartum period, the disease still can increase in its severity for brief periods of time postpartum. For that reason magnesium sulfate therapy should be used in all preeclamptic patients for at least 24 hr postpartum. Similarly, the use of antihypertensives as needed in the postpartum preeclamptic patient remains essential. The criterion for treatment of these patients remains 160 mmHg systolic or 110 mmHg diastolic pressure. Edema, proteinuria, hypertension and oliguria can persist for variable periods of time in the postpartum period. Resolution of pregnancy-induced hypertension is usually heralded by brisk diuresis followed by a marked decrease in edema and an impressive loss of weight, secondary to mobilization of fluid from the extracellular compartment. This usually is followed within several days by resolution of the biochemical changes found in the severe preeclamptic and by a gradual return to normal of the blood pressure. In general, blood pressure changes lag several days behind weight and biochemical changes as evidence of resolution of the pregnancy-induced hypertension.

It is important to try not to place a patient on chronic antihypertensive medications too quickly in the postpartum period. Observation for seven to 14 days is advisable before placing them on an antihypertensive maintenance therapy. Initial follow-up office visits at two to three weeks following hospital discharge will show that a significant number of patients will be normotensive and may be cautiously removed from their antihypertensive medication at that time. Follow-up tests of hepatic and renal function are extremely important in those patients in whom hypertension persists greater than seven to ten days following delivery.

Prognosis
The women with gestational hypertension, i.e., elevated blood pressures without proteinuria or significant edema, are more likely to develop chronic hypertension than those who remain normotensive throughout their pregnancies. In previous statistical reports of the high prevalence of chronic hypertension following preeclampsia and eclampsia, no differentiation was made between primary or secondary pregnancy-induced hypertension. The women, particularly the multipara who develop preeclampsia or eclampsia superimposed on underlying hypertensive or renal disease, are the ones most likely to develop chronic hypertension. The primiparous women who develop primary pregnancy-induced hypertension have the same chance of developing hypertension as those women who remain normotensive throughout their pregnancies [6].

Hypertension and oral contraceptives

The oral contraceptives (OC) were developed in the late 1950s and introduced into clinical use as a high-dose combination estrogen and progestogen product in the early 1960s [31]. The original formulation contained 150 μg of estrogen and 9.85 mg of progestin [32]. During the first decade, the investigations focused on the benefit of pregnancy prevention and the risk of abnormal cycle bleeding. The problem of giving potent steroids to basically healthy women became quickly apparent. One of the most dramatic and significant side effects was the increased frequency of venous thrombosis and thromboembolic disease. Data from several epidemiological studies pointed out the estrogen content as the culprit. The 1970s were spent in reducing the estrogen content to the current 30- to 50-μg level. Concurrent with the reduction in the estrogen formulation, research has been focused on the effect of OCs on a variety of blood clotting factors, platelet function, abnormalities in lipid and glucose metabolism and the persistant incidence of arterial blood pressure elevations and hypertension. All of the above are among now-accepted risk factors in the development of arteriosclerotic cardiovascular disease, such as myocardial infarction, stroke and peripheral vascular disease. It has become apparent that not only the estrogens but also the progestational agents in the OC play important roles in producing the above-mentioned side effects [33, 34].

Incidence
The first case of OC-induced hypertension was reported by Brownrigg in 1962 [35]. This was followed by several more case reports in 1967 by Laragh [36] and

Woods [37]. Tyson et al. [38] in 1968 reported hypertension associated with OC in 15.5% of 45 women, and Saruta [39] and his co-workers found its occurrence in 18% of 56 women. On the other hand, Weir [40] in 1971 reported on a series of 60 users followed over a period of a year and found only a mean systolic pressure elevation of 6.6. mmHg. In no case was the pressure above 140/90 mmHg.

In 1968, three prospective studies were initiated:
1. The Walnut Creek study under the auspices of the National Institute of Health at the Kaiser Permanente Medical Center in Walnut Creek, California.
2. The Royal College Study covering data on a group of patients collected by 1400 general practitioners in Great Britain.
3. The Oxford Study, undertaken by a group of family-planning clinics in Great Britain and analyzed by the epidemiology unit at Oxford.

All these studies have several problems. They were begun in the era of high-dose OC formulation. No serial blood pressure recordings were done and the frequency and the method of taking blood pressure recordings differed [34].

In 1974, the Royal College [41] report on 23,000 women on OC and 23,000 nonusers reported an incidence of 5% of hypertension after five years of pill use. The rate was 2.5 times higher than among the non-OC users. (It must be noted that blood pressures were measured on a regular basis only on the OC users. The blood pressures of control subjects were measured only at the beginning and end of the five-year period.) Ramcharan et al. [42] reported on 12,000 women in the Walnut Creek study after a three-year follow-up in 1973 and found the incidence rate of hypertension of 1.2 per 1000 among nonusers and 6.8 per 1000 among current users of similar ages.

Fisch and Frank [34] in 1977 did a cross-sectional and longitudinal analysis on the same subset of women used by Ramcharan, with an additional 1358 women collected in the fourth year of the Walnut Creek study. They reported only a mild contraceptive-induced blood pressure elevation: systolic, 5–6 mmHg; diastolic 1–2 mmHg. Women continuing OC use had no appreciably greater change in blood pressure between two visits than persistent nonusers. The age-adjusted proportion of OC users with a blood pressure over 140/90 mmHg was about three times that of nonusers.

There was a much greater incidence of abnormal findings in the first British studies than in the Walnut Creek study. However, the latest publication of the Royal College study agree with the Walnut Creek study that there was no significantly increased incidence of circulatory disease in nonsmoking OC users. The only significant increase occurred in smoking OC users – over the age of 35 in the British study and over the age of 40 in the Walnut Creek study [32].

In March 1981, Vessey and colleagues presented a brief update of the mortality data from the Oxford Family Planning Association study. This project entered more than 17,000 cases during 1968–1974, with 56% using OC, 25% barrier methods and 19% the IUD. With the 81 deaths in OC users, the mortality rate was 12.3 per 100,000 women-years as opposed to a rate f 29.9 in the Royal College study. Plunkett [44] explains this discrepancy by the extension of the Oxford study four years after closing of the Royal College study so that actual subject ages may have been younger.

Clinical features. Whether the pill induces hypertension or simply uncovers an underlying tendency toward essential hypertension is not known. Women with preexisting hypertension do not appear to be particularly more susceptible. There is a positive family history of hypertension in about half of those with pill-induced hypertension. A correlation with obesity and with older age has been found, but not in women with a history of pregnancy-induced hypertension [45].

There are a few single case reports associated with OC use of severe, rapidly accelerating hypertension resulting in irreversible renal damage [46, 47, 48].

Mechanism

The exact mechanism by which the OC causes hypertension has yet to be worked out. Reduction of the estrogen component of the OC to 50 μg or less has resulted in a marked decrease in the incidence of venous thromboembolism [49]. Although the blood pressure readings were higher in nonusers, both Mead et al. and a World Health Organization Study found little or no blood pressure change in women taking 30 μg compared with 50-μg preparations [50]. It appears that the progestins, particularly norethindrone acetate, have a dose-related effect on hypertension (RCGP) [34]. Current evidence implicates the renin-angiotensin-aldosterone system as the major component in the pathogenesis of OC-associated hypertension.

Estrogens, normal and synthetic, increase plasma renin substrate and total renin activity (threefold increase in angiotensin II levels) but cause a fall in total serum renin.

Crane [51] feels that the decrease in plasma renin concentration most likely results from the sodium-retaining effect of the estrogen which, acting through the macula densa portion of the juxtaglomerular apparatus gives rise to suppression of renin secretion. He found that a daily dose of 50 μg of ethinyl estradiol for three weeks caused an average increase in total exchangeable sodium of 226 mEq of sodium in normal female subjects. This effect could be prevented by the simultaneous administration of spironolactone, an aldosterone suppressant. He therefore concludes that the estrogenic component produces a mild to moderate hyperaldosterone state through its effect on renin substrate and renin activity, including sodium retention.

The synthetic progestational agents currently used in the OC formulations have a mineralcorticoid effect on the body, causing varying degrees of sodium retention. Norethindrone has been shown to slightly increase renin substrate and renin activity, while norgestrel causes a drop in aldosterone levels. Crane postulates that individuals who have a predisposition to develop hypertension from mineralcorticoids or from a chronic excess of body sodium should be expected to develop an increase in blood pressure.

Other mechanisms that may play a part [45]:
1. Tapia et al. found that women on the OC who became hypertensive did not maintain an initial twofold increase in the enzyme angiotensinase which inactivates angiotensin II, as it did the women who remained normotensive.
2. Rockson and associates found that the women on the OC who developed a significant increase in arterial pressure had a 50% increase in dopamine beta-hydroxylase activity in the plasma. This is believed to represent an increase in catecholamines or sympathetic nervous system activity.
3. Hollenberg [57] found that in most women on OC, there was a mean fall in renal blood flow of 25%. However, in some it was as high as 50%. A greater degree of vasoconstriction may parallel the drop in renal blood flow.

Comment

It has become apparent that not only the estrogen component of the OC, but also the progestins, particularly those with androgenic action, such as levonorgesterol, play a role in the production of hypertension and may adversely affect glucose and lipid metabolism, which have been implicated as risk factors in the production of atherosclerotic cardiovascular disease along with age, smoking, obesity and stress. The negative effect of the progestins appears to be dose related. Each progestin must be considered separately. The chemical classification does not necessarily parallel its biological activity, affinity for hormonal receptors and most importantly its effect in clinical use [52].

The OC is the single most effective reversible method of contraception available today. Oral contraceptives have been useful in the treatment of dysmenorrhea, functional uterine bleeding, benign fibrocystic disease of the breast and functional ovarian cysts. In women using OC, the incidence of salpingitis, anemia due to excessive menstrual bleeding and endometrial hyperplasia have been decreased as well as that of rheumatoid arthritis [53].

In our own practice, we have found that the incidence of OC-induced hypertension is relatively small and readily reversible when the pill is stopped. We use primarily a low-dose formulation of estrogen and avoid the norsteroidal progestational agents.

Contrary to the report of Leiman [53] we find that depo-medroxyprogesterone, when used to suppress, for example, anovulatory bleeding in women on renal dialysis, does not cause hypertension. We also use depo-medroxyprogesterone in high doses (400 mg and above) in the treatment of women with endometrial cancer. In this particular cohort of postmenopausal women, there is a high incidence of obesity, diabetes mellitus and hypertension. On administration of depo-methoxyprogesterone, the blood pressure remains the same or may actually fall. However, patients with a previous history of congestive heart failure may again decompensate due to the retention of salt and fluids.

Our experience with medroxyprogesterone is borne out by Nachtigall et al., who report a ten-year study of 84 matched pairs of menopausal women in which those treated with 2.5 mg of conjugated equine estrogen in cycles with seven days of medroxyprogesterone of 10 mg, showed that the mean blood pressure did not vary significantly, nor did the body weight or glucose levels. The beta lipoproteins were lowered by estrogen, and there were three myocardial infarctions among the controls and only one in the treated group. Again, the authors make no claim for estrogen protective effect, but there was no increased risk. These and many other studies have failed to demonstrate a significant risk of vascular disease during menopausal estrogen therapy [44].

There are many estimates of mortality risks particularly due to cardiovascular events in reponse to OC use. In 1979, Tietze and Lewit pointed out the increasing risk associated with pregnancy and increasing age. Maternal mortality rate ranges between 9.5 and 12.1 per 100,000 live births in women 15–29 years of age, and increases to 43.7 in the late 30s and to 68.2 in the 40- to 44-year-old group. Nonsmoking users of OC between ages 15 and 19 years exhibit a mortality rate between 0.6 and 1.6 per 100,000 women-years. This increases to 9 and 17.7 in the 35- to 39-year and 40- to 44-year age groups, respectively. When smoking and pill use are combined, however, the rates in the latter two groups increase to 31.3 and 60.9 respectively. Tietze and Lewit therefore concluded that barrier contraception and the intrauterine contraceptive device (IUD), with therapeutic abortion as 'back-up' represent the safest approach to contraception in the women aged 35 and over who smoke [44].

The bottom line is risk-benefit ratio to the individual patient. Admittedly there was a high incidence of hypertension reported in the earlier studies, all of which involved high-dose combinations of estrogen and progestens. In young women, particularly those who smoke, blood pressures must be monitored carefully. Blood pressures should be checked every six months with patients having underlying renal disease followed even more carefully. Should the patient's blood pressure rise significantly, that is, a MAP of 105 or above, a lower-dose formulation can be tried. If in spite of this the patient's pressure remains up, the pill should be stopped and another form of contraception should be used. At present, for women 35 and older, it appears that surgical sterilization is likely the safest and most practical approach [44]. Further studies are needed to more carefully assess the role played by the various progestational agents in the present low-dose OC formulation [32].

It is of interest that the Fertility and Maternal Health Drug Advisory Committee of the Food and Drug Administration has recently recommended that the hypertension warning be modified on the OC labeling for both physician and patient, and also recommend that the package insert reflect the possible benefits which may be gained from the use of the oral contraceptives.

References

1. Chesley LC: Hypertensive disorders in pregnancy. New York, Appleton-Century-Crofts, 1978.
2. Welt SI, Crenshaw M, Carlyle MC Jr: Concurrent hypertension and pregnancy. In: Osofsky HJ (ed) Clinical obstetrics and gynecology. 21:619, 1978.
3. Hughes EC (ed): Obstetric-gynecologic terminology. Philadelphia, Davis, 1972, pp 442–423.
4. Friedman EA, Neff RR: Pregnancy outcome as related to hypertension, edema and proteinuria. In: Underheimer M, Katz A, Zuspan F (eds) Hypertension in pregnancy. New York, John Wiley, 1976.
5. Kaplan NM: Clinical hypertension, 2nd Ed. Baltimore, Williams & Wilkins, 1978, p 325.
6. Chesley LC: The remote prognostic significance of the level of blood pressure in pregnancy. Clin Exp Hypertens 2:777–801, 1980.
7. Zuspan FP, Shaugnessy R: Maternal physiology and diseases: chronic hypertension in pregnancy. In: Pithin RM, Zlatnick FJ (eds) Yearbook of obstetrics and gynecology. Chicago, Year Book Medical Publishers, 1979.
8. Barnes CA: Nontoxemic hypertension. In: Barnes CA (ed) Medical disorders in obstetrics practice. London, Blackwell Scientific Publications, 1974.
9. Spargo BH, Lichtig C, Luger AM, Katz AI, Lindheimer MD: Renal lesion in preeclampsia. In: Lindheimer MD, Katz AI, Zuspan FP (eds) Hypertension in pregnancy. New York, John Wiley, 1977.
10. Smythe CM, Bradham WS, Dennis EJ, McIver FA, Horol HG: Renal arteriolar disease in young primigravias. J Lab Clin Med 63:562–573, 1964.
11. DeAlvarez RR: Preeclampsia-eclampsia and renal disease in pregnancy. Clin Obstet Gynecol 21:881–905, 1978.
12. Dunlop JCH: Chronic hypertension and prenatal mortality. Proc R Soc Med 59:838, 1966.
13. Ferris TF: Medical complications of pregnancy. In: Burrows GN, Ferris TF (eds) Medical complications during pregnancy. Philadelphia, Saunders, 1975.
14. Wingate MD et al: Diseases specific to pregnancy. In: Romney SL et al (eds) The health care of women. New York, McGraw-Hill, 1975.
15. Page EW, Christianson R: The impact of mean arterial pressure, in middle trimester upon the outcome of pregnancy. Am J Obstet Gynecol 125:740, 1976.
16. Marchant DJ: Laboratory values and diagnostic tests. Clin Obstet Gynecol 21: 937–944, 1978.
17. Chesley LC, Annitto JE: Pregnancy in the patient with hypertensive disease. Am J Obstet Gynecol 53:372–381, 1947.
18. Arias F, Zamora J: Antihypertensive treatment and pregnancy outcome in patients with mild chronic hypertension. Obstet Gynecol 53:489–494, 1979.
19. Hodari AA: Chronic uterine ischemia and reversible experimental 'toxemia of pregnancy'. Am J Obstet Gynecol 97:597–607, 1967.
20. Gant NF, Madden JD, Siiteri PK, MacDonald PC: The metabolic clearance rate of dehydroisoandrosterone sulfate. IV. Acute effects of induced hypertension, hypotension, and natriuresis in normal and hypertensive pregnancies. Am J Obstet Gynecol 124:143–148, 1976.

21. Petrucco OM, Thompson NM, Lawrence JR, Weldon MW: Immunoflurescent studies in renal biopsies in pre-eclampsia. Br Med J 1:473–476, 1974.
22. Berkowitz RL: Antihypertensive drugs in the pregnant patient. Obstet Gynecol Surv 35(4): 191–204, 1980.
23. Gant NF, Madden JD, Siiteri PK, MacDonald PC: The metabolic clearance rate of dehydroandrosterone sulfate III. The effect of thiazide diuretics in normal and future preeclamptic pregnancies. Am J Obstet Gynecol 123:159–163, 1975.
24. Arias F: Expansion in intravascular volume in patients with chronic hypertension and pregnancy. Am J Obstet Gynecol 123:610, 1975.
25. Soffronoff EC, Kaufmann BM, Connaughton JF: Intravascular volume determination and fetal outcome in hypertensives diseases of pregnancy. Am J Obstet Gynecol 127:4, 1977.
26. Goodman LS, Gillman A: The pharmacological basis of therapeutics. London, Macmillan Publishing, 1977.
27. Rubin PC: Beta-blockers in pregnancy. N Engl J Med 305:1323–1326, 1981.
28. Ueland K, McNulty JH, Ueland FR, Metcalf J: Cardiovascular diseases in pregnancy: special considerations in the use of cardiovascular drugs. Clin Obstet Gynecol 24:809–823, 1981.
29. Ounsted MD, Moar VA, Good FJ, Redman CWG: Hypertension during pregnancy with and with specific treatment: the development of the children at the age of four years. Br J Obstet Gynaecol 87:19–24, 1980.
30. Kopta MM, Tomich PG, Crane JP: Ultrasonic methods of predicting the estimated date of confinement. Obstet Gynecol 57:657–660, 1981.
31. Spellacy WN: A perspective on progestogens in oral contraceptives. Am J Obstet Gynecol 142(6) (part 2):717, 1982.
32. Wied GL et al (ed): Mishell DR (moderator): Dialogue one: an overview of oral contraception. J Reprod Med 27(4) (Suppl):237, 1982.
33. Wynn V: Cardiovascular effects and progestins in oral contraceptives. Am J Obstet Gynecol 142(6) (part 2):718, 1982.
34. Kay CR: Oral contraceptives and health – some recent observations. In: Haspels AA, Kay CR (eds) Internation Symposium on Hormonal Contraception. Proceedings of a symposium held in Utrecht, The Netherlands, 10th Sept 1977. Amsterdam-Oxford, Excerpta Medica, 1978.
35. Brownrigg GM: Toxemia in hormone-induced pseudopregnancy. Can Med Assoc J 87:408, 1962.
36. Laragh JH, Sealey JE, Ledingham JJG, Newton MA: Oral contraceptives: renin aldosterone, and high blood pressure JAMA 201:918, 1967.
37. Woods JW: Oral contraceptives and hypertension. Lancet 2:653, 1967.
38. Tyson JEA: Oral contraception and elevated blood pressure. Am J Obstet Gynecol 100:875, 1968.
39. Saruta T, Saade GA, Kaplan NM: A possible mechanism for hypertension induced by oral contraceptives. Arch Intern Med 126:621, 1970.
40. Weir RJ, Briggs E, Brownrigg J et al: Blood pressure in women after one year of oral contraception. Lancet 1:467–470, 1966.
41. Royal College of General Practitioners: Oral contraceptives and health. London, Pitman Medical, 1974.
42. Ramcharan S, Pellegrin FA, Hoag E: In: Fregly MJ (ed) Oral contraceptives and high blood pressure. Dolphin Press, Gainesville, 1973.
43. Fisch IR, and Frank J: Oral contraceptives and blood pressure. JAMA 237:2499–2503, 1977.
44. Plunkett ER: Contraceptive steroids, age, and the cardiovascular system. Am J Obstet Gynecol 142:747 751, 1982.
45. Kaplan NM: Clinical hypertension, 2nd Ed. Baltimore, Williams & Wilkins, 1978, pp 343–351.
46. Harris PWR: Malignant hypertension associated with oral contraceptives. Lancet 4:466–467, 1969.

47. Zacherle BJ, Richardson JA: Irreversible renal failure secondary to hypertension induced by oral contraceptives. Ann Intern Med 77:83, 1972.
48. Schoolwerth AC, Sandler RS, Klahr S, Kissane JM: Nephrosclerosis postpartum and in women taking oral contraceptives. A report of two cases. Arch Intern Med 136:178, 1976.
49. Meade TW: Oral contraceptives, clotting factors and thrombosis. Am J Obstet Gynecol 142(6) (part 2):758–766, 1982.
50. Meade TW: Effects of progestyogens on the cardiovascular system. Am J Obstet Gynecol 142(6) (part 2):776–780, 1982.
51. Crane MG: Iateogenic hypertension and contraceptive pills. In: Genest J et al (eds) Hypertension. New York, McGraw-Hill, 1977, pp 855–866.
52. Rozenbaum H; Relationships between chemical structures and biologic progestogens. Am J Obstet Gynecol 142(6) (part 2):719–724, 1982.
53. Leiman G: Depomedroxy progesterone acetate as a contraceptive agent: its effect on weight and blood pressure. Am J Obstet Gynecol 114:97, 1972.
54. Mishell DR: Noncontraceptive health benefits of oral steroidal contraceptives. Am J Obstet Gynecol 142(6) (part 2):809, 1982.
55. Schmidt RR (ed): Physicians' Washington Report. Philadelphia, PWR Corporation, 1982.
56. Page EW: On the pathogenesis of pre-eclampsia and eclampsia. Am J Obstet Gynecol 79:883, 1972.
57. Hollenberg NK, Williams GH, Berger B et al: Renal blood flow and its response to angiotensin II, an interaction between oral contraceptive agents, sodium intake and the renin-angiotensin system in healthy young women. Circ Res 38:35, 1976.

14. Systolic hypertension in the elderly

W. McFATE SMITH

Hypertension in the elderly is, of course, not a disease entity as such, and the condition is not uniform in either its manifestation or prognosis. First of all, there is a continuation of ordinary essential hypertension manifest by elevated diastolic pressure and usually accompanied by at least a proportionate rise in systolic blood pressure. The pathophysiology and prognostic risk of this hypertension in the elderly is well known and is certainly not better than for younger people. Moreover, the VA Cooperative Study and the Hypertension Detection and Follow-up Program (for the age group 60–69) demonstrated benefit from treatment which lowered such pressures [1, 2].

Cross-sectional population studies indicate that systolic blood pressure rises throughout life, with females attaining higher levels for comparable ages over 60 (Figure 1). Diastolic blood pressure levels out in the mid to late fifties and declines slightly thereafter [3]. Thus, in those over 60 it is much more common to see systolic elevation without concomitant diastolic elevation, and the prevalence of this disproportion rises with age.

Hypertension in the elderly can be defined as 'pure' or 'isolated' systolic hypertension (ISH); for example, with systolics equal to or greater than 160 mmHg and diastolics less than 90 mmHg, that is, normal or below. As shown in Table 1, approximately 23% of men and 36% of women between the ages of 65 and 79 have systolic blood pressures equal to or greater than 160 mmHg and diastolic blood pressures less than 95 mmHg. The prevalence is somewhat higher in black females and lower in white males [4].

Hypertension in the elderly may also be defined as 'predominantly' systolic hypertension where the systolic blood pressure is disproportionately high relative to mild diastolic elevation. Characteristically, such subjects have a wide pulse pressure (greater than 70 mmHg) and an elevated mean arterial pressure, and peripheral resistance is only mildly elevated. This is the type observed in elderly persons with inelastic large arteries; that is, the systolic pressure is elevated due to structural changes with no, or only minimal, elevation of diastolic blood pressure.

Thus, predominantly systolic hypertension in the elderly begins to appear with

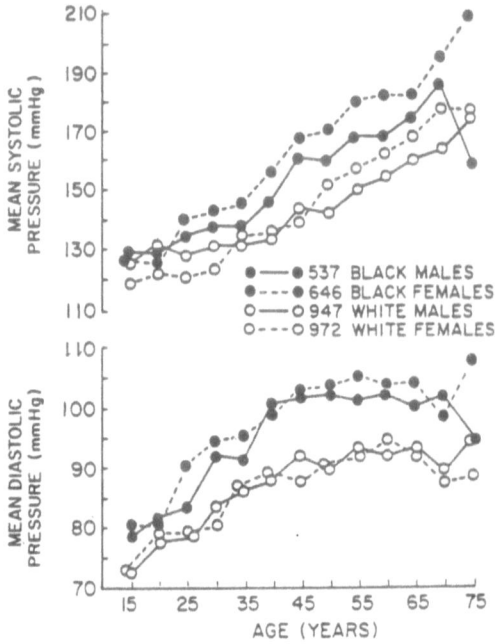

Figure 1. Blood pressure in Evans County Cardiovascular Study, 1960–1962.

Table 1. Prevalence of isolated systolic hypertension in men and women (U.S. 1960–1962)

Age	% Pure systolic hypertension*			
	Men		Women	
	White	Black	White	Black
25–34	0.3	1.0	0.2	0.0
35–44	0.9	0.6	0.9	1.5
45–54	3.5	1.3	4.6	7.6
55–64	9.5	13.0	15.6	4.3
65–74	15.0	25.5	30.7	38.9
75–79	26.9	38.6	32.9	43.1

* Systolic ≥ 160; diastolic < 95, National Health Survey, Series 11, No 5, 1964.

significant frequency around age 60, with an ever increasing prevalence with advancing age. However, systolic hypertension in the elderly is a problem not only because of its prevalence, but because of the ever increasing number and percentage of our citizens that are in this age group.

For example, between now and the end of the century, the population 65 and over will increase by nearly 40%; from 23 million in 1976 to 32 million in the year 2000. It is expected to approximately double between 1976 and 2020 when there should be about 45 million elderly persons. As a percentage of the total population, it will rise from 11% in 1976, to 12% in 2000 and 15.5% in 2020. In this period (1976–2020), all age segments of the elderly population are expected to grow rapidly, but particularly the extremely aged [5]. In fact, the percent changes show a regular progression by age for the 1976–2000 period (Figure 2). The population of 65–74 should increase by about 23%, the population of 75–84 by about 57%, and the population 85 and over by about 91%.

These changes in proportions for various age categories occur differentially in males and females. The rates of increase will generally be greater for elderly females than males in the next few decades, but not as great as the differences in the growth rate between the sexes that we have seen in recent decades. In 1976 there were 69 males for every 100 females in the age group 65 and over, and this deficit of males increases sharply with advancing age.

These age and sex differences, of course, are also reflected in mortality and survival. By 1976 the difference in the life expectancy at birth of males (69 years) and females (76,7 years) had reached 7.7 years. It was only 4.3 years in 1950.

Are there risks associated with isolated and predominantly systolic hypertension? This question has had comparatively limited attention; nonetheless, it

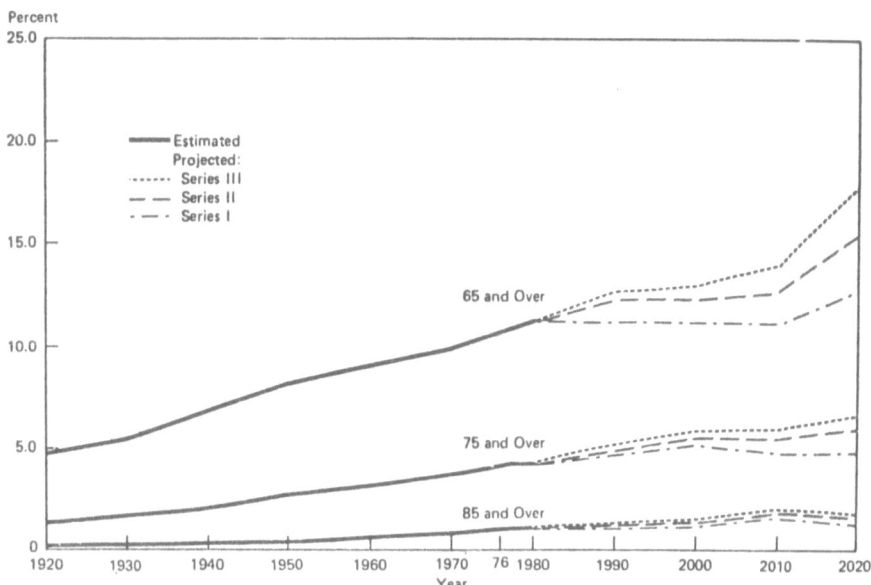

Note: Points are plotted for years ending in zero except for 1976.
Source: Table 2 and Current Population Reports, Series P-25, No. 311, 519, 614, 643, and 704.

Figure 2. Percent of the total population in the older ages: 1920–2020.

seems clear from actuarial data, and from the Framingham Study [6] and the People's Gas Study [7] and Heart Association Detection Project [8] (the latter two in Chicago), that elevated systolic pressure is associated with excess cardiovascular risk, at least up to age 65. Certainly this is true for males, though somewhat less certain for women.

The prospective study of ISH in Seal Beach, California, compared 72 men and women with 72 matched normotensives of average age 69 [9]. In nearly every category, cardiovascular morbidity and mortality were higher in the hypertensives (Table 2).

The Chicago Stroke Study found that when controlling for diastolic blood pressure at levels less than 95 mmHg, the risk of stroke rose as systolic blood pressure increased and that at levels of 180 mmHg and above, the risk ratio for death due to stroke was 2.5 [7] (Table 3).

Table 2. Findings among systolic hypertensives and normotensive controls (72 in each group: av. age – 69 yrs.)

Findings	Percent of pts.	
	>159 / < 90	140 <—— 90
Myo. infarct.	12.5	5.6
Angina	18.1	6.9
Stroke	8.3	2.8
Diabetes	26.4*	9.7*
C-V mortality	9.7*	1.4*
Aortic calcif.	44.4*	22.2*

* Statistically significant (Colandrea et al., Circulation 41:239, 1970).

Table 3. Blood pressure and three-year risk of stroke (men and women, white and black, age 65–74)

Blood pressure status	N	Rate (per 1000) adjusted for age, sex and race	
		Stroke	ABI
1. S<180			
D<95	1,973	53	31
2. D≥95	493	88	63
3. S≥180			
D<95	224	134	51
Rate ratio: 3 vs 1		2.5	1.7

Chicago Stroke Study (Dyer AR et al. Med Clin North Am 61:513, 1977).

Figure 3 illustrates mortality in the Framingham Study according to blood pressure category for men and women ages 45–74 [6]. Note that these rates are not for ISH but for combined or proportionate systolic-diastolic hypertension. Comparing the mortality for men and women who have no hypertension with those who have definite hypertension, it is evident that even in the 65–74 year age group, elevated blood pressure is associated with a significant increase in mortality for both sexes. This is particularly so for women who have a very narrow gradient at younger ages. Note also that for men in the upper age group, even borderline elevations of pressure carry a relatively greater mortality compared to normotensives than they do for men in either of the younger age groups.

Figure 4 illustrates that the probability of developing coronary heart disease (CHD) is predicted by the level of systolic blood pressure and is clearly higher for older people, especially men. Moreover, the risk of various manifestations of coronary heart disease also rises in direct proportion to the systolic blood pressure in both men and women ages 45–75. Thus, it is clear that high blood pressure is bad for the older person, just as it is bad at younger ages.

Is this risk reducible? There is limited information on the value of antihypertensive therapy in the elderly, and what exists is either not persuasive or conflicting. A prevalent view has been that such treatment, while effective in middle-aged hypertensives, is of limited value at best, and being fraught with some risks itself, should be given cautiously if at all. This view was supported by the observations of Adams in 1965 [10], who found no benefit for hemiplegic hypertensives from lowering their blood pressures. Carter in 1970 [11], in a prospective, randomized controlled trial, likewise found that for mortality rate and nonfatal stroke recurrence, no benefit accrued to those over 65, particularly those with only systolic elevations.

Merrett and Adams [12], in a comparative study of mortality rates in elderly

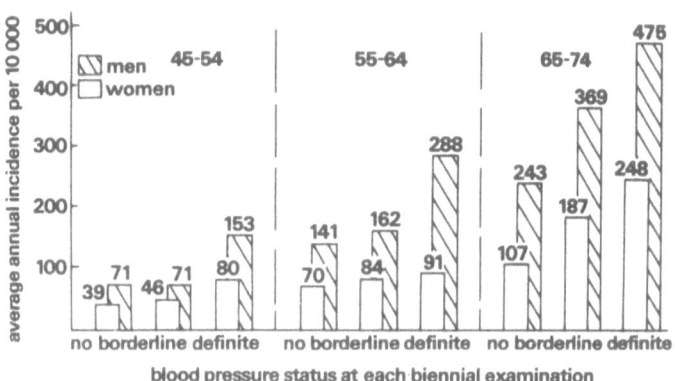

Figure 3. Mortality according to hypertensive status: men and women 45–74 (Framingham Study, 18-year follow-up from Framingham Monograph, 1974).

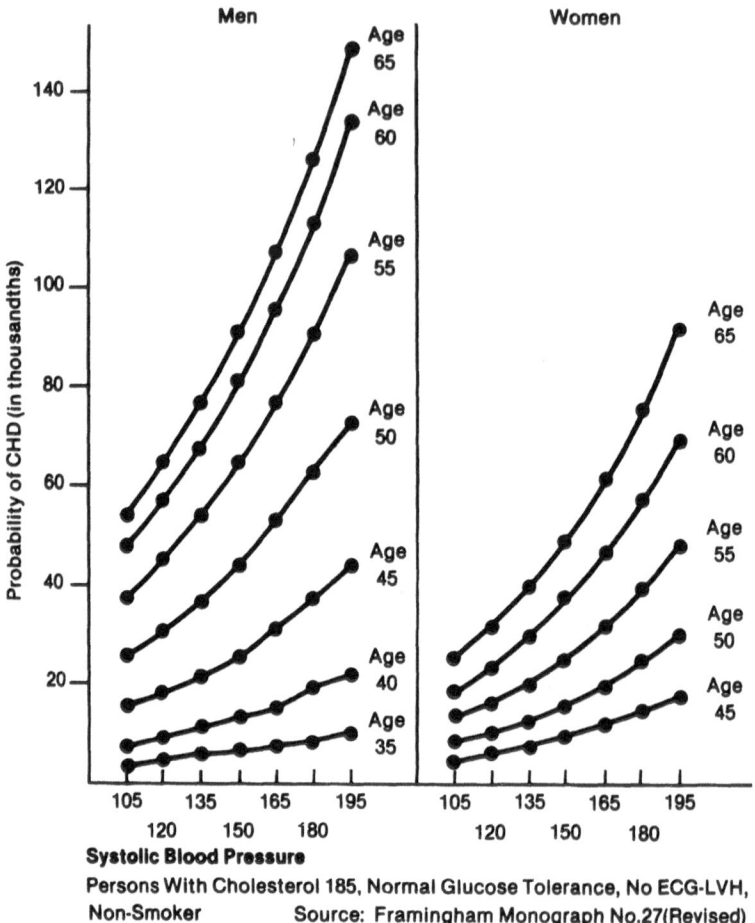

Figure 4. Probability of developing coronary heart disease in 6 years according to systolic blood pressure. Low risk persons 35–65. Framingham Study: 16-year follow-up.

hypertensive and normotensive patients, could demonstrate no adverse effect of elevated blood pressure on stroke survivors.

On the other hand, in 1973, Beevers [13] reported that stroke recurrence, but not myocardial infarction or angina pectoris, was significantly reduced when hypertension was well controlled by therapy. Baker (1968) [14], who studied 430 stroke survivors at the Wadsworth VA Hospital in Los Angeles, found the prognosis to be better in non-hypertensive patients. Priddle reported in 1968 [15] on studies in Toronto that in subjects with diastolic blood pressure less than 100 mmHg and systolics up to 180 mmHg, that diuretic therapy reduced mortality rate by 50 percent.

The Hypertension-Stroke Cooperative Study Group (1974) [16], while not demonstrating a significant reduction in stroke recurrence associated with blood pressure control, noted a reduction in cardiac failure. Moreover, they concluded that there was no evidence that lowering blood pressure was harmful – at least in terms of inducing cerebral infarction. Thus, as indicated above, the data on benefit from therapy is mixed, but no one has reported harmful effects.

Let's turn then to a consideration of the pathophysiologic characteristics of hypertension in the elderly as an approach to understanding why management may be more difficult than in younger hypertensives. The heart rate and cardiac output are not increased. The cardiac output if anything is lower than normal [17]. The rate of left ventricular ejection is decreased, and the peripheral resistance is elevated [18]. Plasma volume tends to be low. Also well known is the fact that systolic hypertension puts an increased workload on the left ventricle. Cardiac work is highly related to the peak systolic pressure. The actual workload is one of the major factors in determining the myocardial oxygen requirements. Hence, the older person with systolic hypertension has a greater workload on his left ventricle at a time when his capacity to deliver oxygen may be compromised by coronary atherosclerosis.

It should also be noted that aortic distensibility is markedly reduced. Illustrated in Figure 5 is the influence of age on the pressure–volume relationship of

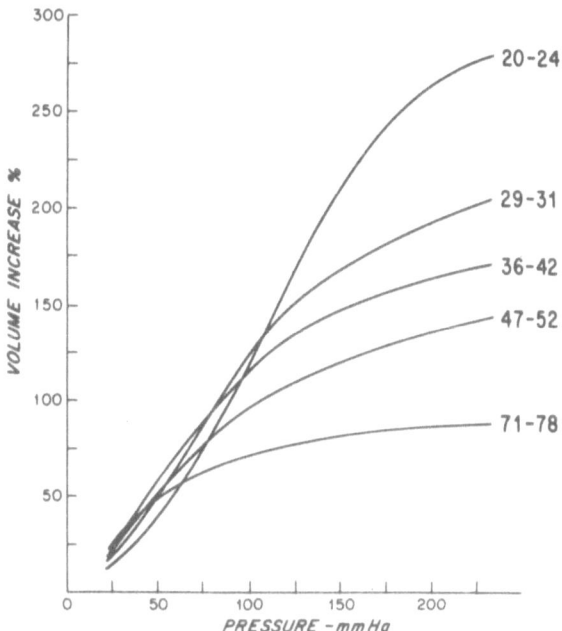

Figure 5. Influence of age on pressure-volume relation of human aortas obtained at autopsy (age in years indicated in each curve). Hallock and Benson. J Clin Invest 16:595, 1937.

the human aorta [19]. The investigator took sections of the thoracic aorta at autopsy from various age groups. The aorta was then distended with fluid to determine the pressure–volume curves. In the 71–78 year age group, small increases in volume were associated with a rapid rise in pressure. By contrast, in the young the volume was more than quadrupled before peak pressures were obtained. What this means, of course, is that for the same amount of blood ejected by the heart, a higher pressure results when it is ejected against a rigid, unyielding atherosclerotic aorta.

The question obviously arises as to whether elderly subjects with isolated or predominantly systolic hypertension should be treated with blood pressure-reducing drugs. My answer to this is that we don't know if they will benefit because the risk may be associated with the advanced atherosclerotic state rather than the pressure elevations per se, and its lowering may not alter the risk. It is an issue which is of great importance. There is an urgent need for a prospective controlled clinical trial to establish the answer.

In the absence of such an answer, my advice is to proceed cautiously. This means avoiding agents which are primarily postural in their action, for example, ganglion blockers, guanethidine, pargyline and perhaps prazosin, all of which can cause marked orthostatic changes in blood pressure. Older patients do not tolerate a sudden drop in pressure upon assuming the upright posture as well as younger patients do.

One should also start with small doses of whatever agent is used, smaller than one would ordinarily use and then proceed to increase the dosage very slowly if tolerated.

I don't think one should try to completely normalize systolic pressure, but to settle for one in the range of 140–160 mmHg. Many elderly patients are a bit sensitive to antihypertensive agents, but this isn't necessarily the rule because some are also somewhat resistant. The reasons for the increased sensitivity are shown in Table 4 and include the decreased aortic distensibility which means that with slight changes in cardiac output, there can be considerable change in systolic blood pressure.

Also since the blood volume tends to be low, and the sympathetic tone in these

Table 4. Pathophysiologic characteristics of hypertension in the elderly

Cardiac index	↓
Peripheral resistance	+
Ventricular ejection rate	↓
* Plasma volume	↓
* Aortic distensibility	↓
* Sympathetic tone	↑
* Baroceptor reflexes	↓

patients tends to be high, further decrease in the blood volume may precipitate hypotension. There is also evidence that the baroreceptor reflexes, those activated in the carotid sinus, are less active in older patients (Figure 6). Hence, they cannot compensate for sudden decreases in blood pressure as is the case for younger people.

When it comes to the choice of drugs, I recommend starting with a diuretic in small doses. One could certainly raise the question about this choice in view of the marginal to decreased blood volume of elderly subjects, but practically speaking, it works well and trouble is infrequent if you begin cautiously with small doses. Frequently this is the only medication necessary to reduce the blood pressure to the desired range.

If a second drug is added, there are many to choose from and no good studies to indicate a preference. Methyldopa is probably the most widely used, and in the European Working Party on High Blood Pressure in the Elderly [20], it appears to have been well tolerated and associated with satisfactory responses of the pressure. Others have indicated their pleasure with using hydralazine as a second or, in some instances, as a third drug in older subjects. There is some logic to this since it is not associated with a postural fall in blood pressure, and, moreover, since the carotid sinus reflexes are less active, they are not as likely to get a reflex tachycardia from the drug.

In conclusion, let me once again focus on the crucial importance on addressing ourselves seriously to the problems of hypertension in the elderly, including the

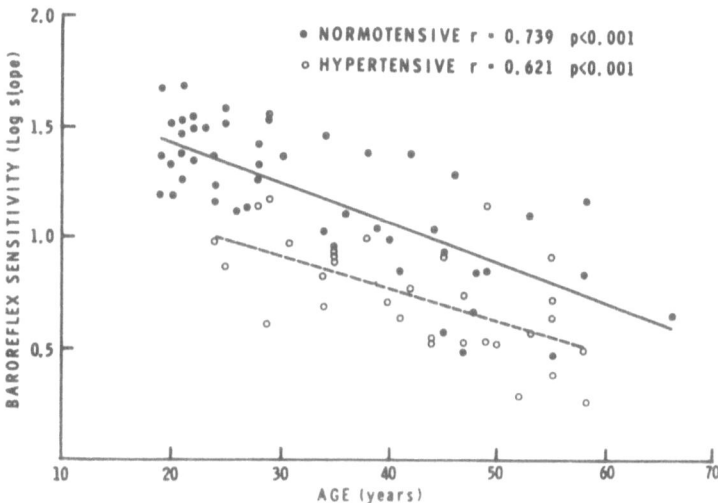

Figure 6. Effect of age on human baroreflex sensitivity. The solid and broken lines are for mormotensives and hypertensives respectively. (From Gribbin B, Pickering TG, Steight P, Peto R. Circ Res 29:424–431, 1971, by permission of the American Heart Association).

238

need for a controlled clinical trial of sufficient size and design to provide definitive answers. (1) There is a steadily and rapidly rising proportion of our population over the age of 60; (2) the prevalence of elevated blood pressure, particularly systolic, rises rapidly over age 60 and is at least 25%; (3) there is no doubt about the excess risk associated with this pressure elevation; and, finally, there remains uncertainty of the risk/benefit of treatment.

References

1. Veterans Administration Cooperative Study Group: Effects of treatment on morbidity in hypertension. II. Results in patients with diastolic blood pressure averaging 90 though 114 mmHg. JAMA 213:1143–1152, 1970.
2. Hypertension Detection and Follow-up Program Cooperative Group: Five-year findings of the Hypertension Detection and Follow-up Program. II. Mortality by race-sex and age. JAMA 242:2572–2577, 1979.
3. Tyroler HA, Heyden S, Hames CG: Weight and hypertension: Evans County studies of blacks and whites. In: Paul O (ed) Epidemiology and control of hypertension. Miami, Symposia Specialists, 1975, p 177.
4. National Center for Health Statistics: Blood pressure of adults by race and area: United States, 1960–1962. Public Health Service Publication No 1000, Series 11, No 5. Washington DC, Government Printing Office, 1964.
5. U.S. Bureau of the Census: Current population reports, Series P-25, No 704, 1977.
6. Kannel WB, Dawber TR: Hypertension as an ingredient of a cardiovascular risk profile. Br J Hosp Med 2:508, 1974.
7. Dyer AR, Stamler J, Shekelle RB, et al: Hypertension in the elderly. Med Clin North Am 61:513–529, 1977.
8. Schoenberger JA, Stamler J, Shekelle RB et al: Current status of hypertension control in an industrial population. JAMA 222:559–562, 1972.
9. Colandrea MA, Freidman GD, Nichaman MZ et al: Systolic hypertension in the elderly: an epidemiologic assessment. Circulation 41:239–245, 1970.
10. Adams GF: Prospects for patients with strokes, with special reference to the hypertensive hemiplegic. Br Med J 2:253–259, 1965.
11. Carter AB: Hypertensive therapy in stroke survivors. Lancet 1:485–489, 1970.
12. Merrett JD, Adams GF: Comparison of mortality rates in elderly hypertensive and normotensive hemiplegic patients. Br Med J 2:802–805, 1966.
13. Beevers DG, Fairman MJ, Hamilton M et al: Antihypertensive treatment and the course of established cerebral vascular disease. Lancet 1:1407–1409, 1973.
14. Baker RN, Schwartz WS, Ramseyer JC: Prognosis among survivors of ischemic stroke. Neurology 18:933–941, 1968.
15. Priddle WW, Liu SF, Breithaupt DJ et al: Amelioration of high blood pressure in the elderly. J Am Geriatr Soc 16:887–892, 1968.
16. Hypertension-Stroke Cooperative Study Group: Effect of antihypertensive treatment on stroke recurrence. JAMA 229(4):409–418, 1974.
17. Brandfonbrener M, Landowne M, Shock NW: Changes in cardiac output with age. Circulation 12:557–566, 1955.
18. Landowne M, Brandfonbrener M, Shock NW: The relation of age to certain measures of performance of the heart and circulation. Circulation 12:567–576, 1955.

19. Hallock P, Benson IC: Studies on elastic properties of human isolated aorta. J Clin Invest 16:595–602, 1937.
20. Amery A, Berthaux P, Birkenhager W et al: Antihypertensive therapy in patients above age 60. Acta Cardiol T 33:113–134, 1978.

15. Paramedical personnel and adherence to antihypertensive regimens

HAROLD W. SCHNAPER

The formal federally supported efforts to attack the problems of the detection and treatment of hypertension date from the publication of the classic Veterans Administration (VA) Hypertension Cooperative Trials in 1967 and 1970 [1–3]. Until then, although hypertension had been linked by insurance data [4] and by risk factor detection programs [5] to increased cardiovascular morbidity and mortality, the attitude toward blood pressure elevation was generally rather casual. The exceptions to this attitude were those patients with accelerated or malignant hypertension and those seen with other hypertensive emergencies, e.g., hypertensive encelphalopathy, acute myocardial infarction, acute left ventricular failure with pulmonary edema, congestive heart failure, progressive azotemia, dissecting aneurysm and other conditions. With these conditions and with some individuals with frighteningly high diastolic pressures, an intensive effort was made to lower the blood pressure during the acute clinical phase; once the problem had subsided and the situation was no longer medically urgent, the focus on maintaining lowered blood pressures usually diminished.

The failure to move before the 1970s in a more forceful manner to control hypertension was not related to any inadequate availability of effective medication. The basis of the stepped-care approach to treatment was the demonstration in the 1950s and early 1960s that pressure could be effectively lowered with few serious side effects [6, 7]. Two totally different factors were responsible. First was a lack of appreciation on the part of both the therapist and the general public of the initial prolonged symptom-free period of target organ deterioration that occurs with hypertension, during which hypertension could be detected only with a sphygmomanometer; these blood pressure measuring devices were almost exclusively available only in the physician's office. The second factor was the failure of both therapist and the general public to appreciate the magnitude of the increased risk of cardiovascular catastrophe that accompanies untreated hypertension and the degree of protection resulting from elevated blood pressure being controlled at normotensive levels.

With the definitive demonstration by the Freis-VA trials [1–3] of significantly greater protection against cardiovascular illness when blood pressure is controlled at normotensive levels, demonstrated first in those with seriously elevated diastolic pressures (115 mmHg and up) [1] and later in those with more modest elevation (105 mmHg and up) [2], the Department of Health, Education and Welfare (now Health and Human Services) became involved in this public health problem. The National Heart, Lung and Blood Institute (NHLBI) established the High Blood Pressure Education Program (NHBPEP) in 1971 with the primary objective of educating the public on the dangers of untreated hypertension and the need for having one's blood pressure measured as the only means of discovering the existence of hypertension. A secondary objective was to emphasize to physicians and others responsible for health care the high level of increased risk with hypertension and the protection of effective lifelong treatment. Admirable progress has been made in both these areas, thanks to the NHBPEP program [8].

The goal of the effective control of blood pressure, however, has not been reached with a large majority of individuals with hypertension. In 1972 only one of six hypertensives was under effective treatment and normotensive; by 1980 this number had risen to one out of four. The differences between the 1972 cohort and the 1980 cohort show that the NHBPEP has effectively accomplished one of its goals: Fewer than one in four individuals with hypertension now are unaware they have high blood pressure, compared with one of every two in 1972 [9]. These gains have been offset to a large extent, however, by an increase in the numbers of hypertensive individuals who are not under treatment or, if under treatment, are not following a prescribed antihypertensive regimen sufficiently faithfully to contain their pressures within normal ranges. Here again, the problem is primarily not the manner in which the medications are prescribed. Therapists by and large now practice the medical routines necessary for gradually building the dosage and types of medication to the appropriate level for blood pressure control. The primary problem is patient compliance with and adherence to the routine prescribed. This is the major hypertension bottleneck and the subject of this chapter, which addresses the impact on this problem of paramedical personnel trained as hypertension specialists.

The compliance problem

The problem of hypertensive patients failing to comply over the long term with their prescribed medical regimen is not, of course, unique in health care. Physicians and public health therapists have long been familiar with the high rate of compliance failures among free-living tuberculosis patients who do not renew their medication supply, among diabetic patients who fail to control their weight and food selection, among mothers who fail to administer daily a prophylactic antibiotic to their rheumatic children to guard against infection recurrence with devastating results and so on. Over the last two decades this general compliance problem has been increasingly appreciated, resulting in an increasing number of studies designed to determine compliance levels and factors involved in non-compliance. The conclusions of these studies vary in terms of what factors help to increase patient compliance, but the overall magnitude of the compliance problem among hypertensive patients is generally agreed upon [10].

Controlled trials have shown that hypertensive patients on a medical regimen need not take 100% of their medication – every dose, every day – to achieve a good level of control [11]. On the average an individual taking approximately 80% of his prescribed medication has his blood pressure controlled at normotensive levels. It is not known whether this success with only 80% of the dosage results from a general tendency among physicians to overprescribe dosages, from a variance in dosage effectiveness among individuals depending on absorption and other circumstances or from some other factor. On the basis of the observation, however, patients can be defined as compliant if they take 80% or more of their prescribed dosages on a regular basis. The real problem is with those hypertensive patients who become very erratic in taking their medication or after a time fail to take it at all.

Measuring levels of compliance and noncompliance involves other issues as well. The 1960 study by Caron and Roth [12] on compliance among peptic ulcer patients involved adding chemical markers to the prescribed medication and drawing blood samples on surprise visits to the patient's home to determine levels of compliance; such a method is now not considered acceptable in terms of medical ethics. There are obvious problems, however, with simply asking patients if they are continuing to comply with their medical regimen. In 1974 a Harris poll was conducted at the request of the National Heart, Blood and Lung Institute to investigate compliance levels among hypertensive patients [13]. The poll drew its sample from the more than 16 million hypertensive patients in the U.S. taking antihypertensive medication. With only slight variations according to socioeconomic factors and race, two-thirds of the sample group stated they took their medication in 100% of the dosage. One fourth said they never took their medication; this group, for obvious reasons, can be considered more reliable in their report than the two thirds. Of this group taking no medication, most said that their physicians had told them to stop the regimen, followed by those who said they no longer had hypertension and had no need for further medication. There is no way of knowing, of course, whether in fact their physicians had ordered the regimen stopped. Only a very small percentage of those not taking their medication complained about side effects or the cost of the medication. Of the two-thirds who claimed full compliance, allowing for an amount of natural exaggeration, the true figure is probably closer to 50%.

The Harris poll measured only the compliance level of those individuals whose hypertension had already been diagnosed and who had been put on a prescribed medical regimen. Before an individual reaches this point, however, he or she generally passes through earlier phases of compliance. In the Hypertension Detection and Follow-Up Program [13] there were three phases of compliance. Of the more than 150,000 individuals screened as potentially having hypertension, a representative sample of 1000 was studied in terms of compliance. The first goal was for a trained interviewer to enter each of these households and measure the blood pressure of adults to determine whether they were hypertensive and should be referred for follow-up. In this first phase of compliance there was an 11% failure, varying by socioeconomic groups; these individuals would not allow the interviewer into their homes to take blood pressure measurement. Of those who did allow this measurement, 14% were found to be hypertensive at a level at which they were requested to obtain follow-up at a university clinic. In this second phase of compliance, approximately one-fourth failed to report for follow-up to detect whether they were in fact hypertensive or had merely experienced a transient rise in blood pressure during the initial interview. In total, then, about one-third of potentially hypertensive individuals failed to comply even before being diagnosed and put on an antihypertensive regimen.

Once patients begin an antihypertensive regimen, the third phase of compliance is still lower: fewer than 50% of these individuals remain on the regimen after six months [10]. According to our experience this is a conservative figure, with the actual rate of noncompliance closer to 65%.

Factors in compliance

In the study by Roth and Caron of compliance among peptide ulcer patients on a medical regimen, the initial noncompliance rate among sample patients was 50%, similar to the rate with hypertensive patients. The sample group was randomly divided and half underwent intensive education about peptic ulcer disease, including anatomy and physiology, the effects and expected benefits of a medication treatment regimen and the serious results of allowing the disease to progress untreated. The control group continued in the treatment program but received no education. After six months, of those patients remaining in the treatment program, there was no significant difference in compliance between the two groups; educating the patients apparently had no effect. In fact, the number of patients who dropped out of the treatment program altogether was greater in the group receiving this education, and in this respect the educational efforts seem actually to have had a deleterious effect [12].

Among other studies of factors affecting the rate of compliance, a series of trials conducted in Ontario has produced the most significant data [10, 11, 14–16]. Several different treatment approaches and factors were tested in an attempt to improve patient compliance. As in the Roth and Caron Study [12], education was considered as a variable, which the Ontario group, using a series of educational steps, referred to as mastery learning. The patients were instructed gradually and had to demonstrate mastery of one phase of educational material before moving on to the next; the process ended only when each patient showed complete understading of the presented information about hypertension. As with earlier studies, education proved to have no effect on compliance levels. There was no difference, moreover, between patients receiving the education while on company time and those reporting to private physicians on their own time.

A second tested factor involved tailoring the individual's medication schedule to patterns of activity to increase the likelihood of compliance. In some cases, for example, the medication was attached to a personal item such as a razor to ensure that the patient would not simply forget to take it. The process of tailoring the medication regimen to the individual's level and pattern of activity was shown to increase compliance only for a brief period, after which the levels of compliance in this group returned to control levels.

Other factors investigated in this study show more promise. Two factors that apparently increase the patient's level of compliance – although the relationships are still being tested and have not been proven – involve the frequency of the patient's dose and the seriousness with which the physician or therapist views the importance of the patient's staying with the regimen [17]. Among patients otherwise unlikely to comply regularly with the medication regimen, patients who take the daily dose at one time have a significantly higher level of compliance than those taking the dose at multiple times through the day. Similarly, the level of compliance is higher among patients to whom the physician or therapist expresses a very serious attitude about the eventual results of uncontrolled hypertension, stressing the morbidity and mortality of the disease, than among those to whom a more casual and routine attitude is expressed.

Two other factors were demonstrated in the Ontario study to have a more dramatic impact on compliance levels: the duration and frequency of patient visits [17]. Although this has yet to be conclusively proven, the greater amount of time the patient spends in the clinic or other health care setting, the more likely the patient is to comply with his treatment, regardless of whether this longer interaction with the patient involves a physician, nurse or receptionist. The greater personalization of the treatment seems to have this positive effect. The frequency of visits has an even greater effect; the study conclusively demonstrated the benefit of this factor. Patients seeing a physician twice a month had higher levels of compliance than those with one visit a month, and the same was true of patients seen once a week rather than every two weeks. There were no significant differences among patient groups seeing a physician, a pharmacist or a nurse practitioner, as long as in each case the need for continuing the medication was stressed. The compliance level in each of these groups was more than twice that of the corresponding control group. This benefit lasted only as long as the greater frequency of visits was maintained, however: patients returned to control levels of compliance within six months after returning to a schedule of less frequent routine visits.

Reducing noncompliance: use of paramedical personnel

The two most promising methods of improving patient compliance, increased duration and frequency of patient visits, will both put an increasing strain on the health care system, which is already over-burdened in terms of physician availability. Two-thirds of the 46 million visits by patients to physicians in 1976 were for the control of hypertension [18], a percentage that has been steadily increasing. Estimates of the total number of hypertensive individuals in the United States vary from 22 to 64 million. On the basis of the most conservative estimate of this number, the total resources required to treat only hypertensive patients involve the full-time work of some 35,000 physicians; such resources simply are not available. Presently only approximately one-third of the conservatively estimated number of hypertensive individuals are under treatment, and even this third, with the present system and present physician resources, cannot be seen with the increased frequency of visits necessary for greater compliance levels.

One solution to the problem of resources currently being explored is a greater use of trained nonphysician hypertension specialists working under the direction of physicians but qualified to assume a number of treatment functions previously considered the sole prerogative of the physician. The adjunctive role of paramedical personnel is not new but can be traced at least as far back as the use of medical corpsmen in World War II, who unburdened physicians of many functions including medical work-up and routine therapy; more recently, the military has developed a training program for physicians' assistants to assume still more responsibilities. In the area of public health care as well there is a long tradition of public health nurses providing care in isolated areas. In the last two decades larger numbers of nurse specialists have emerged in many areas of medical care, including nurse practitioners who are assuming increasing responsibility in the care of patients with chronic disease, diabetes, and arthritis and rheumatism, as well as hypertension. The specialized training of these nurse practitioners is equivalent to that of physicians' assistants.

In the area of hypertension treatment these paramedical personnel are being trained to take on an even greater role, including diagnostic work-ups, physical examinations and recommendations for treatment to the supervising physician. The major remaining issue in the shifting of these responsibilities to paramedical personnel involves the degree of physician supervision that should be required;

to this end most medical programs making extensive use of such personnel utilize a written protocol of very specific diagnostic and treatment algorithms. Effective guidelines for the management of hypertensive patients have been set forth by the National High Blood Pressure Education Group [9], the guidelines of which are a model for the protocols adapted in many hypertensive clinics.

Several different programs have over the last two decades been exploring this adjunctive use of paramedical personnel in the treatment of hypertension. One of the earliest groups, operating out of 15 clinics in and about Memphis, extended the role of nurses in the delivery of long-term medical care for selected chronic diseases, including hypertension [19]. Specially trained nurses under physician supervision have managed the majority of treatment responsibilities for over 8000 patients in the first ten years in these clinics, with more than 32,000 patient visits and 3000 home visits. There has been growing interest in this program's series of workshops on expanding traditional nurse roles.

As a second example, in 1972 the Georgia Department of Human Resources began operation of a hypertension clinic run principally by nurse practitioners trained to assume much of the physician's role in treatment [20]. These nurses, already experienced in a screening and follow-up program, underwent additional formal education for 12 weeks followed by six months of seeing patients together with a physician. The training was directed to the use of a standardized treatment protocol based on a step-care plan. In all, these allied health professionals assumed eight responsibilities in the management of hypertensive patients:

1. Initial patient assessment, in which the nurse together with the physician determine the diagnosis and plan for treatment;
2. Follow-up of patient on return visits, using a problem-oriented medical record approach reviewed by the physician;
3. Adjustment of medication according to standardized algorithms, reviewed by the physician;
4. Continued monitoring of the treatment in terms of its effectiveness and side effects;
5. Surveillance of patient for other health problems;
6. Continued education of the patient;
7. Continued efforts to improve patient compliance; and
8. Careful follow-up if the patient misses an appointment.

In all areas of the patient's management the physician is available for consultation; after this program became established, the physician was consulted on the average in only one of six patient visits. After 18 months' experience this system was shown to be highly successful in terms of both compliance and control, in comparison with hypertension management in a private physician's office and hospital outpatient clinic: 81% of patients regularly returned for follow-up visits to this nurse-run clinic, compared to 41% to the physician's office and 55% to the hospital clinic, and 52.5% achieved good control of their hypertension, compared to 26% in the physician's office and 23% in the hospital clinic. Additionally, this nurse-managed clinic operates with greater cost-effectiveness than traditional clinics operated by physicians.

The Veterans Administration Pilot Hypertension Screening and Treatment Program, begun in 1972, represents the most extensive approach in the use of specially trained nonphysician therapists in the primary treatment of hypertensive patients [21]. The goals of this program, put into effect at 32 VA clinics, were to assess the effectiveness of clinics operated principally by nurses and physician assistants in controlling hypertension and increasing patient compliance at a minimum cost. On the average each clinic is run by a team of two nonphysician therapists, a clerk-receptionist trained to measure blood pressure and a supervising part-time physician. The therapists have undergone intensive four-week training sessions [22]. The treatment program follows a step-care protocol based on the report of the National High Blood Pressure Education Advisory Committee [19] but can be modified by the supervising physician. According to general guidelines established for these clinics, the supervising physician sees the patient in a minimum of four conditions:

1. To establish the patient's treatment;
2. If the maximum drug dosage following the established protocol is reached without the patient achieving good control;
3. If significant drug toxicity occurs;
4. If a significant hypertensive complication occurs.

The physician is always available, moreover, for consultation by the therapists. The nonphysician personnel provide approximately 85% of the total time involved in patient treatment and clinic management.

The results of the Pilot Program have been significant. Of over 6000 patients in all categories of hypertension receiving five or more treatment visits, the average treated diastolic pressure was below 90 mmHg in half of all patients and below 100 mmHg in four-fifths, control results markedly better than are generally reported. The compliance results are even more significant: 72% of moderately and severely hypertensive patients (105 or greater mmHg) and 62% of mildly hypertensive patients (90–104 mmHg) were still complying with their medical regimen after an average of 2.5 years of treatment. These results as well are significantly higher than those generally reported. As an added dividend, these clinics provided care at an average annual cost per patient of only approximately $220 (fiscal 1979) by means of simplified office and treatment procedures in routine cases of therapeutic control in addition to the use of nonphysician paramedical personnel [21].

Conclusion

Because an increasing number of hypertensive individuals are being identified and brought into treatment programs, and because the most effective methods currently known for improving the often very low levels of patient compliance demand that still more time be spent in working with patients, alternative approaches must be put into use to take the burden off the already overburdened traditional health care system. Physician resources cannot now adequately meet the needs of the current number of hypertensive patients under treatment, much less so in the future. Experience demonstrates that many of the responsibilities of this treatment can be given to specially trained paramedical personnel in a system that can both increase compliance levels and allow a significant cost savings.

In my own experience as a supervising physician in a Veterans Administration nurse-run hypertension clinic, the quality of medical care in this area has been equivalent to that of physicians. In any one series of patient visits between 85% and 90% of hypertensive patients under treatment have their blood pressure under control. The concern presently involves how far this approach can go in delegating responsibility to nonphysicians with specialized training, an issue debated by state health care licensing organizations. It is thus an aspect of our protocol that I review the records of all patient visits and sign all prescriptions, in addition to becoming involved in any cases that do not fit the treatment algorithms, occurring in fewer than 1% of cases. I have always found that these nurse practitioners respond more than adequately to the needs of patient management. This method is, I think, the only practical means currently available by which the goal of controlling hypertension throughout the U.S. can be met.

References

1. Veterans Administration Cooperative Study Group: Effects of treatment on morbidity in hypertension. I. Results in patients with diastolic blood pressures averaging 115 through 129 mmHg. JAMA 202:116, 1967.
2. Veterans Administration Cooperative Study Group: Effects of treatment on morbidity in hypertension. II. Results in patients with diastolic pressures averaging 90 through 114 mmHg. JAMA 213:1143, 1970.
3. Veterans Administration Cooperative Study Group: Effects of treatment on morbidity in hypertension. III. Influence of age, diastolic pressure, and prior cardiovascular disease: further analysis of side effects. Circulation 45:991, 1972.
4. Society of Actuaries: Build and blood pressure study, Vols I & II, 1959.
5. Dawber TR: The Framingham Study. Cambridge, Mass, Harvard University Press, 1980.
6. Perry HM Jr, Schroeder HA: A comparison of mortality rates in severe hypertension treated by medical and surgical regimens, A.M.A. Arch Intern Med 102:418, 1958.
7. Perry HM Jr, Schroeder HA, Catanzaro FJ, Moore-Jones D, Camel GH: Studies on the control of hypertension. VIII. Mortality, morbidity and remissions during twelve years intensive therapy. Circulation 33:958, 1966.

8. National High Blood Pressure Education Program, National Heart and Lung Institute: Professional education. Report of task force II to the hypertension information and education advisory committee, Sept 1, 1973.

9. The 1980 Report of the Joint National Committee on Detection, Evaluation, and Treatment of High Blood Pressure, Arch Intern Med 140:1280, 1980.

10. Sackett RL, Haynes RB (eds): Compliance with therapeutic regimens Baltimore, Johns Hopkins University Press, pp 9–25.

11. Sackett DL, Hayes RB, Gibson ES, Hackett B, Taylor DW, Roberts RS, Johnson AL: Randomized clinical trial of strategies for improving medication compliance in primary hypertension. Lancet i:1205–1207, 1975.

12. Caron HS Roth HP: Objective assessment of cooperation with an ulcer diet. Am J Med Sci 261:61–66, 1971.

13. HDFP Cooperative Group: Blood pressure from fourteen communities: A four stage screen for hypertension. JAMA 237:2385–2391, 1977.

14. Sackett DL, Haynes RB, Gibson ES, Taylor DW, Roberts RS, Johnson AL, Hackett BC, Turford C, Mossey J: Randomized trials of complicance-improving strategies in hypertension. In: Lasgna L (ed) Patient compliance. Mt. Kisco, NY, Futura Publishing, 1976, pp 1–19.

15. Sackett DL, Haynes RB, Gibson ES, Hackett BC, Taylor DW, Roberts RS, Johnson AL: Randomized clinical trial of strategies for improving medication compliance in primary hypertension. Lancet 1: 1205:1207, 1975.

16. Haynes RB, Sackett DL, Gibson ES, Taylor DW, Hackett BC, Roberts RS, Johnson AL: Improvement of medication complication in uncontrolled hypertension. Lancet i:1265–1268, 1976.

17. Taylor DW, Sackett DL, Haynes RB et al: Compliance with antihypertensive drug therapy. In: Perry HM Jr, Smith WM (eds) Mild hypertension: to treat or not to treat. Ann NY Acad Sci 304:390, 1978.

18. Schnaper HW: Use of paramedical personnel in routine antihypertensive treatment In: Perry HM Jr, Smith WM (eds) Mild hypertension: to treat or not to treat. Ann NY Acad Sci 304:381–385, 1978.

19. Ambulatory Care Services Protocols: ACS diabetes and hypertension form (5/72). Copyright by Beth Israel Hospital and Massachusetts Institute of Technology.

20. Wilber JA, McCoombs NJ: The allied health professional's role. Drug Therapy 21:83, 1975.

21. Perry HM Jr, Schnaper HW, Meyer G, Swatzell R: Clinical program for screening and treatment of hypertension in veterans. J Nat Med Assoc 74:433, 1982.

22. Carlson JH, Perry AG: Hypertension specialist training program. Washington DC, US Government Printing Office O-311-644/3253, 1979.

16. Economics of hypertension

WILLIAM B. STASON

Hypertension is, without doubt, one of the major challenges facing American medicine. Whether we accept 25 million (>95 mmHg), 36 million (>90 mmHg) or some other number as the true prevalence of hypertension requiring attention, it clearly affects a very large number of people. Furthermore, its impact, on morbidity and mortality in the form of increased risks of congestive heart failure (4 ×), strokes (3 ×) and heart attacks (2 ×) and renal failure is enormous. Finally, treatment is available which, *if properly applied*, can substantially reduce those risks. It is this constellation of factors that both makes hypertension the significant challenge it is for the practitioner and, at the same time, underlies the importance of examining the economic implications of that challenge.

The economics of health care has come, in recent years, to be equated with cost containment and the ogre of increased governmental regulation. This is unfortunate. Though concern over the cost of health care is most certainly with us and is likely to remain with us for some time to come, I would like to argue that proper recognition of the cost implications of disease and its treatment can work to the benefit of all of us – physician, patient and society alike. In particular, I believe that application of the principles of economics to health care decisions can help all of us to set better priorities for use of our scarce resources, be these public dollars for hypertension programs, time in the case of the busy physician or the resources of the uninsured patient, employer or purveyor of National Health Insurance.

There are two basic ways in which information on the costs of illness and the costs of medical care can be, and have been, used to influence health care decisions. The first is the use of aggregate cost figures to describe the magnitude of a particular health care problem or the importance of a particular health care initiative. The second is cost-effectiveness analysis, a technique that can provide guidance in selecting between alternative approaches to treatment or between alternative uses of health care.

Definition of certain key terms will provide the basis for discussion. All of these terms are simple in concept. All too often, however, they tend to be misunderstood or misused.

Cost-effectiveness. This expression has become a buzzword in recent years. Very simply, the cost-effectiveness of a health care practice or procedure is the net cost in dollars per unit of health benefits gained. Usually benefits are expressed in years of life and/or some measure of the extent of morbidity or the quality of life. Alternatively, health benefits might be expressed in less definitive terms such as the number of millimeters of mercury reduction in blood pressure. Hence, cost-effectiveness considers the effectiveness, and hence the quality of health care services, as well as their costs. The lower the ratio of costs to effectiveness, the more cost-effective a given health program or procedure is. If resources are limited, one might use the cost-effectiveness ratio to set priorities by providing the most cost-effective services first and then by proceeding down a priority list until resources are exhausted. Some claim that use of the cost-effectiveness criterion to determine whether or not a given health care service should be provided is antithetical to the medical ethic of doing everything possible for every patient. I would respond in two ways. First, I would argue that, in fact, you already employ cost-effectiveness principles, albeit implicitly and perhaps inconsistently. Second, I would agree that the cost-effectiveness criterion should be only one element among several in resource allocation decisions. Risk–benefit issues and equity considerations may be of overriding importance. *Cost–benefit analysis* is very similar to *cost-effectiveness analysis* except that health benefits are translated into dollar terms. Wages lost as a result of absenteeism or premature death are the most commonly used measures. The results of cost–benefit analyses can be presented either as differences or ratios. If the benefits exceed the costs, the case can be made that the program is worth doing. A recent report from the National High Blood Pressure Education Program indicated that the benefits of treating high blood pressure exceeded the costs by 20–30%. These results have been used to support arguments for increased activity in the treatment of high blood pressure.

Direct and indirect costs. Medical care costs include the costs of hospitalization, office visits, medications and laboratory examinations. A variety of indirect costs, such as wages lost, the time and expense required on the part of patient to keep office appointments and medical expenses that are generated or induced as the result of a special program, also need to be considered. Induced costs would include the costs of diagnosing or treating a disease discovered incidentally during a program aimed primarily at hypertension.

Cost versus charges. The distinction is important. Charges for medical services do not always reflect their true costs of production. Hospital laboratory charges, for example, frequently exceed their costs by a factor of two or three; while other hospital services break even or run at a deficit.

Average costs versus marginal costs. Average costs are determined by dividing the total costs of delivering a service by the number of units of service produced. The average cost of an office visit, for example, would be total operating expenses divided by the number of office visits that were provided. Marginal costs, on the other hand, assume that a health care program or practice is already in existence and examine only the incremental costs of providing a new program or additional services. Marginal (or incremental) costs then must be compared to marginal (or incremental) benefits.

Opportunity costs. These represent the value of the best alternative use of resources. If a doctor considers taking more patients with hypertension into his practice, he must weigh the value of so doing against whatever he may have to give up as a result. If the office schedule is already full, he must either reduce the number of patients with other types of illness or expand the number of hours worked per day and, hence, cut into leisure time. If, on the other hand, the doctor's practice is not as busy as he or she would like, then the value, or opportunity costs, of underused time is something much lower.

With these basic definitions in hand, let us examine some of the economic ramifications of hypertension, first in terms of the economic costs of hypertension to society and then from the cost-effectiveness perspective.

It is the economic costs of illness to which we are most often exposed in the media. These figures usually describe both the medical and nonmedical costs of a disease. Under medical care costs are included the costs of ambulatory care (office visits, medications, laboratory examinations) and the costs of hospitalizations attributable to the disease or its complications. Under nonmedical costs are economic valuations of premature deaths and morbidity from strokes, heart attacks, renal failure or other complications attributable to the disease. One problem in estimating the economic impact of hypertension is the very real difficulty of separating the effects of elevated blood pressure from those of other risk factors for cardiovascular and renal diseases. Another is the dilemma of how to value human life or economic productivity. Using conservative assumptions the total medical treatment cost for ambulatory and hospital care for hypertension, at present, appears to be about $ 5 billion a year nationally; compared to about $ 11 billion a year for losses in economic productivity that would occur in the absence of treatment. At very least these figures are impressive indicators of the importance of hypertension as a public health problem. Advocates of hypertension programs use similar figures very effectively to gain community support at the local level and public and Congressional support at a national level. What these dollar amounts don't tell you, however, is the costs and benefits that would result from an all-out effort to treat hypertension. Stated differently, they give no insights into what the marginal costs and marginal benefits of such an effort might be. Optimistic estimates suggest that, for an additional $ 3.2 billion per year, we might gain something in excess of $ 5 billion in savings from the mortality and morbidity prevented. These estimates are highly optimistic, however, in the sense that they assume, not only that the control of mild hypertension and systolic hypertension is effective in reducing the risks of untoward events to those experienced by normotensive persons, but also that the effort would be 100% successful in reaching and achieving long-term blood pressure control in the target population. These assumptions, obviously, are open to question. The balance between benefits and costs, correspondingly, would be affected, with the greater effect probably being a reduction of benefits.

Examination of the cost-effectiveness of hypertension treatment provides a complementary perspective. We believe that careful cost-effectiveness analyses, coupled with further research into critical questions bearing on both the cost and the effectiveness sides of the ratio, can make important contributions to achieving a better allocation of health care resources.

There are two basic principles underlying cost-effectiveness analysis. The first is that health care resources are, in fact, limited. Historically in the United States, we have never acted as if they were, and the credo of 'Do everything for every patient' has been widely accepted. If this country were willing to spend 15–20% of the Gross National Product on health, compared to the present 9%, there would be no issue of cost containment even today, and assessment of the cost-effectiveness of health care programs would be irrelevant. Treatment decisions would require only that the benefits exceed the risks. Such is not the case, however. The costs of health services have risen dramatically in the past 20 years and at a rate much greater than other sectors of the economy. The consequence has been a groundswell of opinion and activities aimed at limiting growth of the health industry. Resources are limited!

The second basic principle is that costs to one decision-maker may be very different from costs to another; measures of effectiveness likewise may differ. Physicians, patients, employers and leaders of society each view the world from varying vantage points.

The physician's cost–benefit agenda is depicted in Table 1. On the cost side, the physician is concerned with the expenses of running a practice; salaries for office personnel, overhead and material expenses. Many physicians also take into account the patient's out-of-pocket expenses and try to minimize these for patients wih limited financial means. Inflationary pressures of liberal utilization of health care services on health insurance premiums are not particularly germane, however, unless the physician is a member of an HMO in which there is a financial incentive for reducing unnecessary use of health services. On the benefit side, the physician is concerned both with the welfare of the patient and with his own welfare. Net income, professional satisfaction, and peer recognition are very real benefits in the eyes of the physician; and rightly so. Cost-effectiveness assessment for the physician might relate to the allocation of his

Table 1. Costs and benefits of hypertension treatment from the physician's perspective

Physician's perspective

Costs:	Direct expenses of practice		
	Concern for patients' out-of-pocket expenses		
Benefits:	For patient	–	Lower BP
			Reduced risk of morbid and mortal events
			Relief of symptoms
			Minimize medication side effects
	For physician	–	Net income
			Professional satisfaction
			Peer support

time between the different patients. Decisions on appropriate frequency of visits for a given patient and the substitution of generic drugs for trade-name drugs, or reserpine for propranolol or alpha-methyl dopa in the treatment of hypertension, might turn on both benefit and cost considerations. Likewise, the decision whether to hire a nurse practitioner to assume responsibility for the follow-up of hypertensive patients also might be based on cost-effectiveness considerations.

The patient has a very different set of priorities (Table 2). Out-of-pocket expenses are a major concern and may adversely influence compliance if they are a major burden. Lost wages and lost leisure time as a result either of disability or the need to be absent from work to visit the physician are real considerations; while the cost of a health insurance premium is perceived as a cost only to the extent that it is not provided as a benefit of employment. On the benefit side, relief of symptoms is the primary concern. Reduction of future risk is less tangible and somehow less important. Because hypertension is usually asymptomatic and the reduction in risk of stroke or myocardial infarction is both a

Table 2. Costs and benefits of hypertension treatment from the patient's perspective

Patient's perspective

Costs:	Out-of-pocket expenses
	Health insurance premium
	Lost wages
	Lost leisure time
Benefits:	Relief of symptoms
	Reduced future risk
	Side effects of treatment
	Effects on job security
	Effects on anxiety/self image

statistical phenomenon and in the future, the negative impact of medication side effects and the inconvenience of treatment may weigh heavily against the benefits. Job security is another issue: some employers, either consciously or unconsciously, may be biased against a hypertensive person in terms of promotion or hiring practices. The demands of labor unions for strict confidentiality of medical information in worksite treatment programs is one manifestation of this concern. The psychological effects of labeling and treatment also must be considered. In my experience the decision of a patient whether or not to remain on treatment for hypertension is, very much, a cost-effectiveness one. Often the balance is a very narrow one.

Finally, society has still another perspective. For society, total costs, direct and indirect, and total benefits are relevant. Private and public dollar costs, economic costs, and the personal consequences of mortality and morbidity all must be considered. The cost-effectiveness analysis of hypertension management that we have performed [1] takes a societal point of view.

Conceptually, this study is based on the fact that a patient first must be made aware that his or her blood pressure is elevated. Then, sequentially, he/she must be confirmed to be a hypertensive by repetitive blood pressure measurements, started on medications and maintained on long-term treatment. This sequence of events is summarized in Figure 1. Benefits result only if sustained blood pressure reductions are achieved. Recent evidence indicates that short-term therapy confers short-term benefits, though long-term control is the ultimate goal. Because of the attrition that occurs at each step in the process of detection and management, money spent on screening, evaluation and even on initiating treatment may not be productive of long-term benefits. Public screening is a case in point. Unless a person is screened, and screened reliably, and then referred and treated, benefits will not accrue; costs will, however.

To develop our model for hypertension management, we first specified costs (Table 3). The direct costs of treating hypertension included doctor visits, laboratory examinations and medications. Subtracted from treatment costs were savings in the costs of hospitalizations for heart attacks and strokes prevented

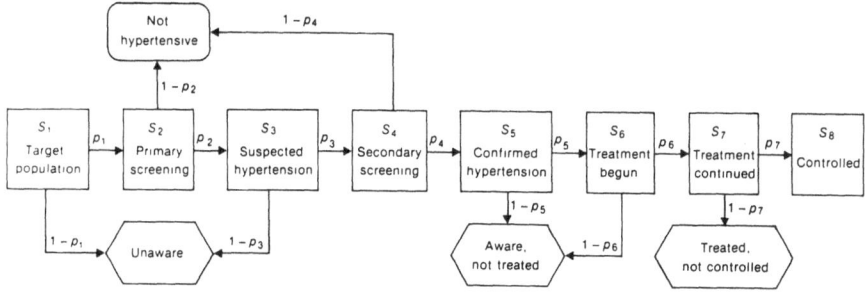

Figure 1. Multistage model for the management of hypertension (adapted from [1]).

Table 3. Categories of cost considered in the cost-effectiveness model for hypertension treatment. All costs discounted at 5% per year

Net costs

Direct medical care costs
- Physician visits
- Medications
- Laboratory examinations

Indirect costs
- Savings in morbidity from strokes and myocardial infarctions prevented
- Costs of treating medication side effects
- Costs of health care in added years of life

as a result of treatment. Added were the costs of treating medication side effects; for example, hyperuricemia or acute gout. Finally, we considered the costs of health care that would have been incurred in the years of life that would not have been lived had the patient died of a heart attack or stroke due to untreated hypertension. This last point, though numerically inconsequential as far as the results of our analysis are concerned, has important health planning implications. As the incidence of strokes and myocardial infarctions is reduced as a result of the treatment of hypertension, relatively larger numbers of patients with cancer and other disabling conditions of old age will present to health care facilities. The health care delivery system will have to accommodate to needs for treatment of this changing spectrum of chronic and life-threatening disease.

Measures of effectiveness (or benefits) are shown in Table 4. Improved life expectancy and prevention of morbidity from heart attacks, angina pectoris or heart failure and strokes are the major goals of treatment. These must be balanced against medication side effects. Adjustments to estimated life expectancy for the quality of life were based on the concept that a year of life with angina, with the residuum of a stroke or with gout is worth something less to an individual than a year of life with full health. Though quantitation of effects of disease on the quality of life is controversial, there can be little disagreement that the concept is an important one.

Table 4. Measures of effectiveness considered in the cost-effectiveness model. Results are expressed in years of life expectancy adjusted for decrements in the quality of life. Net effectivenes, like costs, discounted at 5% per year

Net effectiveness

Increased life expectancy
Improved quality of life from morbidity prevented
Adverse effects of treatment on the quality of life

Estimates for both costs and measures of effectiveness were based on information drawn widely from the clinical, epidemiological and health statistics literature. Reliance was placed on the Framingham Heart Study for estimates of excess morbidity and mortality from elevated blood pressure. Where data were sparse the effects of alternative assumptions were tested in sensitivity analyses. This approach permitted identification of variables that heavily influence the results and which, therefore, should serve as targets for future research. The most important of these is our inadequate knowledge of benefits to be expected from treating hypertension and, especially, mild hypertension and systolic hypertension.

Cost-effectiveness results are presented in terms of the net dollar cost per year of increased quality adjusted life expectancy gained. Figure 2 shows this cost-effectiveness ratio for different levels of pretreatment diastolic blood pressure for men and for women. Similar curves could have been constructed for systolic blood pressure. What can be seen is that the cost-effectiveness ratio is lower (or treatment is more cost-effective) at higher pretreatment diastolic pressures. This result, certainly, is not surprising. What is less obvious, however, is the finding that the cost-effectiveness of treatment at any given level of blood

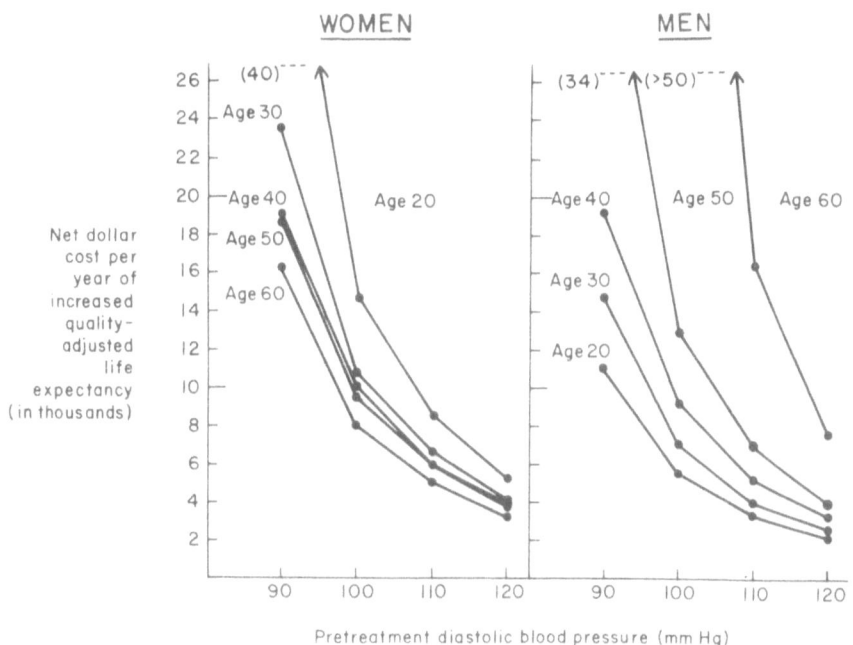

Figure 2. Cost-effectiveness of hypertension treatment according to age, sex and pretreatment levels of diastolic blood pressure. Estimates assume full adherence to medical regimens and discount both costs and benefits at 5% per year (adapted from [1]).

258

pressure rises with age in women, while treatment of younger men appears to be more cost-effective than treatment of older men. The explanation for this lies in the fact that men suffer cardiovascular complications at earlier ages than do women.

Figure 3 demonstrates the importance of patient compliance to the cost-effectiveness of treatment. Levels of noncompliance usually encountered in clinical practice about double the cost-effectiveness ratio. For persons with initial diastolic pressures between 95 and 104 mmHg it increases from $10,000 to about $20,000 per year of life saved and for pressures of 105 mmHg and above it increases from about $5000 to $10,000. Because of problems with compliance, resources may be better spent improving the compliance of patients currently under care than encouraging widespread public screening programs.

Additional expenditures for hypertensive care are extremely unlikely to reduce total health care costs. We estimate that, at best, only slightly more than 20% of the cost of treating hypertensives with initial diastolic blood pressures of 105 mmHg and above will be recovered through savings from reduced hospitalizations for strokes or heart attacks. For mild hypertensives this figure is of the order of 10%. This does not mean that hypertension programs are not cost-effective, or that they should not be undertaken, but only that their values to society must be argued in human terms or in broader economic terms than on the basis of expected medical cost savings.

How might cost-effectiveness results such as ours be used? First, they can be used by the clinician to help set priorities in his own practice. Time spent with a young man with a high diastolic pressure, who has had difficulty adhering to his three or four times a day drug regimen because it interferes with his work day, would very likely represent a better investment than time spent with a sixty- or seventy-year-old man with a blood pressure of 180/95.

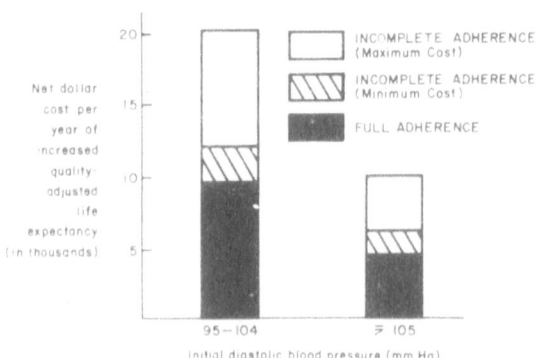

Figure 3. Effects of alternative adherence assumptions on the cost-effectiveness of treatment for mild (DBP 95–104 mmHg) and moderate or severe (105 mmHg and above) hypertension. Results are for 40-year-old persons and are discounted at 5% per year (adapted from [1]).

Second, from a policy point of view, cost-effectiveness estimates can be, and increasingly are being, used to influence decisions in the allocation of health care resources; within hypertension and between hypertension, cholesterol screening, coronary bypass surgery, CAT scanning and so forth. For this purpose comparable analyses of these other health care practices are needed. Some of these have been done, some are in progress, and others, no doubt, will be done in the future.

Finally, it is my opinion that the major potential of cost effectiveness analyses lies not so much in details of their results, but more in the indirect effects they can have on health care delivery. Policy decisions have been, and will continue to be, based on an array of factors, political imperatives not the least of these. Cost-effectiveness results, by themselves, can be expected to have only limited impact. As physicians, hospital administrators, employers and others become familiar with and accept cost-effectiveness principles, however, the indirect effects may become far-reaching. Increased cost awareness alone will achieve a great deal. Explicit consideration of the trade-offs of risks versus benefits, on one hand, and costs versus benefits, on the other, will achieve even more in the direction of controlling health care costs and preserving high quality health care.

DR. PERRY: I listen with amazement as Dr. Stason presents and I still have difficulty accepting it. What I am curious about, Bill, is that there must be some break point at which treatment of hypertension becomes effective. The black man with a diastolic pressure of 140 and twenty years old – how can one fix a break point at which treatment would become cost-effective? I hear you constantly say that it really isn't cost-effective. I guess I philosophically have difficulty accepting this.

DR. STASON: The only real break points in cost-effectiveness results are either where the numerator of the cost-effectiveness ratio (net costs) becomes zero or negative indicating that more costs are saved than are incurred; or if the denominator (net effectiveness) becomes zero or negative. Obviously any net costs divided by zero is infinity. With these exceptions the cost-effectiveness ratio is a continuum. 'Cost-effectiveness' is not an absolute, but, instead has to be reasoned in terms of the comparison of one health care practice to another. For example, a cost-effectiveness ratio of $10,000 per year of life saved for hypertension looks very, very good indeed in relation to the cost-effectiveness ratio of $50,000 per year of life saved which we have estimated for some types of patients receiving coronary bypass surgery. In this example treatment of hypertension is more 'cost-effective' than coronary bypass surgery. Still, the costs saved as a result of treating hypertension are not equal to the costs of treatment. Whether the costs of treatment exceed savings for the specific case of 20-year-old blacks with a diastolic blood pressures of 140 mmHg, I don't know. At some point, one would expect net savings would be achieved.

Reference

1. Weinstein MC, Stason WB: Hypertension: a policy perspective. Cambridge, Mass, Harvard University Press, 1976.

Subject Index